Neuroimaging

A Teaching File

Neuroimaging

A Teaching File

Matthew F. Omojola, MD, FRCPC
Professor, Radiology and Neurological Sciences
Division of Neuroradiology
Department of Radiology
University of Nebraska Medical Center
Omaha, Nebraska

Mauricio Castillo, MD, FACR
Professor of Radiology
Chief, Division of Neuroradiology
Department of Radiology
University of North Carolina
Chapel Hill, North Carolina

. Wolters Kluwer

Philadelphia • Baltimore • New York • London
Buenos Aires • Hong Kong • Sydney • Tokyo

Acquisitions Editor: Ryan Shaw
Product Development Editor: Amy G. Dinkel
Production Project Manager: Priscilla Crater
Design Coordinator: Stephen Druding
Prepress Vendor: Integra Software Services Pvt. Ltd.

Library of Congress Cataloging-in-Publication Data

Neuroimaging (Omojola)
  Neuroimaging : a teaching file / [edited by] Matthew F. Omojola, Mauricio Castillo.
    p. ; cm.
  Includes bibliographical references and index.
  ISBN 978-1-4511-7328-4
  I. Omojola, Matthew F., editor. II. Castillo, Mauricio., editor. III. Title.
  [DNLM: 1. Neuroimaging—Case Reports.   2. Central Nervous System—pathology—Case Reports.   3. Central Nervous System Diseases—diagnosis—Case Reports.   WL 141.5.N47]
  RC386.6.D52
  616.8'04754—dc23
                                    2014023085

LWW.com

For Omoniyi, Olufemi, Ayokunle, Oluwadamilola, Temitope, and Opeyemi; the best children in the world.

MFO

Stephen Bagg, MD
Fellow in Neuroradiology
Division of Neuroradiology
Department of Radiology
University of North Carolina
Chapel Hill, North Carolina

Mauricio Castillo, MD, FACR
Professor of Radiology
Chief, Division of Neuroradiology
Department of Radiology
University of North Carolina
Chapel Hill, North Carolina

Alin Chirindel, MD
Fellow, Russell H Morgan Department of Radiology
    and Radiological Science,
Johns Hopkins Medical Institutions
Baltimore, Maryland

Karen Ragland Cole, MD, MPH, MBA
Vice Director, Pediatric Radiology
Long Beach Memorial Hospital
Clinical Professor Radiology
Department Neuroradiology
University of Southern California
Keck School of Medicine
Long Beach, California

John M. Collins, MD, PhD
Assistant Professor of Radiology
Department of Radiology
The University of Chicago Medicine
Chicago, Illinois

Felipe Espinoza, MD
Fellow in Neuroradiology
Division of Neuroradiology
Department of Radiology
University of North Carolina
Chapel Hill, North Carolina

Pierre Fayad, MD, FAHA, FAA
Reynolds Centennial Professor of Neurology
Department of Neurological Sciences
Director, UNMC-CU Neurology Residency Program
Director, Stroke Center
The Nebraska Medical Center
University of Nebraska Medical Center (UNMC)
Omaha, Nebraska

Diana F. Florescu, MD
Associate Professor
Department of Medicine
Transplant Infectious Diseases Program
University of Nebraska Medical Center
Omaha, Nebraska

J. Gibson, MD
Fellow in Neuroradiology
Division of Neuroradiology
Department of Radiology
University of North Carolina
Chapel Hill, North Carolina

Bryan S. Jeun, MD
Fellow in Neuroradiology
Department of Diagnostic Radiology
Yale University School of Medicine
New Haven, Connecticut

Michele H. Johnson, MD
Associate Professor
Department of Diagnostic Radiology
Yale University School of Medicine
New Haven, Connecticut

Syed A. Jaffar Kazmi, MD
Assistant Professor
Departments of Pathology and Microbiology
University of Nebraska Medical Center
Omaha, Nebraska

Matthew Kruse, MD
Resident, Russell H Morgan Department of Radiology
    and Radiological Science,
Johns Hopkins Medical Institutions
Baltimore, Maryland

Miguel Lemus, MD
Staff Radiologist
Department of Radiology
Hospital University of Bellvitge
l'Hospitalet de Llobregat,
Spain

Ajay Malhotra, MD
Assistant Professor
Department of Diagnostic Radiology
Yale University School of Medicine
New Haven, Connecticut

Robert D. Messina, MD
Assistant Professor
Department of Diagnostic Radiology
Yale University School of Medicine
New Haven, Connecticut

Frank J. Minja, MD
Assistant Professor
Department of Diagnostic Radiology
Yale University School of Medicine
New Haven, Connecticut

Matthew F. Omojola, MD, FRCPC
Professor, Radiology and Neurological Sciences
Division of Neuroradiology
Department of Radiology
University of Nebraska Medical Center
Omaha, Nebraska

Ray Peeples, MD
Fellow in Neuroradiology
Division of Neuroradiology
Department of Radiology
University of North Carolina
Chapel Hill, North Carolina

Sofia Pina, MD
Staff Neuroradiologist
Department of Neuroradiology
Hospital Santo António – CHP
Porto, Portugal

Colin S. Poon, MD, PhD, FRCPC
Staff Radiologist
Department of Radiology
Orillia Soldiers' Memorial Hospital
Orillia, Ontario. Canada
Adjunct Assistant Professor of Radiology
Yale University School of Medicine
New Haven, Connecticut

Noelia Silva Priegue, MD
Staff Neuroradiologist
Hospital Povisa
Vigo, Spain

Samer Salhab, MD
Fellow in Neuroradiology
Department of Diagnostic Radiology
Yale University School of Medicine
New Haven, Connecticut

Rathan Subramaniam, MD
Visiting Associate Professor of Radiology
Russell H Morgan Department of Radiology and
    Radiological Sciences
Johns Hopkins University School of Medicine
Adjunct Associate Professor of Radiology
Boston University School of Medicine
Boston, Massachusetts

Matthew L. White, MD
Professor of Radiology
Division Chief Neuroradiology
University of Nebraska Medical Center
Omaha, Nebraska

David Yousem, MD
Professor of Radiology and Radiological Science
Russell H Morgan Department of Radiology
    and Radiological Science,
Johns Hopkins Medical Institutions
Baltimore, Maryland

Rana K. Zabad, MD
Assistant Professor and Director
Multiple Sclerosis Program
Department of Neurological Sciences
University of Nebraska Medical Center
Omaha, Nebraska

Elcin Zan, MD
Fellow, Russell H Morgan Department of Radiology
    and Radiological Science,
Johns Hopkins Medical Institutions
Baltimore, Maryland

Vahe M. Zohrabian, MD
Assistant Professor
Department of Diagnostic Radiology
Yale University School of Medicine
New Haven, Connecticut

William B. Zucconi, DO
Assistant Professor
Department of Diagnostic Radiology
Yale University School of Medicine
New Haven, Connecticut

Teaching files are one of the hallmarks of education in radiology. When there was a need for a comprehensive series to provide the resident and practicing radiologist with the kind of personal consultation with the experts normally found only in the setting of a teaching hospital, Wolters Kluwer was proud to have created a series that answers this need.

Actual cases have been culled from extensive teaching files in major medical centers. The discussions presented mimic those performed on a daily basis between residents and faculty members in all radiology departments.

This series is designed so that each case can be studied as an unknown. A consistent format is used to present each case. A brief clinical history is given, followed by several images. Then, relevant findings, differential diagnosis, and final diagnosis are given, followed by a discussion of the case. The authors thereby guide the reader through the interpretation of each case.

Last year we made additional changes to the series. Cases have been randomized to better prepare the reader for the challenges of the clinical setting. In addition, to answer the growing demand for electronic content, we have included more cases online, which has left us, in turn, able to offer a more cost-effective product.

We hope that this series will continue to be a trusted teaching tool for radiologists at any stage of training or practice and that it will also be a benefit to clinicians whose patients undergo these imaging studies.

The Publisher

I have always maintained a teaching file from my days as a radiology resident. My teaching materials always came from these files which are updated from time to time. It is therefore a great privilege to be asked to lead a group of great contributors to put together some of these cases that we share with you here in a teaching file format. The presentation follows the new format of the teaching file in the Wolters Kluwer series, incorporating the relevant imaging findings with the clinical information in a case-based format. The Question-and-Answer segments, the Reporting Responsibilities, and the "What the Treating Physician Needs to Know" segments were the most difficult for me to write. I actually enjoyed doing them. These sections have turned out to be as informative as the Discussion section. I have tried to use the ACR communication guide as a guide in composing the Reporting Responsibilities. However, communication continues to evolve in clinical practice with the emergence of the electronic medical record. Individual practice should decide what is feasible with regard to the communication practice. Where possible we have included the specific clinical scenario leading to the diagnosis in each case so that the path to diagnosis would be clear. While this is a guide, the path to diagnosis may not necessarily be the same in your own practice. This may change from time to time depending on the available clinical information. We have collaborated with our colleagues from the clinical services and pathology where possible in some of the chapters. I believe that we get the best result through interdisciplinary collaborations in the management of our patients.

This title should be useful to residents in radiology and the busy general radiologists who want to quickly look up a case similar to a problem case they may have. In this regard, we have elected to present each case discussion starting with the imaging findings and discussion of the differential diagnosis to be closely followed by the pathology, clinical presentation, and treatment where necessary so that our readers would be able to first compare the imaging findings with their cases before diving into the clinical findings. I also think this book will be useful to the neurology and psychiatry residents doing elective rotations in neuroimaging. Students doing observership in neuroimaging and medical students doing neuroscience rotation may also find this book useful. I have been privileged to mentor many of these residents and students. We have included some cases on normal anatomy. We have also covered how advanced imaging could be helpful in the differential diagnosis in relevant situations. We have been as comprehensive as possible in each case considering the constraint of space. I think we have covered most of the common cases in neuroimaging practice. Several cases with several imaging features are discussed in several places resulting in some form of duplication which I consider necessary in order to do justice to the more common imaging features of such cases.

Matthew F. Omojola

This book is the work of several contributors. I am therefore grateful to my contributors for making this book a reality. I would like to thank Dr. Justin Tran for reading through the section on traumatic brain lesions and for his suggestions. Dr. Najib Murr read through the section on hippocampal malrotation and made suggestions.

My special thanks to my colleagues in the department of Neurological Sciences at the University of Nebraska Medical Center for their support throughout my time at the UNMC. They have contributed immensely to my longevity at this institution. I would like to thank the many Neurology and Psychiatry residents who took electives with me for the impetus to be a part of this project. I am grateful to all our colleagues, who took care of the patients presented here, for their contributions to the well-being of our patients.

I want to remember the late Jonathan Pine, with whom I started out this project at LWW, for his kindness, support, and dedication to duty while he was under tremendous burden, which I was not aware off until the very end. I'd also like to thank Charley Mitchell, who originated the project but left LWW before we could actualize it. Charley was very supportive of this project, and I thank him for his comforting words during the initial break in the project. This project could not have been completed without the support of many people at LWW, including Amy Dinkel and her group. I learned a lot from my development editor, Mary Beth Murphy.

Deborah Klein sought and pulled most of the references for this book. Drs. Terri Love and Lisa Wheelock supplied some images on posterior fossa congenital lesions, some of which I used in this book. I am also grateful to many other colleagues who contributed images.

I owe a debt of gratitude to my co-editor Dr. Mauricio Castillo, my mentor and a great friend without whom this work could not have been done. Mauricio has served our profession and specialty with distinction in so many ways. Those of us who have benefited from his knowledge, leadership and wisdom should be thankful for knowing him. I would like to thank Allan Fox, MD for my foundation in Neuroradiology. I am indebted to my children, Omoniyi, Olufemi, Ayokunle, Oluwadamilola, Temitope and Opeyemi; my cheerleaders for their love, constant encouragement and support. I don't know what I could have done without them! I am grateful to my wife, Jumoke, for her support.

Matthew F. Omojola

CLINICAL HISTORY *8-year-old male with malignant astrocytoma of the corpus callosum treated with combination therapy.*

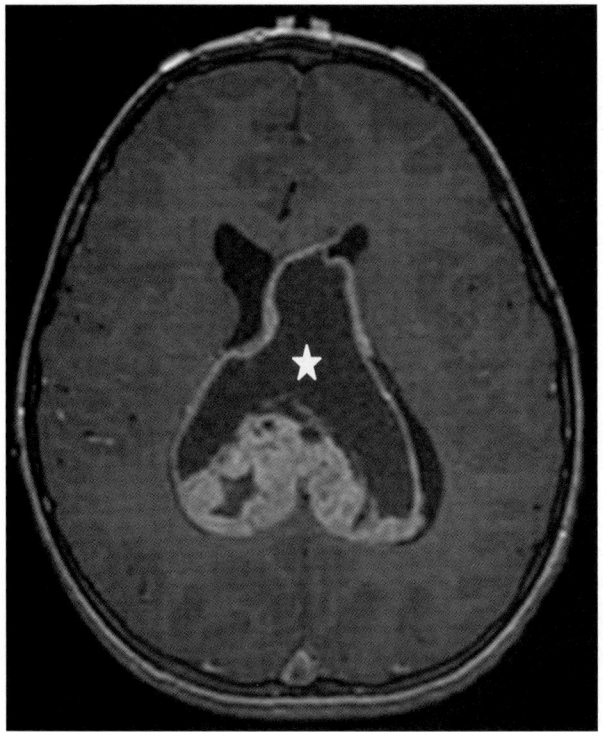

FIGURE 1-1

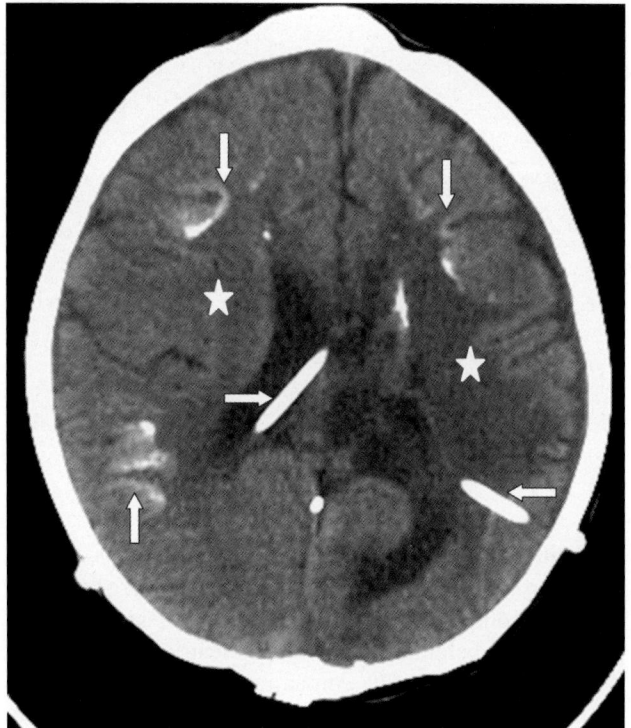

FIGURE 1-2

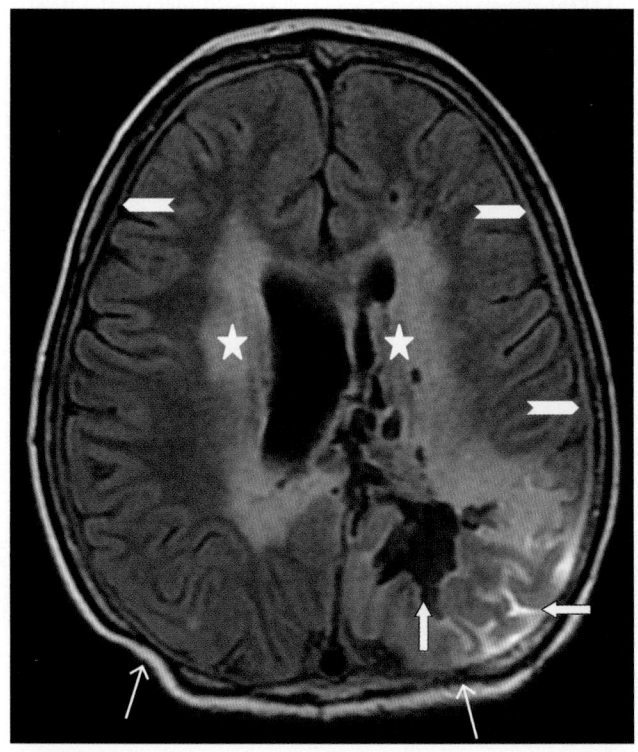

FIGURE 1-3

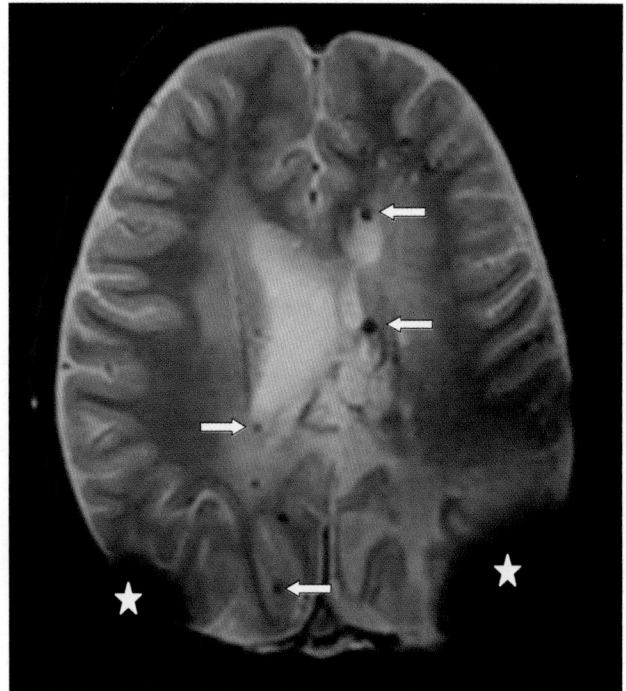

FIGURE 1-4

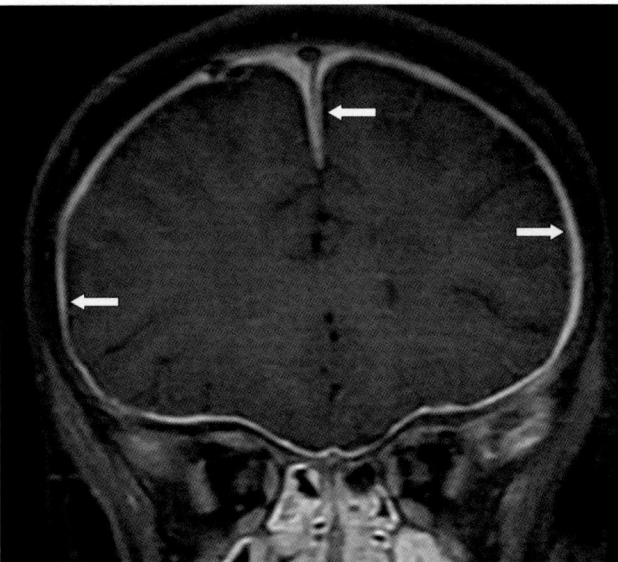

FIGURE 1-5

FINDINGS Figure 1-1. Axial treatment planning post-contrast T1WI through the lateral ventricles. There is a large partially cystic and solid mass (WHO IV) astrocytoma (star) of the corpus callosum bulging into the lateral ventricles. Figure 1-2. Axial NCCT through the corona radiata about 2 years into his treatment which included surgical removal of the tumor via bilateral parietal craniotomies, radiation treatment, and chemotherapy. There are bilateral ventriculoperitoneal (VP) shunts (transverse arrows), multifocal subcortical calcifications (vertical arrows), and bilateral periventricular smudgy white matter (WM) hypodensities (stars). Figure 1-3. Axial FLAIR through the corona radiata. There is bilateral confluent WM hyperintensity (stars). The left parasagittal parietal surgical cavity (vertical arrow) represents part of the surgical tract to the original tumor. There are hyperintensities in the left parietal sulci (transverse arrow) produced by the VP shunt susceptibility artifact. There is thickening of the dura (chevrons). The craniotomy flap is present posteriorly (line arrows). Figure 1-4. Axial GRE through the centrum semiovale. There are bilateral large signal void artifacts from the VP shunts (stars). There are multiple punctate hypointensities in bilateral centrum semiovale WM (transverse arrows) consistent with telangiectasia or microhemorrhages or calcifications. Figure 1-5. Coronal post-contrast T1WI through the frontal lobes. There is smooth pachymeningeal enhancement (arrows) which is circumferential around the cerebral and cerebellar hemispheres.

DIFFERENTIAL DIAGNOSIS N/A.

DIAGNOSIS Treatment-related changes.

DISCUSSION This case illustrates some of the changes that can occur following intervention in the management of intracranial pathology. Multimodal interventions happen very frequently in clinical management, and we have to be familiar with the effects of these on images. Some of these may mimic abnormalities, some are abnormalities, and some are just life support instruments casting artifacts. Surgical intervention usually starts with a craniotomy (a cranial vault bone flap raised to allow entry and replaced at the end of the intervention) or craniectomy (a bone flap raised and not replaced or may be replaced at a later date). The margins of these flaps are seen as defects in the cranial vault. The craniectomy could produce a sunken effect on the scalp. Because of foreign bodies at the margins of the craniotomy, it is easier to identify on the GRE sequence where the susceptibility effect is greatest. These margins are usually easy to see on CT bone windows.

If there is hydrocephalus or one is expected, a ventricular drain or a VP shunt may be placed. The drain or shunt should pass through the lateral ventricle for it to function properly. Shunt complications may include malfunction such as overdrainage or inadequate drainage which could result in slit ventricles or hydrocephalus, respectively, shunt infection with ventriculitis and ependymal contrast enhancement with intraventricular debris, extraaxial collections particularly with overdrainage and intraventricular hematoma (IVH) during insertion or revision of the shunt. The valve of the shunt may produce signal void artifacts peripherally on the cranial vault particularly on the GRE and DWI, and sulcal hyperintensities on FLAIR images.

Confluent WM T2 hyperintensity or leukoencephalopathy is a fairly common complication of radiation treatment and chemotherapy. In the acute phase, this probably relates to edema, while on the long term, there are demyelination, axonal loss, spongiosis, gliosis, and vasculopathy. Decreased N-acetyl aspartate (NAA) has been demonstrated on MR spectroscopy within the WM hyperintensity. Brain necrosis presenting with contrast enhancement could mimic neoplasm. MRI perfusion study may be useful for distinguishing radiation necrosis (low to poor relative Cerebral Blood Volume [rCBV]) from tumor (high rCBV). Brain volume loss with widening of the sulci and enlargement of the ventricles is not uncommon following treatment. Punctate GRE hypointensities within the WM may represent calcifications, microhemorrhage, or telangiectasia. CT usually differentiates calcifications (dense on CT) from microhemorrhages and telangiectasia (usually not seen on CT). Mineralizing angiopathy resulting in calcifications is a common complication of tumor treatment. All these changes begin as early as within 3 months of completion of treatment. Mild pachymeningeal enhancement may be seen following surgery, and this could disappear subsequently. Avid and robust pachymeningeal enhancement may suggest intracranial hypotension particularly if there is associated hind brain sagging or pseudo Chiari I. Nodular pachymeningeal configuration may indicate tumor seeding. Some of these changes may or may not be symptomatic.

Question for Further Thought

1. Which is the best imaging technique for the evaluation of treatment changes?

Reporting Responsibilities

Significant changes following brain tumor treatment should be reported directly. Complications of shunts usually require immediate attention. New tumors or new areas of contrast enhancement usually require further evaluation with DWI if one has not been obtained, perfusion studies, and MR spectroscopy.

What the Treating Physician Needs to Know

- What is new? Where and how severe?
- Are life support tubes doing what they should be doing?
- What other investigations should be done to clarify the new findings?

Answer

1. While CT may be able to demonstrate all the changes discussed here, MRI offers the best imaging technique to evaluate posttreatment changes. If the consideration is whether a shunt or EVD is functioning or not, CT is adequate. Parenchymal changes, however, are best evaluated by MRI particularly with other available procedures such as MR spectroscopy, perfusion, and the multiplanar capability of MRI.

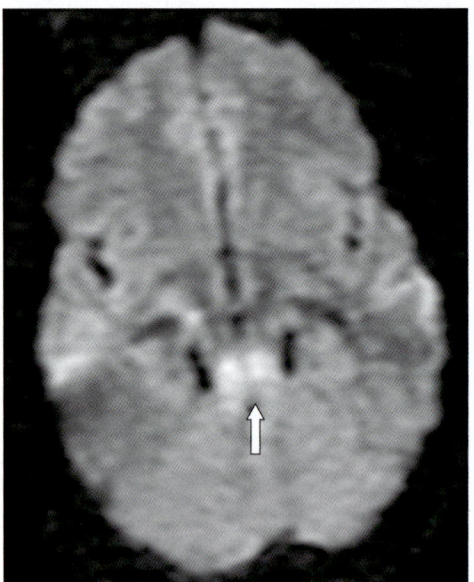

FIGURE 2-1

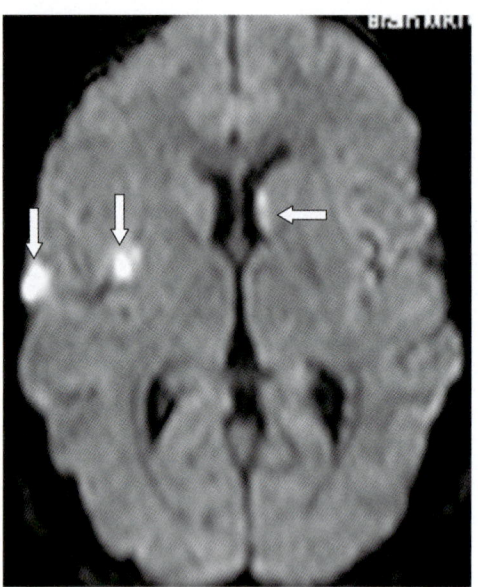

FIGURE 2-2

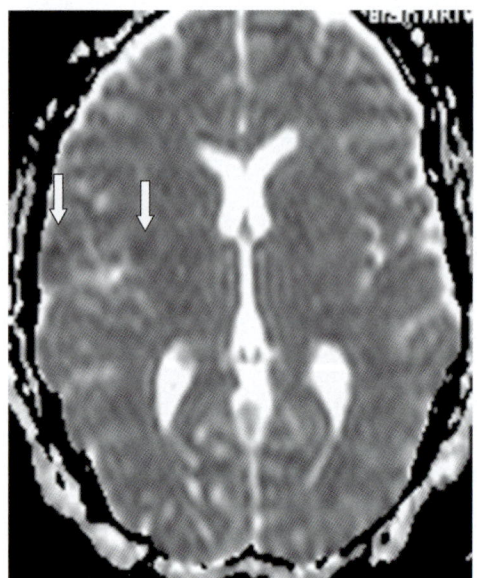

FIGURE 2-3

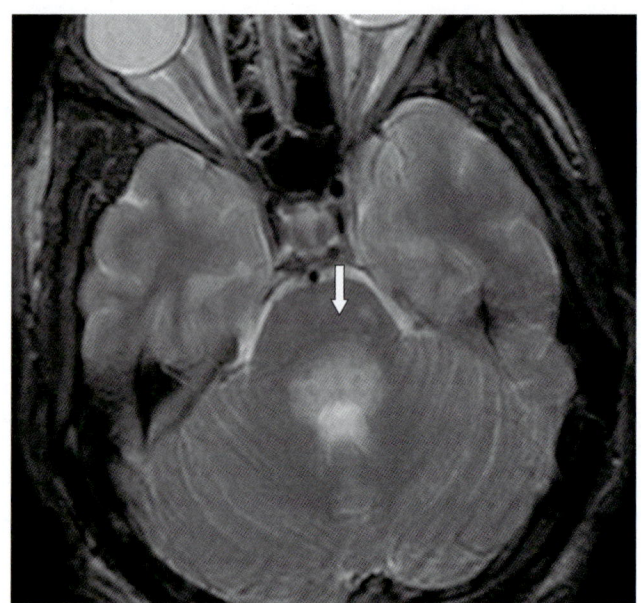

FIGURE 2-4

FINDINGS Figure 2-1. Axial DWI through the midbrain. There is hyperintensity posteriorly in the midbrain (arrow). ADC map (not shown) did not show low ADC. Figures 2-2 and 2-3. Axial DWI with corresponding ADC map through the basal ganglia. There are multifocal areas of restricted diffusion (arrows) in the left caudate nucleus, right insula, and operculum. Figures 2-4 and 2-5. Axial T2WI through the pons and midbrain, respectively. There is confluent hyperintensity in the pontine tegmentum extending into midbrain tegmentum and tectum (arrows).

Inferior extension of the lesion to the medulla is present (not shown). Figure 2-6. Axial FLAIR through the pons 4 months later. There is minimal residual hyperintensity in the tegmentum (arrow). There is no contrast enhancement on the initial and follow-up images in any of the areas involved.

DIFFERENTIAL DIAGNOSIS Multifocal infarcts, demyelinating process, encephalitis, brainstem glioma, osmotic demyelination.

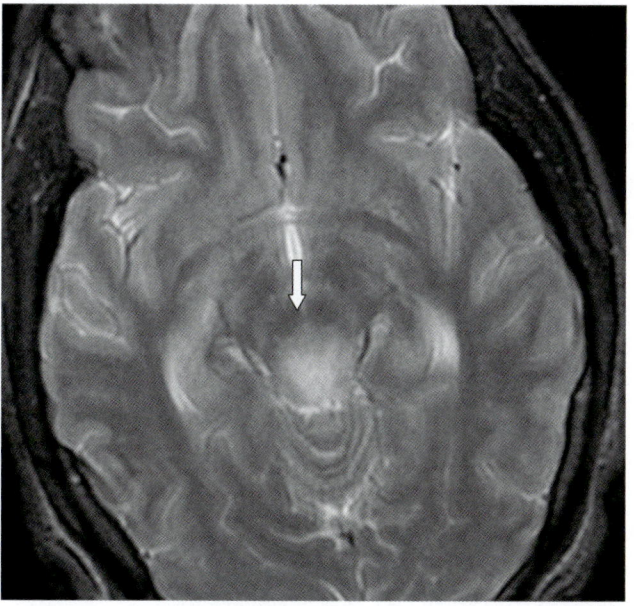

FIGURE 2-5

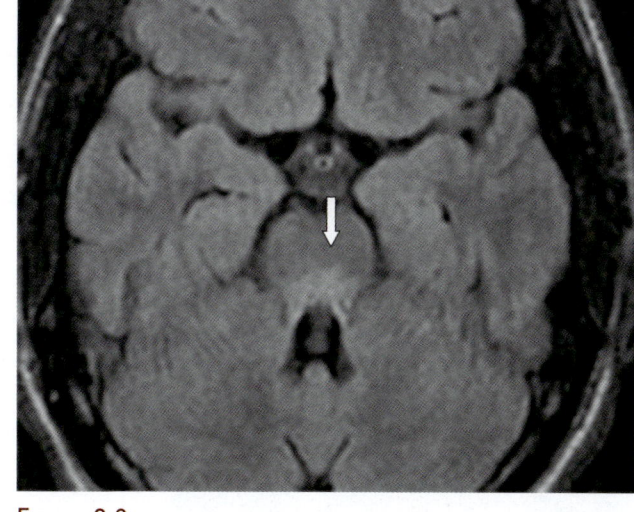

FIGURE 2-6

DIAGNOSIS Brainstem encephalitis (presumed Bickerstaff brainstem encephalitis [BBE]).

DISCUSSION BBE is a rare autoimmune brainstem encephalitis of unknown etiology. The MRI changes of BBE which is present in about 30% of the patients are a longitudinal confluent T2 hyperintensity in the brainstem extending from the medulla to the midbrain, usually without restricted diffusion or contrast enhancement, but some expansion of the brainstem. It has been described by some as vasogenic edema, while some have reported areas of restricted diffusion in some cases. In most of the images published, the tegmentum has been the region most affected. Concomitant involvement of the cerebellum and supratentorial structures has been reported. A negative MRI does not exclude the diagnosis if the clinical criteria are met. The diffuse nature of the changes and lack of restricted diffusion exclude brainstem infarct. It may be difficult to completely exclude other demyelinating processes. The wide age range does not fit with brainstem glioma. Osmotic myelinolysis usually spares the periphery and is mostly confined to the pons. Usually there is complete recovery with resolution of the signal changes in BBE as in this case.

The clinical criteria for BBE include ataxia with bilateral ophthalmoplegia. There is usually disturbed consciousness, bulbar palsy, pupillary changes, facial weakness, and hyperreflexia. Tetraparesis could be present in about 50% of the patients. The diagnosis is supported by the presence of anti-GQ1b antibodies and an abnormal brain MRI. However, absence of these does not exclude the diagnosis. There is clinical overlap between BBE, Miller Fisher syndrome (MFS), Guillain-Barré syndrome (GBS), and acute demyelinating encephalomyelitis (ADEM). There is usually a preceding infection resulting in a prodromal stage. Treatment is by corticosteroids, airways management, intravenous immunoglobulin, and plasmapheresis.

Question for Further Thought

1. Which are the organisms implicated in the prodromal phase of BBE?

Reporting Responsibilities

Direct reporting is indicated in view of the differential and the necessity for aggressive management in this otherwise curable illness.

What the Treating Physician Needs to Know

- Extent of disease
- Reasonable differential diagnosis

Answer

1. BBE has been reported following infection with several organisms including *Mycoplasma pneumoniae*, *cytomegalovirus*, *Haemophilus influenzae*, and *Campylobacter jejuni*. The exact pathogenesis is unknown. BBE is associated with the presence of antiganglioside antibody, (anti-GQ1b), which is also present in other diseases with similar prodromal phase such as MFS, ADEM, and GBS indicating similar pathogenetic mechanism of these diseases.

CLINICAL HISTORY *54-year-old female presenting with headache and right facial nerve weakness.*

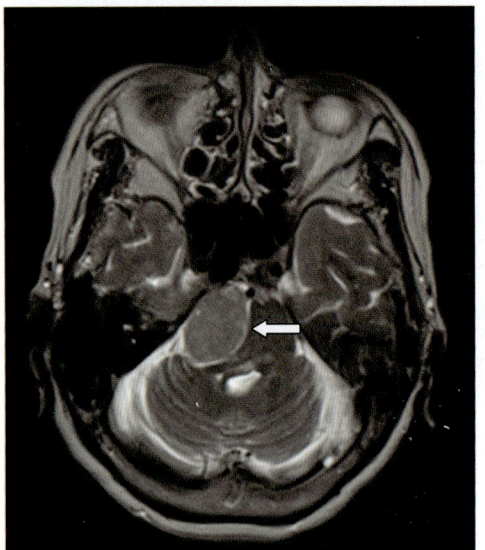

FIGURE 3-1

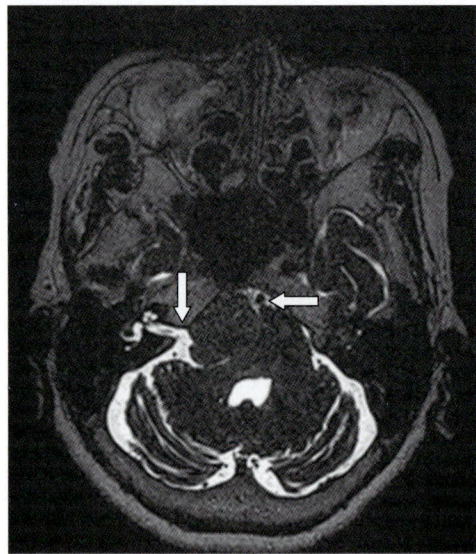

FIGURE 3-2

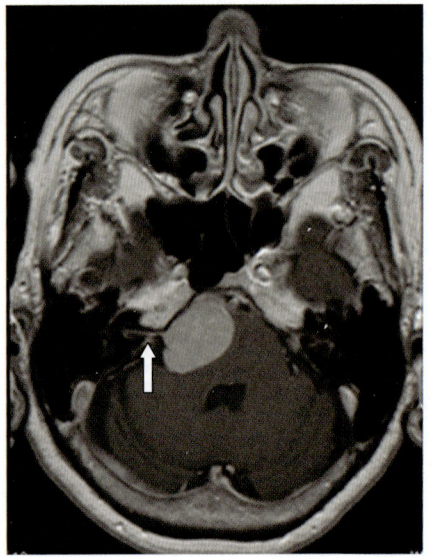

FIGURE 3-3

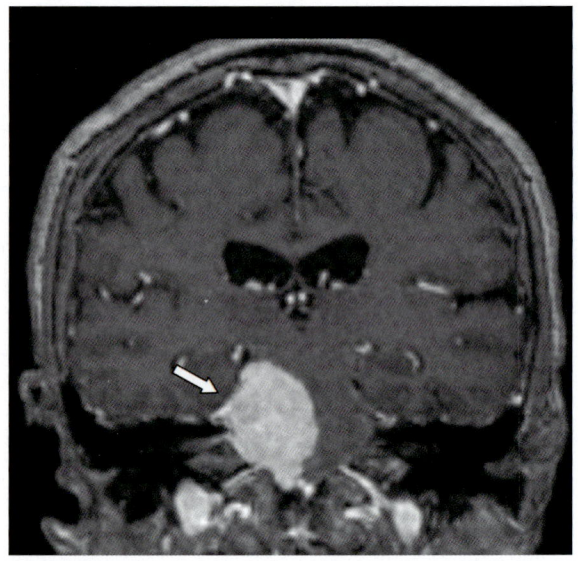

FIGURE 3-4

FINDINGS Figure 3-1. Axial T2WI through the cerebellopontine angle (CPA). There is a mass at the right CPA with a cleft of cerebrospinal fluid (CSF) separating it from the brainstem (arrow), confirming its extraaxial location. The adjacent brainstem is compressed and displaced to the left, demonstrating mild edema. The mass is ovoid, sharply circumscribed, and hypointense. Figure 3-2. Axial 3D volumetric heavily T2WI. This better demonstrates the relationship of the mass to the adjacent neural and vascular structures including cranial nerves VII and VIII (vertical arrow) and the basilar artery (BA) (transverse arrow). Figure 3-3. Axial post-contrast T1WI reveals a broad-based mass with intense, homogeneous enhancement with a dural tail extending into the right internal auditory canal (IAC) (arrow). Figure 3-4. Coronal post-contrast T1WI confirms the dural-based lesion along the tentorium cerebelli (arrow).

DIFFERENTIAL DIAGNOSIS Vestibular schwannoma, dural metastasis, hemangiopericytoma, meningioma and epidermoid.

DIAGNOSIS   CPA meningioma.

DISCUSSION   Meningioma is a well-circumscribed, extraaxial mass that is typically hyperdense or isodense on CT, often with hyperostosis on bone window images. Meningioma is isointense to hypointense on T2WI and usually shows intense, homogeneous enhancement. A broad dural base is common, with a "dural tail" more commonly seen with meningioma than other dural-based lesions. Dural enhancement can extend into the IAC as in this case but usually does not widen the IAC or blunt the bony margin of the porus acusticus. In contrast, vestibular schwannoma frequently widens the IAC and tends to present an acute angle to the petrous bone. Larger schwannomas are often heterogeneous and show areas of hemorrhage and cyst formation, less commonly seen in meningioma. A dural tail is uncommonly seen with schwannomas. Dural metastases are often nodular and multiple and have a more aggressive appearance than meningioma, often with edema in the adjacent brain. Epidermoid tumor demonstrates restricted diffusion, encases rather than displaces adjacent structures, and rarely enhances. Hemangiopericytoma is an aggressive lesion often with bone erosion and destruction rather than hyperostosis. It may present extracalvarial component.

Meningioma is most commonly benign and WHO I. Atypical and/or malignant meningiomas, although rare, typically show more aggressive imaging features. CPA meningioma is the second most common CPA tumor after vestibular schwannoma (which accounts for 75% to 80% of CPA masses). Meningioma occurs in middle age and is more common in females. Meningioma often remains asymptomatic until large and presents with mass effect on adjacent neural or vascular structures.

Questions for Further Thought
1. What is the choice of therapy?
2. Is the "dural tail" malignant infiltration?

Reporting Responsibilities
Findings of significant edema and mass effect upon the brainstem and/or compression of neural or vascular structures must be urgently reported. Images should be scrutinized for the presence of multiple dural-based lesions that may suggest neurofibromatosis type II or meningiomatosis.

What the Treating Physician Needs to Know
- Location and size
- Relationship to adjacent neural and vascular structures including cranial nerves V, VII, and VIII, BA, or the anterior inferior cerebellar artery loop within the IAC
- Extension of the mass anteriorly into Meckel cave, inferiorly into the jugular fossa or extension to the level of the foramen magnum

Answers
1. Surgery is the treatment of choice, when possible. Stereotactic radiosurgery is considered for surgically inoperable lesions or following incomplete resection.
2. The "dural tail" usually represents hypervascular dural reaction rather than actual tumoral infiltration. The "dural tail" sign is not specific for meningioma. It does not indicate malignancy.

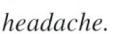

CLINICAL HISTORY *14-year-old female with 1-year history of worsening headache.*

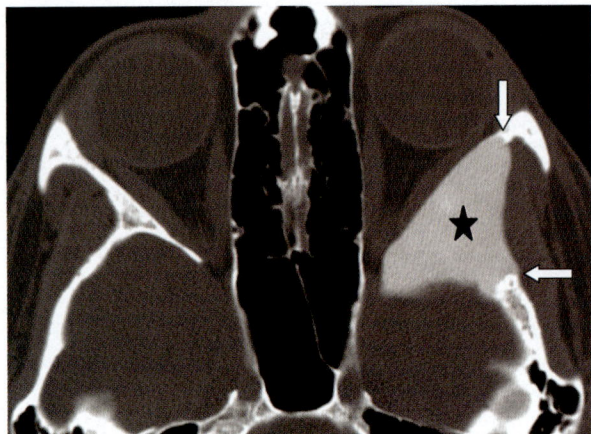

FIGURE 4-1

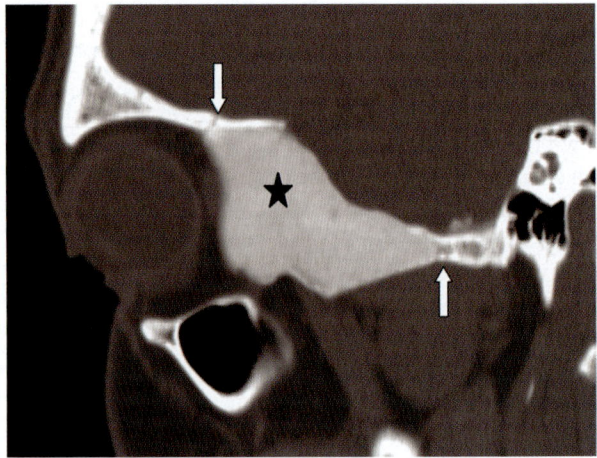

FIGURE 4-2

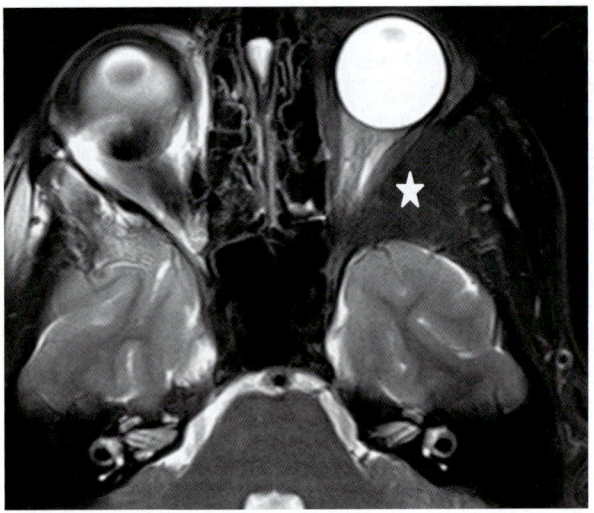

FIGURE 4-3

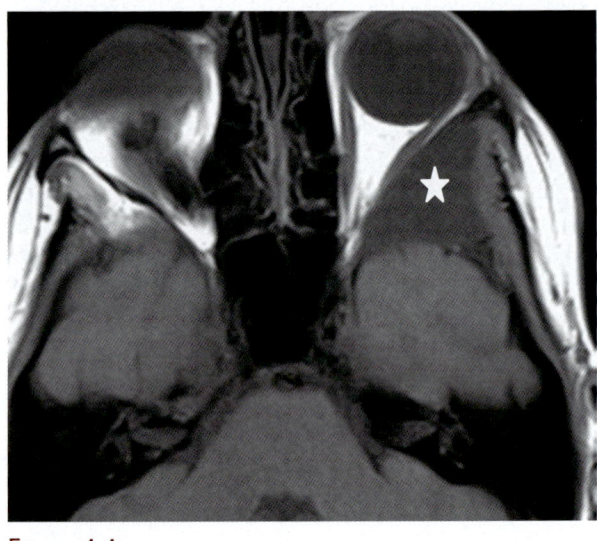

FIGURE 4-4

FINDINGS Figures 4-1 and 4-2. Axial and reformatted sagittal NCCT through the orbits. There is expansion and sclerotic (ground-glass) appearance of the left greater wing of sphenoid bone (stars). There is abrupt sharp transition between the lesion and surrounding bone (arrows). There is mild encroachment on the left orbit with mild proptosis. Figures 4-3 and 4-4. Axial T2WI and T1WI, respectively, through the lesion. There is homogeneous hypointensity of expanded thickened left greater wing of sphenoid bone (stars). There is compression of the left lateral rectus and narrowing of the left orbital apex. Figure 4-5. Axial post-contrast T1WI through the lesion. There is almost homogeneous contrast enhancement of the lesion with two tiny poorly enhancing foci (arrows).

DIFFERENTIAL DIAGNOSIS Osteoblastic metastasis, fibrous dysplasia (FD), Paget disease, intraosseous meningioma.

DIAGNOSIS Fibrous dysplasia (FD).

DISCUSSION The classical imaging findings of FD are best depicted on the NCCT. Monostotic and polyostotic forms of the disease exist. The cranial vault and skull base are affected in up to 25% of cases, with the monostotic being more common. There is expansion of the involved bone. It has a sclerotic, most often homogeneous ground-glass, appearance both on CT and on plain radiograph. Some hypodense foci could be present. The margins are sharply

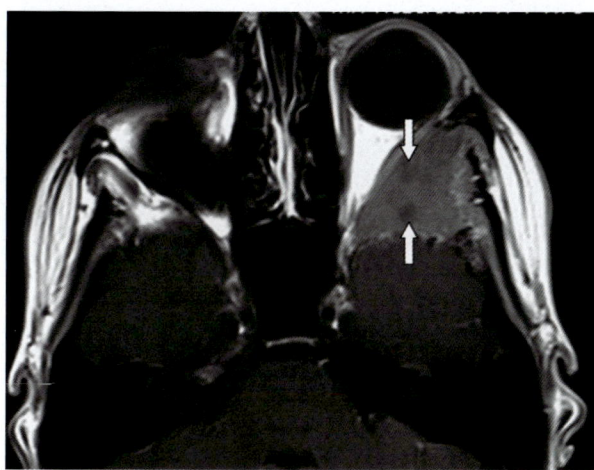

Figure 4-5

demarcated from surrounding bone. It varies in size ranging from a few centimeters to large lesion that may encompass the calvarium and skull base. FD is most common in the ethmoid bones, frontal bones, skull base, maxilla, and zygomatic arch but can affect any cranial bones. It is also found all over the skeleton. It is deforming and can encroach on structures and foramina, thereby impinging cranial nerves. MRI usually demonstrates hypointense lesion on all sequences, sometimes with focal areas of hyperintensity on FLAIR. It enhances avidly homogeneously, but heterogeneity is not uncommon. When it affects the frontal or sphenoid bone, FD could encroach on the orbits causing proptosis and deform the skull base foramina and fissures impinging on cranial nerves. FD is glucose avid on FDG-PET. The sharp margins tend to distinguish FD from its mimics such as osteoblastic metastases, intraosseous meningioma, and Paget disease. The cotton-wool appearance of the bone is typical of Paget. The "pagetoid" FD may resemble Paget! Apart from the pagetoid-type FD, the other two types of FD described are the cystic and sclerotic types.

FD is a rare disease of the young usually presenting under 30 years. It has no gender preference; but the McCune-Albright syndrome has a predilection for girls. Most are monostotic with up to 25% polyostotic and found at multiple sites. The underlying pathology is abnormal formation of fibro-osseous tissue resulting in admixture of woven bone and fibrous tissue and expansion of the bone. The imaging heterogeneity may be due to elements of fat, cystic degeneration, and calcifications within the lesion. Clinical presentations depend on location. Orbital involvement may result in proptosis. Skull base involvement may lead to craniopathies. Facial or skull deformity is common in large lesions, while hearing loss and facial weakness occur in temporal bone involvement. It is generally painless, but craniopathies may produce pain. There is no specific treatment. Surgical excision or curettage may result in recurrence.

Question for Further Thought

1. Is there a genetic or syndromic form of FD?

Reporting Responsibilities

Routine reporting is sufficient in most cases in this benign bone lesion. However, distortion or compression of critical structures and foramina as in this case requires direct reporting.

What the Treating Physician Needs to Know

- Location, extent of lesion, and number if more than one
- Presence of critical structures compression or foraminal deformity
- Certainty of diagnosis

Answer

1. FD is associated with mutation in the *GNAS1* gene, which controls skeleton-forming mesenchymal tissue. The McCune-Albright syndrome is polyostotic FD affecting mainly young girls in their first decade of life with endocrinopathy resulting in precocious puberty, and skin hyperpigmentation otherwise known as "café-au-lait" spots which could be confused with skin changes of neurofibromatosis.

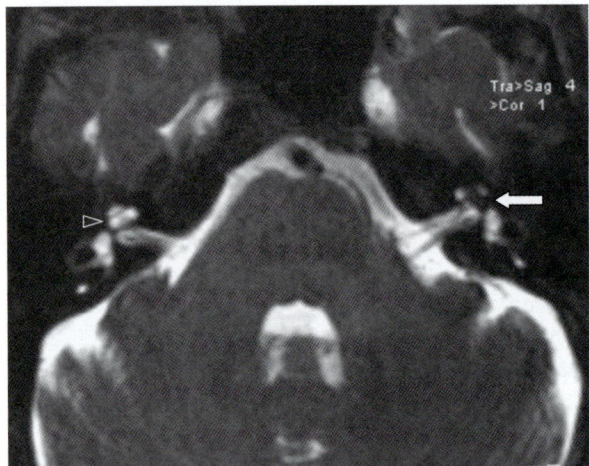

FIGURE 5-1

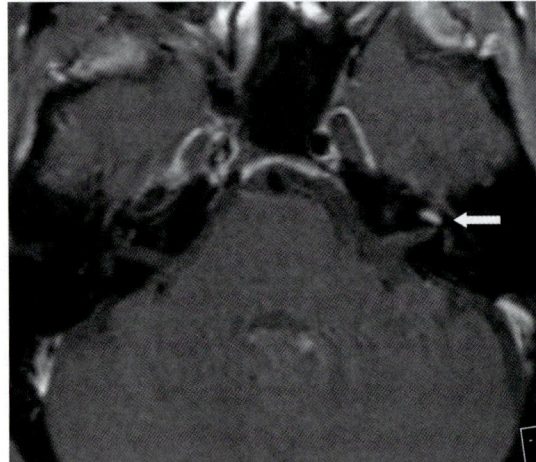

FIGURE 5-2

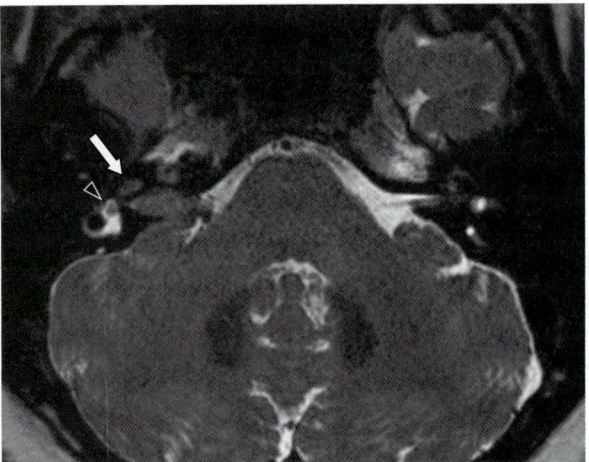

FIGURE 5-3

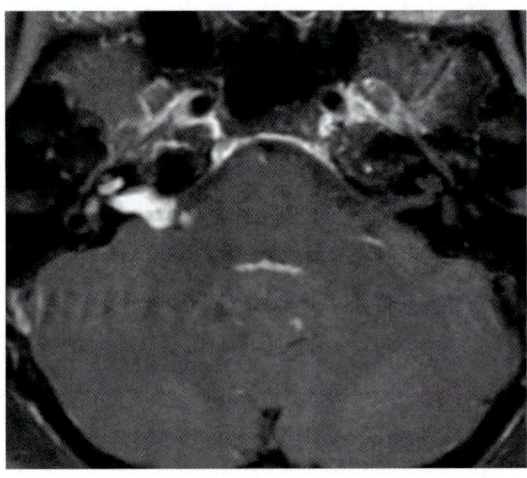

FIGURE 5-4

FINDINGS Figure 5-1. Axial T2WI through the cerebello-pontine angles (CPAs). The normal T2 signal hyperintensity of the fluid (perilymph and endolymph) in the middle turn of the left cochlea has been replaced (arrow) (note the normal cochlea on the right, open arrowhead). Figure 5-2. Axial post-contrast T1WI through same level. There is avid corresponding enhancement (arrow). Figures 5-3 and 5-4. Axial T2WI and corresponding post-contrast T1WI through the internal auditory canal (IAC), respectively, in a companion case. There is avidly contrast-enhancing isointense tumor filling the right IAC and protruding into the CPA cistern with extension into the cochlea (transmodiolar type—arrow in Figure 5-3) and vestibule (transmacular type—arrowhead in Figure 5-3).

DIFFERENTIAL DIAGNOSIS Cochleitis/labyrinthitis, cochlear schwannoma.

DIAGNOSIS Intralabyrinthine (cochlear) schwannoma (ILS).

DISCUSSION A high index of suspicion and a high-resolution MRI are required to make the diagnosis of ILS. ILS originates within the cochlea. It is hyperintense on unenhanced T1WI and enhances avidly following intravenous gadolinium administration. It is sharply circumscribed and hypointense on thin heavily T2W "cisternogram." A recent classification system is based on the anatomic region(s) of tumor involvement. The "intracochlear" type is the most common, where tumor is confined to the turns in the cochlea. The "intravestibular" type has tumor in the vestibule with or without extension into the semicircular canals, whereas "vestibulocochlear" ILS involves both compartments of the inner ear, but not the IAC or middle ear space. Tumors that grow between the IAC and inner ear are "transmodiolar" if they grow across the modiolus to or from the cochlea. A "transmacular" tumor crosses the macula cribrosa and involves the vestibule and IAC. The rarest of all is the "transotic" schwannoma, which spans the IAC and inner and middle ear compartments. Our companion case (Figures 5-3 and 5-4) shows tumor filling the IAC and protruding into the CPA cistern with both transmodiolar and transmacular growth patterns.

The main differential for our case is inflammatory inner ear disease or labyrinthitis. MRI findings in inflammatory disease may be subtle (if present at all) and require careful attention to the signal properties of the inner ear fluid and any corresponding enhancement. The normal T2 fluid hyperintensity in acute labyrinthitis is usually normal, and the degree of enhancement may be mild but is commonly diffuse within the labyrinth. In contrast, the pronounced T2 fluid signal replacement and the corresponding intense contrast enhancement seen in cases of ILS are quite focal. CT is virtually always normal in acute cases of labyrinthitis unless caused by gross middle ear disease (tympanogenic labyrinthitis) or temporal bone fracture. MRI of hemorrhagic or posttraumatic labyrinthitis may demonstrate inherent T1 hyperintensity of the inner ear fluid. If chronic, labyrinthine fibrosis and varying degrees of ossification (labyrinthitis ossificans) may develop, in which case CT is useful in confirming the diagnosis.

Purely ILSs are rare, benign tumors arising from the Schwann cells lining the terminal ends of the cochlear and vestibular nerves. The clinical presentation is nonspecific and variable and may include unilateral sensorineural hearing loss, vertigo, tinnitus, and subjective ear fullness—mimicking many neurootologic diseases.

Question for Further Thought

1. What are the management options for these tumors? When is surgery indicated?

Reporting Responsibilities

Direct reporting is necessary as in any tumor. Anatomic extent of disease must be described, including the IAC and CPA components if present and any corresponding mass effect on the brainstem.

What the Treating Physician Needs to Know

- Anatomic compartments involved (cochlea, vestibule, IAC, middle ear)
- Follow-up recommendations: serial MR surveillance for schwannoma and for cases of indeterminate enhancement/labyrinthitis
- Follow-up MRI and/or concurrent CT in select cases (complicated infection, bone involvement, labyrinthitis ossificans)

Answer

1. In patients with serviceable hearing, these slow-growing tumors may be observed with periodic MRI. Clinical factors supporting surgical intervention include intractable vestibular symptoms, demonstrable tumor growth, tumor presence in the IAC/CPA cistern and absence of serviceable hearing. Hearing preservation is not possible after surgical removal of an intralabyrinthine tumor. Poor surgical candidates have been treated with conventional external beam radiation therapy or stereotactic radiosurgery.

CLINICAL HISTORY *3-year-old male with progressive right-sided hearing loss.*

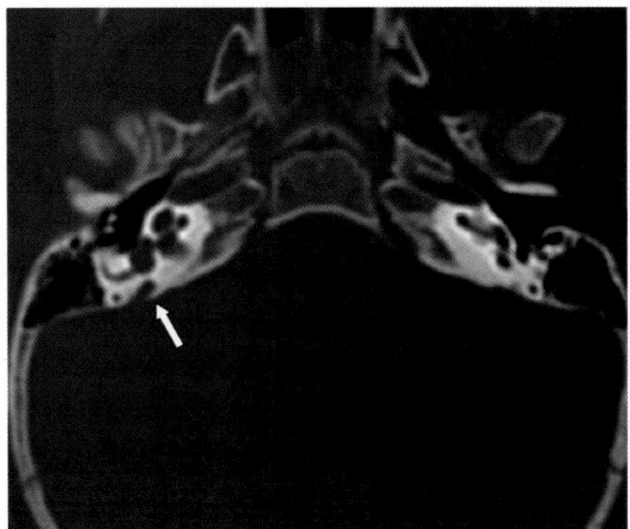

FIGURE 6-1

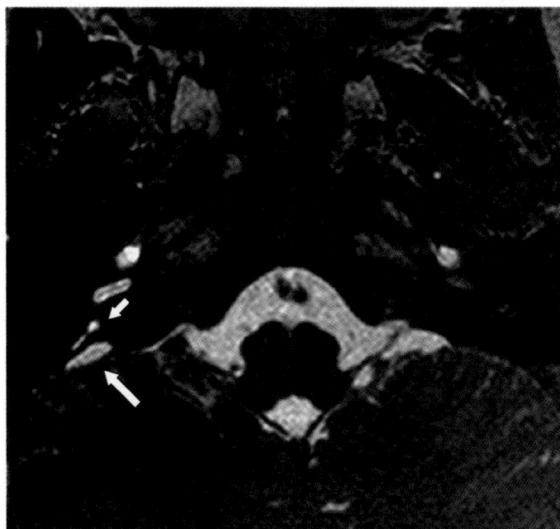

FIGURE 6-2

FINDINGS Figure 6-1. Axial NCCT of the right temporal bone. There is mild enlargement of the right vestibular aqueduct, measuring approximately 1.3 mm (long white arrow). The left vestibular aqueduct is not enlarged. Figure 6-2. Axial T2WI through the temporal bones. There is an enlarged, elongated T2 hyperintense structure (isointense to endolymph of adjacent inner ear structures) along the posterior margin of the right temporal bone consistent with an enlarged endolymphatic sac (long white arrow). The diameter of the right endolymphatic duct/sac is larger than the adjacent semicircular canal (short white arrow). The normal left endolymphatic duct/sac is not visible on MRI, an expected finding.

DIFFERENTIAL DIAGNOSIS Pendred syndrome, endolymphatic sac tumor, enlarged endolymphatic sac.

DIAGNOSIS Enlarged endolymphatic sac syndrome.

DISCUSSION On CT, the normal bony vestibular aqueduct, which contains the endolymphatic duct, has an inverted "J" or hockey stick appearance. The short limb arises along the anteromedial wall of the vestibule and courses posteromedially and parallel to the common crus, descends posterolaterally through the petrous pyramid, and terminates along the posterior temporal bone. On MRI, the normal endolymphatic duct is seen as the union of the utricular and saccular ducts and courses through the bony vestibular aqueduct to terminate as a blind-ending endolymphatic sac in the fovea of the posterior temporal bone, a small recess between layers of dura and adjacent to the sigmoid sinus. The transition between the endolymphatic duct and sac occurs within

the bony vestibular aqueduct, although there is no reliable imaging correlate. A normal endolymphatic sac in the fovea is barely visible as a fluid-filled hyperintense structure on T2WI. The diagnosis on axial thin-section CT of the temporal bone is made by measuring the midpoint of the distal limb in the bony vestibular aqueduct halfway between the bend at the proximal limb and the fovea. A measurement greater than 1.5 mm is defined as abnormal vestibular aqueduct enlargement, although more recent studies have reported a midpoint measurement greater than 1 mm and opercular measurement that is equal to or larger than 2 mm. As a general rule, a vestibular aqueduct diameter that exceeds that of the adjacent posterior semicircular canal or facial nerve canal is considered enlarged. CT may also demonstrate associated cochlear dysplasias and vestibular anomalies, the most common being modiolar deficiency (or absence). Although thin-section CT of the temporal bone is adequate to demonstrate enlargement of the vestibular aqueduct, it cannot show the membranous labyrinth and thus is less sensitive for the detection of associated cochlear anomalies. Enlargement of the endolymphatic sac may occur in the presence of a normal-sized vestibular aqueduct on CT. High-resolution T2WI is the superior imaging tool, even in less-experienced hands, allowing for obvious detection of an elongated fluid-filled T2 hyperintense endolymphatic sac. Precise measurements on axial T2WI are still made at the midpoint between the bend at the proximal limb of the endolymphatic duct and the posterior margin of the temporal bone. Endolymphatic sac tumor presents as a highly vascular retrolabyrinthine mass centered in the fovea of the endolymphatic sac and demonstrates calcification, heterogeneous MRI signal and enhancement, and permeative bony destruction.

Enlargement of the endolymphatic duct and sac is recognized as the most common congenital anomaly of the inner ear on imaging and is one of the most common morphologic findings associated with congenital sensorineural hearing loss. Embryologically described as arrested fetal development of the inner ear due to a nonspecific insult, the trigger of sensorineural hearing loss in this condition may be mild head trauma to an already fragile or structurally deficient cochlea.

Questions for Further Thought

1. Are there any associated genetic alterations?
2. What is the choice of therapy?

Reporting Responsibilities

Routine reporting is sufficient, as this is not an acute disorder unless it is unexpected. Enlargement of the endolymphatic sac may occur in the presence of a normal-sized vestibular aqueduct on CT, and as such, high-resolution MRI should be pursued in the appropriate clinical context. It is important to have a systematic approach in evaluating temporal bone CT, as the diagnosis is easily missed if not carefully scrutinized. It is necessary to report associated cochlear anomalies, cochlear dysmorphisms, scalar asymmetries, as well as vestibular anomalies, such as enlargement of the membranous vestibule, gross vestibular dysplasias, and semicircular canal dysplasias.

What the Treating Physician Needs to Know

- Laterality
- Associated cochlear and vestibular anomalies

Answers

1. Most cases are sporadic, although a familial autosomal recessive inheritance pattern has been reported. Pendred syndrome, an autosomal recessive syndrome seen in 15% of patients with enlarged vestibular aqueduct due to *SLC26A4 Pendrin* gene mutation on chromosome 7, presents with dyshormonogenic goiter and modiolar deficiency.
2. There is no accepted treatment, although physicians may recommend avoidance of contact sports or other activities that may result in head trauma and promote hearing loss in this condition. Surgical occlusion and obliteration of the endolymphatic sac has had limited success. Fortunately, cochlear implantation has been shown to significantly increase quality of life for those with profound bilateral SNHL.

CASE 7

CLINICAL HISTORY *82-year-old female with headache.*

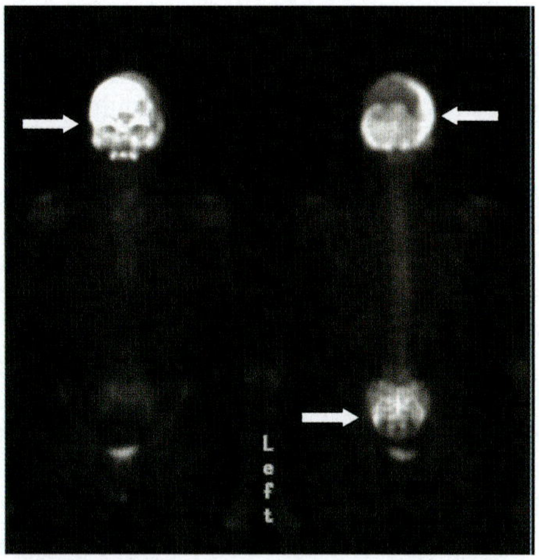

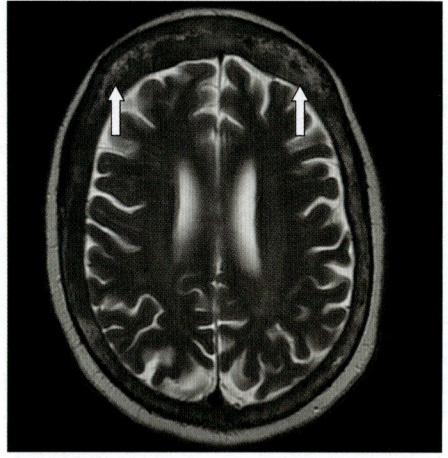

FIGURE 7-1

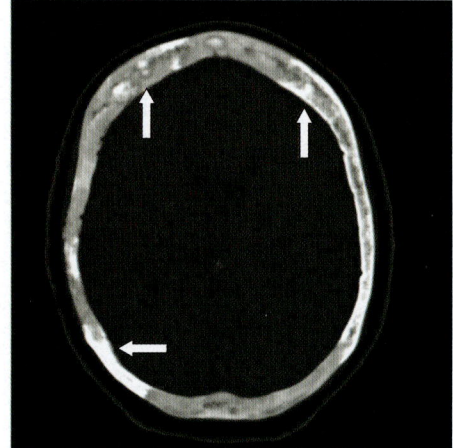

FIGURE 7-2

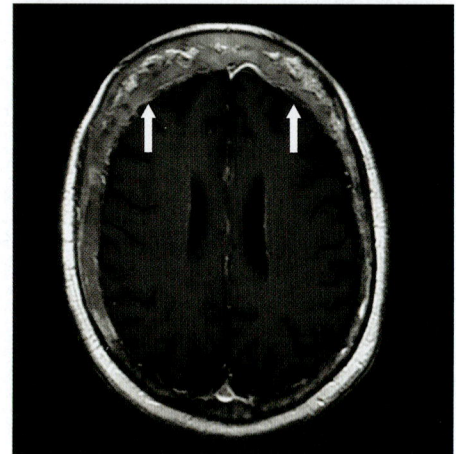

FIGURE 7-3

FIGURE 7-4

FINDINGS Figure 7-1. Bone scintigraphy. There is abnormal tracer uptake in the calvarium, skull base, and pelvis (arrows). Figure 7-2. NCCT head bone window. There are cortical thickening, abnormal bone matrix, and patchy sclerosis (hyperdensity) (arrows). Figure 7-3. Axial T2WI through the cerebral hemispheres. There are diffuse thickening and heterogeneous marrow intensity of the cranial vault (arrows). Figure 7-4. Axial post-contrast T1WI through the cranial vault. There are marrow replacement, expansion of the diploic space, and patchy enhancement (arrows).

DIFFERENTIAL DIAGNOSIS Paget disease, metastases, fibrous dysplasia.

DIAGNOSIS Paget disease.

DISCUSSION Paget disease is a common metabolic condition of the bones which leads to excessive remodeling and deformity. Any bone can be involved, though the skull, spine, and pelvis are common sites. The disease progresses through three phases, each with a distinct imaging appearance. The lytic phase, characterized by predominant osteolytic activity, results in lucent lesions on plain film and CT. In the skull, these can be large and geographic, often referred to as osteoporosis circumscripta. A mixed phase follows which reflects osteoblastic repair. Cortical and trabecular thickening are typical of this stage. Finally, a blastic phase ensues, with development of sclerotic foci, indicating an excessive osteoblastic response. In the skull, this can result in the pathognomonic "cotton-wool" appearance whereby fluffy-appearing sclerotic lesions develop in areas of prior osteoporosis circumscripta resulting in a mixed-density pattern on CT. The diploic space of the skull may widen with considerable deformity of the bony anatomy. MRI T1WI shows areas of hypointensity within thickened cranial vault or skull base with heterogeneous contrast enhancement. It is often heterogeneous intensity on T2WI. Complications include bony weakening with the potential for fracture, accelerated arthritis, neurologic symptoms due to narrowing of the skull base and spinal foramina, and rarely, sarcomatous transformation and giant cell formation.

Paget is a disease of the elderly with a slight male preponderance. It is uncommon in people of African and Asian descent. Paget is due to replacement of bone marrow and bone thickening by fibrovascular tissue which subsequently progresses to calcification and sclerosis. Clinical presentation when symptomatic may include macrocrania, asymmetric deformity of the skull, cranial neuropathy, and pain particularly when complicated by fracture, giant cell tumor formation, or sarcomatous degeneration. There is usually elevated serum alkaline phosphatase. Treatment is by bisphosphonates.

Questions for Further Thought

1. What sort of imaging is most appropriate in the diagnosis and follow-up of Paget disease?
2. How would sarcomatous transformation appear on imaging?

Reporting Responsibilities

Routine reporting is sufficient unless there are complications such as fractures, sarcomatous change, and foraminal narrowing. Recognize the characteristic appearance of Paget disease so as to distinguish it from other more ominous or malignant conditions.

What the Treating Physician Needs to Know

- Paget disease is a common benign condition of the bones which, in most cases, can be diagnosed with certainty based on characteristic imaging features
- Are there any complications?
- What is the extent of the disease?

Answers

1. Plain films and/or bone scintigraphy are usually adequate to make the diagnosis. When the imaging features are not sufficiently specific, for example, with an incidental skull abnormality on head CT, consider imaging the pelvis and long bones. These are frequent sites of concomitant disease where the features may be more typical.
2. Sarcomatous transformation should be highly suspected when areas of new lytic change develop in Pagetoid bone, especially if a soft tissue process can be detected.

CLINICAL HISTORY *46-year-old male with a mass on the head.*

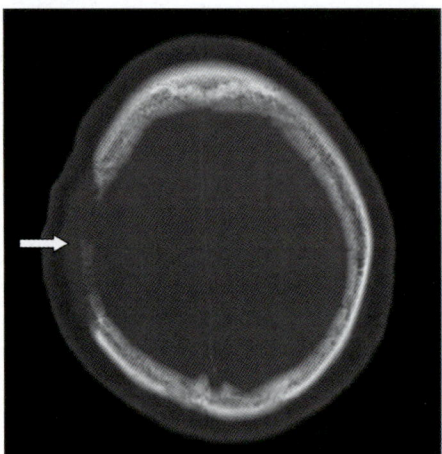

FIGURE 8-1

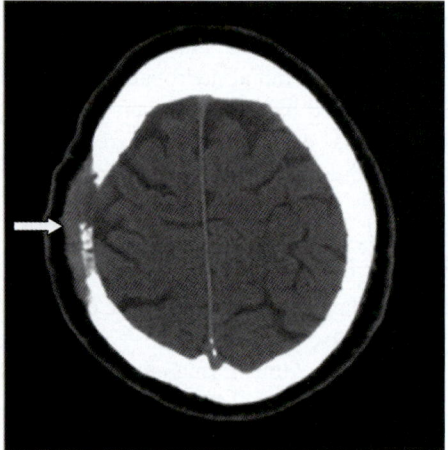

FIGURE 8-2

FINDINGS Figures 8-1 and 8-2. Axial NCCT bone and soft tissue windows, respectively, through the parietal bones. There is a soft tissue mass of the right parietal calvarium (arrows) with through and through cortical erosion with beveled margin.

DIFFERENTIAL DIAGNOSIS Metastatic disease, myeloma, lymphoma, eosinophilic granuloma, hemangioma.

DIAGNOSIS Right parietal bone hemangioma.

DISCUSSION Hemangioma of the bone is a benign lesion of disordered vessels, not a tumor. On CT, hemangioma presents as focal lucency within a bone. Occasionally, an internal texture may be discerned, for example, a honeycomb or spoke-wheel pattern in the skull, or a striated, corduroy pattern in the spine. On MRI, hemangiomas are enhancing lesions that are hyperintense of T2WI and isointense to hyperintense on T1WI depending on the amount of fat present. Cranial vault hemangiomas are usually small and result in cortical thinning and diploic widening, often with greater effect on the outer table rather than the inner table. The large and aggressive appearing lesion in the above case is unusual. This lesion could mimic any of the lesions in the list of differential diagnoses. Tissue sampling will be necessary for the correct diagnosis.

Histologic classification of hemangiomas depends on the histologic type of vessels present. Capillary hemangioma, commonly found in the spine, shows numerous small caliber vessels, often oriented in parallel. Cavernous hemangioma is composed of fewer but larger vessels along with fibrous septa and is more common in the skull. Mixed capillary and cavernous varieties also exist. Regardless of the site, these lesions are most often asymptomatic and detected incidentally.

Question for Further Thought

1. Typical, atypical, and aggressive hemangiomas, what is the difference?

Reporting Responsibilities

Routine reporting is sufficient since most of these are asymptomatic and incidental. Large lesions, however, may require direct reporting for proper management. Recognize the benign nature of the lesion. Many of these lesions may have nonspecific appearance on MRI. When in doubt, suggest CT follow-up, as the classic patterns of lucency noted above will often help to exclude other possibilities.

What the Treating Physician Needs to Know

- Hemangioma of the bone is most often an occult, incidental finding of no significance
- In rare cases, large or atypical lesions may require tissue sampling

Answer

1. These terms are most often used in relation to spine lesions. A typical hemangioma will be hyperintense on T1WI (reflecting fatty material) and T2WI (reflecting slow flow vessels in addition to fatty material). This appearance is highly specific and should lead to a confident diagnosis. An atypical hemangioma remains hyperintense on T2WI but lacks T1 hyperintensity due to scarcity of fat. This is a nonspecific appearance and can be a diagnostic dilemma as metastatic disease or other marrow-replacing processes may present similarly. An aggressive hemangioma will appear as in the case above, with substantial bony deformation and often an extraosseous soft tissue component. Tissue sampling is necessary in these cases to exclude a malignant etiology.

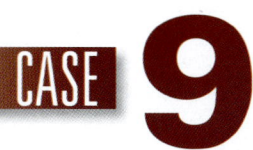

CASE 9

CLINICAL HISTORY *Patient with red and swollen left eye.*

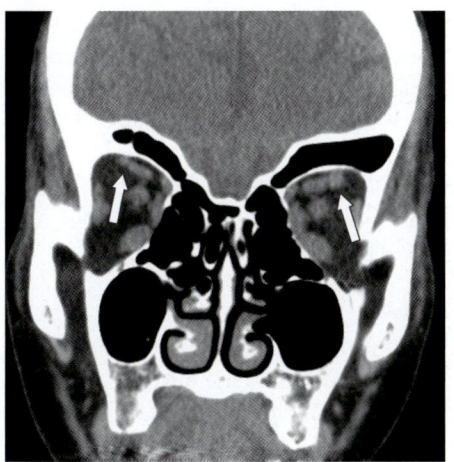

FIGURE 9-1.

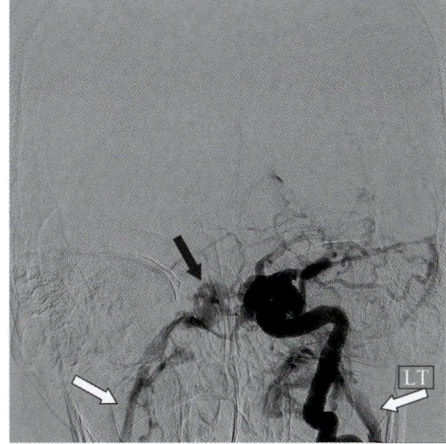

FIGURE 9-2.

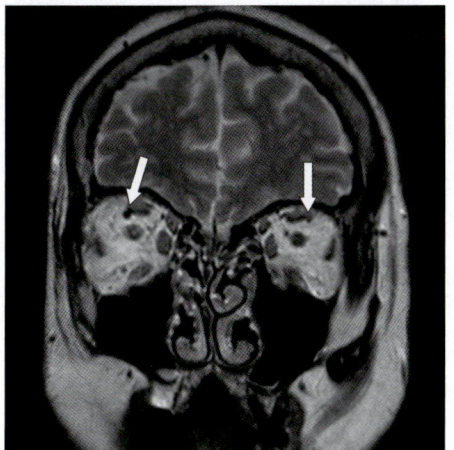

FIGURE 9-3.

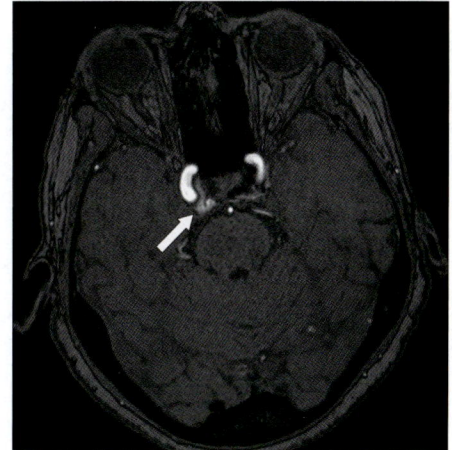

FIGURE 9-4.

FINDINGS Figure 9-1. Coronal NCCT through the orbits. There is enlargement of the left superior ophthalmic vein relative to the right (arrows). Figure 9-2. DSA left internal carotid artery (ICA) PA (posterior-anterior) view. There is abnormal early and dense opacification of the left cavernous sinus with early opacification of the contralateral right cavernous sinus (black arrow) and the bilateral jugular veins (white arrows). Figure 9-3. Coronal T2WI through the orbits in a companion case with incidental findings at imaging for unrelated complaint. There is mild prominence of the right superior ophthalmic vein (arrows). Figure 9-4. Time of flight MRA source images level of the cavernous sinus in the same patient as figure 9-3. There is asymmetric flow-related signal in the right cavernous sinus.

DIFFERENTIAL DIAGNOSIS Cavernous sinus thrombosis, carotid cavernous fistula (CCF), cavernous ICA aneurysm.

DIAGNOSIS Both patients have CCF.

DISCUSSION CCF implies an abnormal communication between the cavernous sinus and some element of the carotid vasculature, either the ICA itself or a branch of the ICA. CT and MRI show enlarged cavernous sinus with corresponding enlargement of the superior ophthalmic vein. The findings could be bilateral in high-flow fistulas with cross communication to the contralateral side. Proptosis with orbital fat stranding and enlarged extraocular muscles may be present. Brain parenchymal and/or subarachnoid hemorrhage from ruptured engorged cortical veins are occasionally present. Retroclival and pterygoid venous plexus enhancement could be present. CT and MR angiography may be diagnostic in showing abnormal early opacification or abnormal flow in the cavernous sinus and prominence of the cavernous sinus outflow pathways. DSA is diagnostic and will reveal the source arteries and full pattern of venous outflow.

CCFs are rare and are classified as being either high flow (direct) or low flow (indirect). High-flow CCFs are typically

17

posttraumatic or secondary to rupture of a cavernous ICA aneurysm. Low-flow CCFs arise from small dural arteriovenous (AV) fistulas involving the cavernous sinus and meningeal branches of the external carotid artery (ECA) and ICA. Standard imaging can suggest the diagnosis when abnormal arterial flow into the cavernous sinus results in expansion of the sinus and its outflow pathways (such as the superior ophthalmic vein).

The most common cause of a direct CCF is trauma, usually high flow and most commonly occurs in the young but could be found in all ages and both gender. Indirect or dural CCF on the other hand tends to occur in elderly women and is usually low flow. Complications of CCF include vision loss due to central retinal vein occlusion or secondary glaucoma, epistaxis that could be fatal, subarachnoid hemorrhage, and intracerebral hemorrhage due to retrograde venous drainage.

Question for Further Thought

1. When and how should CCFs be treated?

Reporting Responsibilities

Direct reporting is required because of the progressive visual complications or fatal hemorrhages if left untreated. Suspect CCF and suggest dedicated imaging when abnormal bulging of one or both cavernous sinuses is seen or when the superior ophthalmic veins are larger than normal.

What the Treating Physician Needs to Know

- CCF is an infrequent but potentially serious condition as sequelae include loss of vision, intracerebral hemorrhage, subarachnoid hemorrhage, and venous thrombosis
- Is it a direct or indirect fistula? This will affect how it is treated
- Are there any complications?
- All arterial feeders and venous outflows should be delineated

Answer

1. All direct or high-flow CCFs should be treated. These are usually of acute onset and result in striking clinical findings including orbital swelling, chemosis, bruit, bulging red eye, and loss of vision. Endovascular embolization is the preferred approach. For low-flow CCFs, particularly asymptomatic or incidental lesions, the need for treatment should be evaluated on an individual basis. A mild CCF may never produce symptoms, and the available treatments are not without substantial risk themselves.

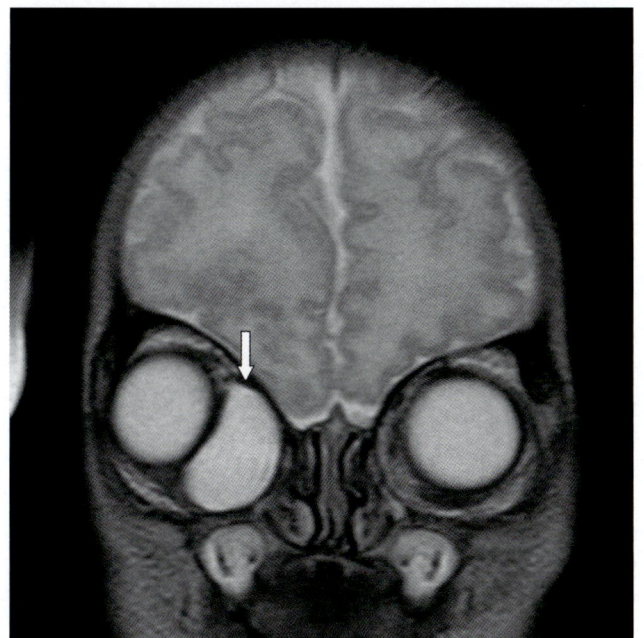

FIGURE 10-1

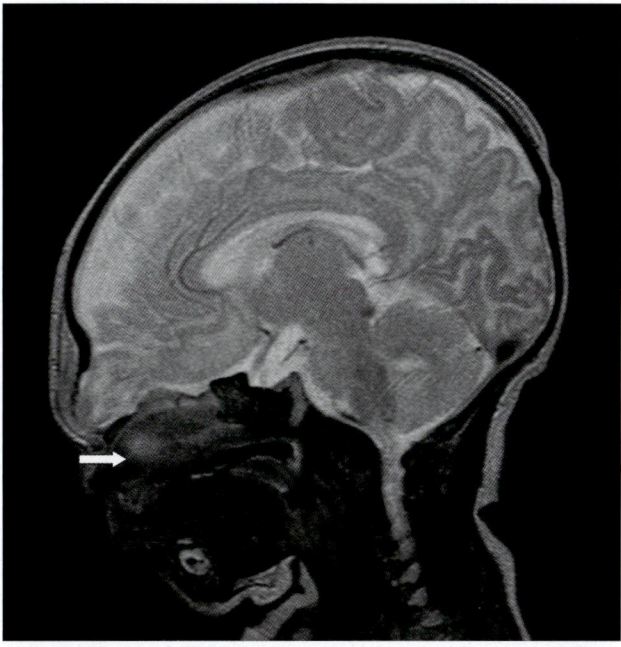

FIGURE 10-2

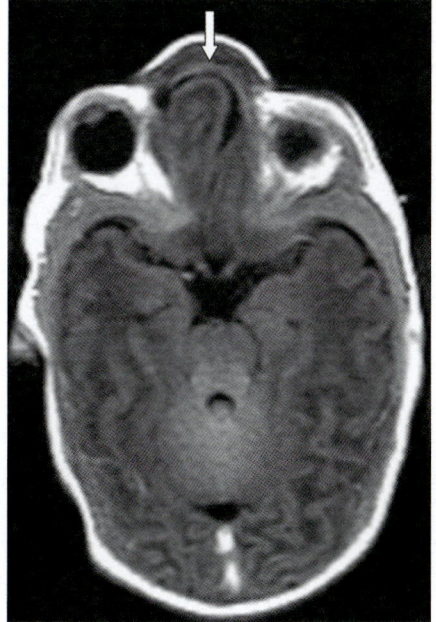

FIGURE 10-3

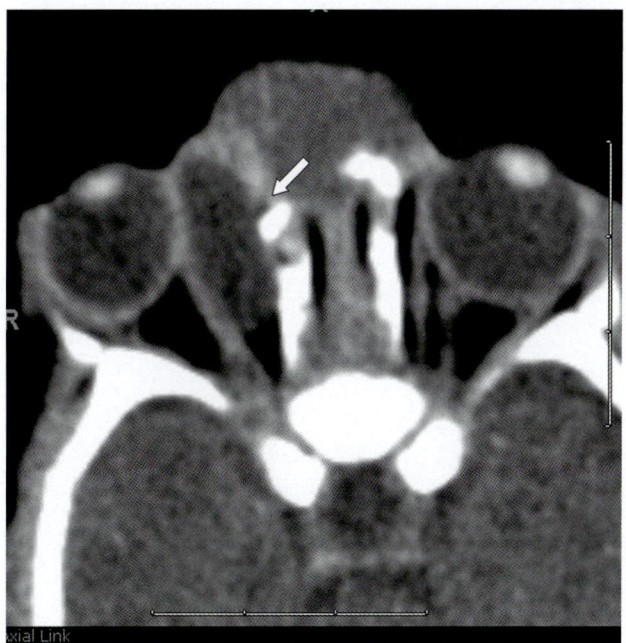

FIGURE 10-4

FINDINGS Figure 10-1. Coronal T2WI through the orbits. There is a cystic mass within the right orbit, medial to the globe, and medial rectus muscle (arrow). Figures 10-2 and 10-3. Sagittal T2WI and axial FLAIR, respectively, through the orbits. There is abnormal protrusion of brain parenchyma into the nasofrontal region (arrows). Figure 10-4.

Axial CECT through the orbits. There is a thin communication (white arrow) between the orbital cyst and the nasal abnormality.

DIFFERENTIAL DIAGNOSIS Mucocele, dermoid/epidermoid, dacryocystocele, meningocele.

DIAGNOSIS Orbital meningocele with nasofrontal meningoencephalocele.

DISCUSSION Cephalocele defines any abnormal protrusion of intracranial contents through cranial vault or skull base defects and is of several types. A cephalocele containing meninges and cerebrospinal fluid (CSF) alone is called a meningocele. A cephalocele containing CSF and brain tissue is called a meningoencephalocele, while an atretic cephalocele contains only meninges and degenerated brain tissue without CSF. Typical CT changes of a skull base meningocele include CSF density structure protruding through the skull base or the orbitofacial region, identifiable defect in the adjacent bone, and displacement of normal structures such as the globe and extraocular muscles as in this case. CT findings of meningoencephalocele on the other hand tend to include some brain material with or without CSF as in the nasofrontal component of the present cephalocele. 3D bone reconstruction may define the bony defect perfectly. Similarly, meningocele follows CSF intensity on all MRI sequences within the abnormal protrusion of the meninges. Brain material is present in meningoencephalocele.

Cephaloceles can be congenital or posttraumatic/postsurgical in nature. Typical locations include the anterior skull base, orbitofrontal, occipital, and parietal regions. A meningocele may be occult and asymptomatic or may produce symptoms related to mass effect. As with any static fluid collection, meningoceles are susceptible to infection. Meningoceles are benign and usually easy to correct at surgery. Meningoencephalocele on the other hand may be a little more complex. When congenital, however, cephaloceles may herald the presence of a more serious underlying syndrome or condition, as in the case presented here.

Question for Further Thought

1. How do you differentiate a skull base meningocele from other common skull base cystic lesions?

Reporting Responsibilities

Direct reporting is essential as the complications could be catastrophic if left untreated. Verify the cystic nature of the lesion and accurately describe the location as well as associated mass effect. Make an effort to identify the site of the bony defect. Thin-section CT may be required as the site of communication with the intracranial space can be extremely small.

What the Treating Physician Needs to Know

- Meningoceles are benign and usually easily corrected. However, when congenital, they are often associated with an underlying syndrome or condition which may be far more problematic
- Location and size
- Content if more than CSF

Answer

1. Mucoceles are typically associated with a paranasal sinus and show evidence of chronic bony remodeling/ expansion. An epidermoid may be suspected based on characteristic high signal on DWI. Dermoids may show characteristics of fatty material on CT and MRI. A meningocele should follow CSF characteristics on any imaging sequence. If a bony defect can be identified, the diagnosis should be offered with confidence.

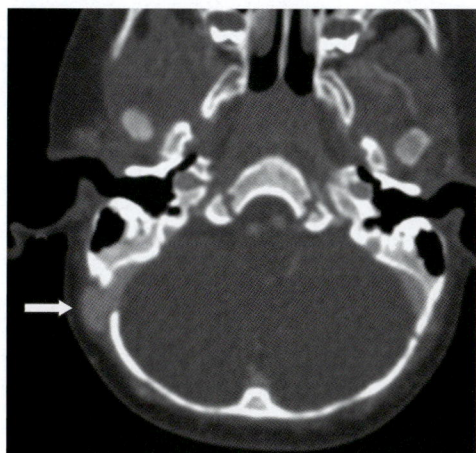

FIGURE 11-1

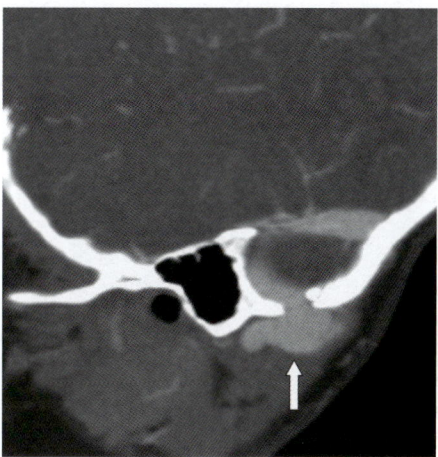

FIGURE 11-2

FINDINGS Figures 11-1 and 11-2. Axial and sagittal CTA images. There is a defect in the right retromastoid occipital bone. An intensely enhancing structure passes through this defect to join the sigmoid sinus (arrow).

DIFFERENTIAL DIAGNOSIS AV malformation, AV fistula, sinus pericranii.

DIAGNOSIS Sinus pericranii.

DISCUSSION Sinus pericranii is an anomalous communication between a scalp vein and a dural venous sinus. The most typical arrangement is communication between a varix, or dilated vein, in the scalp and the superior sagittal sinus via an enlarged transcalvarial emissary vein. Drainage to the other dural sinuses, as in this case, is less common. On noncontrast CT, the calvarial defect may be the only hint of this entity. MRI will better reveal the likely vascular nature of the lesion. Contrast studies and CTA confirm the diagnosis. DSA can also be obtained for confirmation and mapping prior to surgery.

These are very rare almost always congenital lesions, though posttraumatic versions have been reported. On clinical examination, the patient may present with a soft, reducible scalp mass possibly causing a bluish discoloration of the overlying skin. Most of the time, sinus pericranii are small, asymptomatic, and detected incidentally on imaging for some other reason.

Question for Further Thought

1. Is there an association between sinus pericranii and other intracranial vascular anomalies?

Reporting Responsibilities

Direct reporting is essential to prevent inadvertent needling or intervention. Describe the location and nature of the anomalously communicating veins. Search the brain for other venous anomalies.

What the Treating Physician Needs to Know

- Sinus pericranii is, in most cases, an asymptomatic and incidentally detected anomalous communication between the extracranial and intracranial venous systems
- When small, these are often left alone
- Sinus pericranii is associated with a small risk of hemorrhage, and so, when these are large or of concern to the patient, they can be surgically treated without difficulty

Answer

1. Sinus pericranii is often found in conjunction with other venous anomalies, such as developmental venous anomalies, venous malformations, and aberrant development of the dural sinuses.

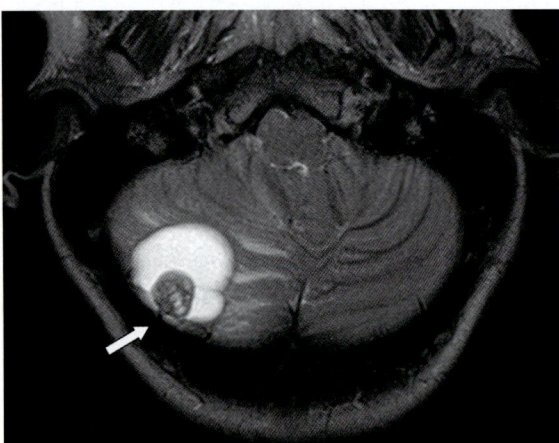

FIGURE 12-1

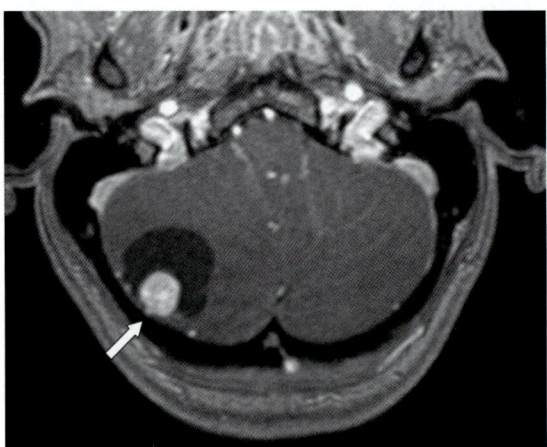

FIGURE 12-2

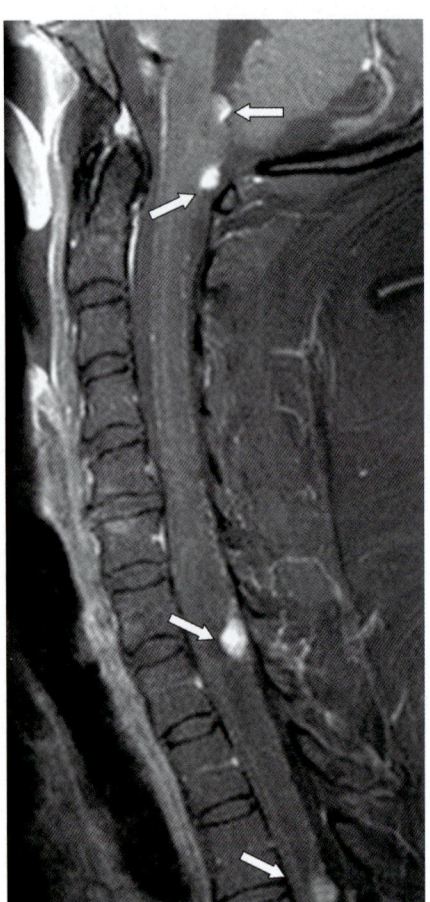

FIGURE 12-3

FINDINGS Figure 12-1. Axial T2WI through the posterior fossa. There is a mixed cystic and solid tumor in the right cerebellar hemisphere. A solid nodule (arrow) abuts the pial surface of the cerebellum. Figure 12-2. Axial post-contrast T1WI through the mass. The solid nodule (arrow) demonstrates intense enhancement, but there is a lack of enhancement of the cyst wall. Figure 12-3. Sagittal post-contrast T1WI in a companion case demonstrates multiple hemangioblastomas (arrows) in the posterior fossa, cervical and thoracic spine, diagnostic of von Hippel-Lindau syndrome.

DIFFERENTIAL DIAGNOSIS Hemangioblastoma, pilocytic astrocytoma, glioblastoma, metastasis.

DIAGNOSIS Hemangioblastoma.

DISCUSSION Hemangioblastoma is most commonly located in the cerebellum, brainstem, or spinal cord. The majority (90%) arises in the posterior fossa, with supratentorial lesions usually limited to patients with von Hippel-Lindau syndrome. The tumor is usually well demarcated, but vasogenic edema may be present. The classic appearance of a cystic mass with mural nodule abutting the pial surface constitutes about 60% of the cases; as much as 40% of the cases manifest as purely solid tumors. There is usually very little or no surrounding edema. Hemangioblastoma is often highly vascular, and hemorrhage may be present. Prominent feeding arteries and draining veins may be visible and seen as flow voids on MRI. These vessels can be well demonstrated on CTA. On angiography, prolonged vascular blush and arterial-venous shunting are commonly present. Some tumors may benefit from preoperative embolization.

Patient age helps to differentiate hemangioblastoma from pilocytic astrocytoma, with the former seen primarily in adults and the latter seen in pediatric patients. When the diagnosis of hemangioblastoma is considered in younger and pediatric patients or when multiple tumors are present, von Hippel-Lindau syndrome needs to be considered.

Glioblastoma usually appears more heterogeneous and infiltrative compared to hemangioblastoma. There is usually substantial vasogenic edema surrounding glioblastoma. Although hemangioblastoma is the most common primary posterior fossa tumor in adults, metastasis is far more common statistically and needs to be excluded.

Most cases of hemangioblastoma are sporadic and are seen in adults older than 30 years. However, approximately 25% of cases arise in patients with von Hippel-Lindau syndrome. Patients with von Hippel-Lindau syndrome often present at younger age (usually over 15 years) and have multiple tumors. Hemangioblastoma is a WHO I tumor. Surgical treatment usually requires en bloc resection, as piecemeal resection can result in excessive hemorrhage.

Question for Further Thought

1. What is the association between patients with hemangioblastoma and polycythemia?

Reporting Responsibilities

Direct reporting is essential for all tumors. Assess the degree of mass effect. It is always necessary to evaluate for vascularity and hemorrhage and to exclude additional or multiple lesions. Additional spine evaluation is necessary to exclude multiple lesions.

What the Treating Physician Needs to Know

- Are there additional lesions in the neuroaxis which will suggest von Hippel-Lindau syndrome and warrant investigation with abdominal imaging?
- Spine evaluation is required to exclude these additional lesions

Answer

1. Upregulation of erythropoietin may be seen in patients with hemangioblastoma, resulting in polycythemia.

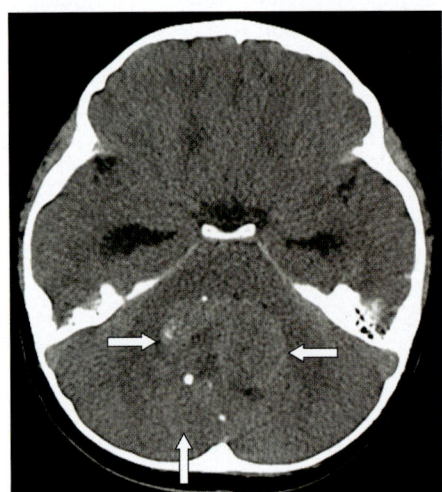

FIGURE 13-1

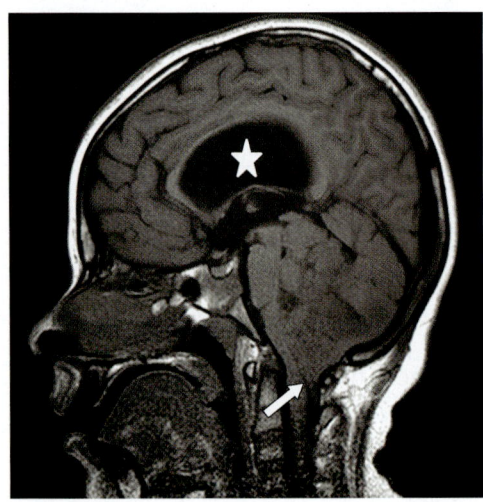

FIGURE 13-2

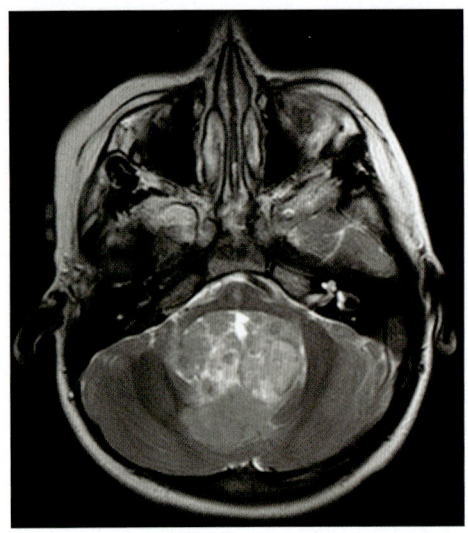

FIGURE 13-3

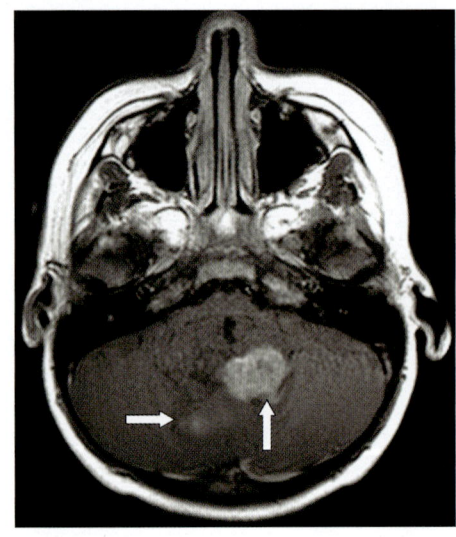

FIGURE 13-4

FINDINGS Figure 13-1. Axial NCCT through the posterior fossa. There is a heterogeneous midline posterior fossa mass with scattered calcifications (arrows). Figure 13-2. Sagittal T1WI. The mass is within the fourth ventricle, with extension of tumor through the midline foramen of Magendie (arrow). Notice stretching of the corpus callosum, indicating hydrocephalus (star). Figure 13-3. Axial T2WI through the mass. The lesion is heterogeneous with some cystic foci. Figure 13-4. Axial post-contrast T1WI through the mass. There are areas of enhancement (arrows) within the mass.

DIFFERENTIAL DIAGNOSIS Medulloblastoma, ependymoma, choroid plexus papilloma.

DIAGNOSIS Ependymoma.

DISCUSSION Ependymoma is a tumor derived from ependymal rest cells. Most are infratentorial and within the fourth ventricle. They are usually well defined and show very heterogeneous characteristics on both CT and MRI, reflecting the presence of tumoral hemorrhage or cysts and calcifications. Supratentorial ependymomas tend to exhibit more cystic component than their posterior fossa counterpart. Enhancement is variable, but most do enhance to some degree. There is usually very little or no perilesional edema. Classically, ependymoma is described as a plastic tumor in that it can insinuate itself and extrude, almost like toothpaste, through small spaces such as the foramina of Luschka and Magendie. When present, this is a very helpful imaging sign to discriminate it from the other posterior fossa masses listed in the differential diagnosis.

Ependymomas are designated WHO II and III tumors, and there is no definite imaging way to separate WHO II lesion from the anaplastic tumor except that grade III lesions are more likely to contrast enhance. The histologic criteria are also very uncertain. The difference is in their biologic and clinical behaviors. The anaplastic lesion grows rather more rapidly causing raised intracranial pressure early in the disease. SV40 virus strain has been identified in ependymomas, raising the possibility of an association with this infection. Ependymomas have no gender preference. Posterior fossa ependymomas are more common in children than adults and invariably present with features of hydrocephalus and raised intracranial pressure such as headache, nausea, and vomiting. Macrocrania is a feature in children under the age of 2 years. Children with posterior fossa ependymomas fare worse than their adult counterpart principally because of the location of their tumors in the posterior fossa and increased incidence of anaplasia. Incomplete resection and cerebrospinal fluid (CSF) disseminations are poor prognostic factors.

Question for Further Thought

1. Where, precisely, is the layer of cells from which an ependymoma arises?

Reporting Responsibilities

Direct reporting is necessary in this obstructive neoplasm. The hydrocephalus should be treated promptly. Identify the tumor as being largely intraventricular as opposed to paraventricular, which can help to limit the differential. Note any associated hydrocephalus as this may need to be addressed urgently. Presence of leptomeningeal tumors should be mentioned.

What the Treating Physician Needs to Know

- Ependymoma is one of several tumors arising within the posterior fossa, often in children or young adults
- Imaging findings can be suggestive of the diagnosis
- There is overlap between the appearances of posterior fossa tumors, and therefore, a differential diagnosis should always be given
- Presence of complications such as herniations, CSF dissemination, and hydrocephalus

Answer

1. Ependymal rest cells can be found anywhere in the periventricular region and even somewhat removed from the ventricle. On rare occasions, ependymomas may even appear to be entirely parenchymal. These are usually supratentorial in location. More typically, posterior fossa ependymomas are often described as arising from the floor of the fourth ventricle. This results in a tumor with a sharp interface along the ventricle roof. On the other hand, medulloblastoma, which would be high on the differential whenever ependymoma is considered, is described as arising from the fourth ventricle roof, giving a sharp interface with the ventricular floor.

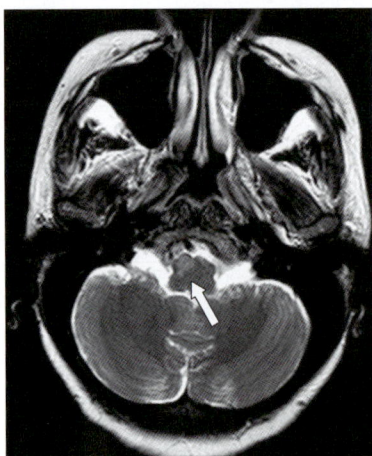

FIGURE **14-1**

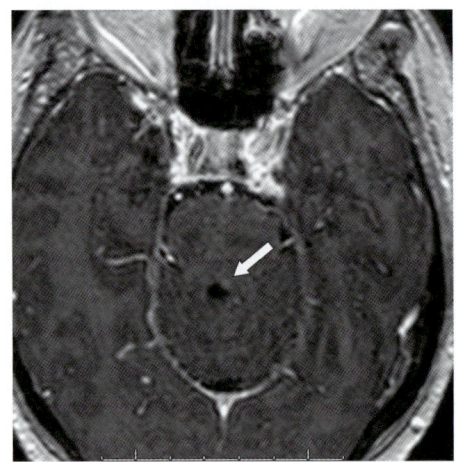

FIGURE **14-2**

FINDINGS Figure 14-1. Axial T2WI through the medulla. There is hyperintensity within the right medullary olive with minimal swelling (white arrow). Figure 14-2. Axial post-contrast T1WI. The lesion does not show pathologic enhancement to suggest the presence of a metastatic lesion. However, more superiorly, at the level of the contralateral superior cerebellar peduncle, there is a small enhancing focus compatible with metastasis (white arrow).

DIFFERENTIAL DIAGNOSIS Metastatic disease, ischemia, demyelination, hypertrophic olivary degeneration (HOD).

DIAGNOSIS Hypertrophic olivary degeneration (HOD).

DISCUSSION HOD results from an insult that interrupts some component of the dentato-rubro-olivary pathway. This pathway, also referred to as the triangle of Guillain-Mollaret, represents a synaptic network connecting the ipsilateral red nucleus via the ipsilateral central tegmental tract to the ipsilateral inferior olivary nucleus within the medulla. The contralateral dentate nucleus also contributes input to this network, to the ipsilateral red nucleus via the contralateral superior cerebellar peduncle, and to the ipsilateral olivary nucleus via the inferior cerebellar peduncles. HOD may be suspected when increased T2 signal with or without hypertrophy is seen in the medullary olive. A search for the offending lesion should then be made, with attention to the ipsilateral central tegmental pathway (red nucleus to olivary nucleus) or within the contralateral dentate nucleus or superior cerebellar peduncle. Histologically, deafferentation of olivary nucleus input results in neuronal loss and a proliferation of glia which may give the affected olive a hypertrophic appearance.

Question for Further Thought

1. Can HOD be detected clinically?

Reporting Responsibilities

Direct reporting is necessary. HOD is a rare condition and should be kept in mind whenever nonspecific signal change is seen in the medullary olive unexplained by something more common (multiple sclerosis [MS], stroke, etc.). HOD may be suggested when a potential causative lesion is found in the dentato-rubro-olivary pathway.

What the Treating Physician Needs to Know

• HOD is a rare entity and likely often missed or misdiagnosed as some more common brainstem pathology

Answer

1. On clinical examination, HOD will present as palatal tremor or myoclonus. This finding, subsequent to a known brainstem insult, is reasonably specific for the diagnosis.

CLINICAL HISTORY *19-year-old male with moyamoya syndrome (proximal internal carotid artery [ICA] occlusion).*

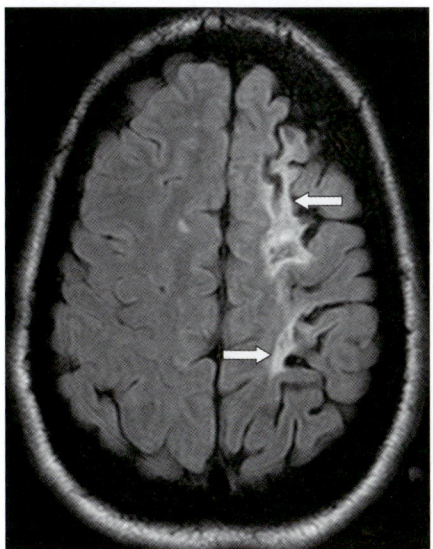

FIGURE 15-1

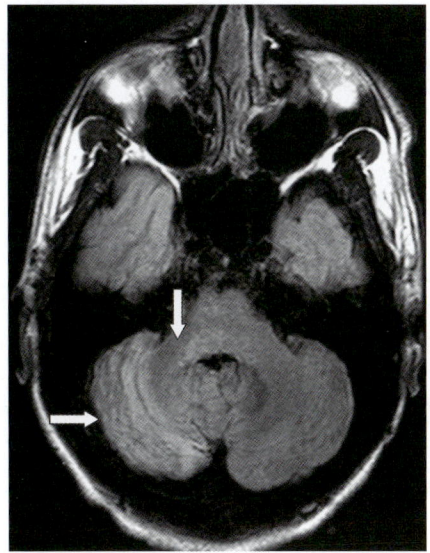

FIGURE 15-2

FINDINGS Figure 15-1. Axial FLAIR image through the cerebrum. There is an old left hemispheric watershed infarct (arrows) with left hemispheric atrophy. Figure 15-2. Axial FLAIR through the cerebellum. There is atrophy and smudgy hyperintensity within the right cerebellar hemisphere, right brachium pontis, and pons (arrows).

DIFFERENTIAL DIAGNOSIS Crossed cerebellar atrophy and diaschisis, primary cerebellar infarct, chronic infection/inflammation of the cerebellum.

DIAGNOSIS Crossed cerebellar atrophy and diaschisis.

DISCUSSION Crossed cerebellar atrophy and diaschisis results from a substantial insult to the cerebrum, usually ischemic and usually in the MCA distribution. This results in loss of neuronal input to the cortico-ponto-cerebellar tract and deafferentation injury to the contralateral cerebellar hemisphere. This results in atrophy of the affected cerebral hemisphere, and over time, the affected cerebellum evolves in a similar way to the infarcted tissue ultimately leading to atrophy.

Question for Further Thought

1. Can crossed cerebellar diaschisis be predicted in the acute phase of a cerebral infarct?

Reporting Responsibilities

This is a chronic situation, and routine reporting is sufficient. When cerebellar atrophy coexists with chronic ischemia in the contralateral cerebrum, crossed cerebellar diaschisis and atrophy should be suggested rather than invoking a separate cerebellar insult.

What the Treating Physician Needs to Know

• Crossed cerebellar atrophy is an occasional secondary finding following a substantial infarct to the contralateral cerebral hemisphere

Answer

1. In the acute phase, the cerebellar hemisphere contralateral to an acute cerebral infarct may show abnormal perfusion parameters (decreased blood flow, increased transit time) which are predictive of developing crossed cerebellar diaschisis and atrophy in the long term.

CLINICAL HISTORY *2-week-old male with increasing head circumference.*

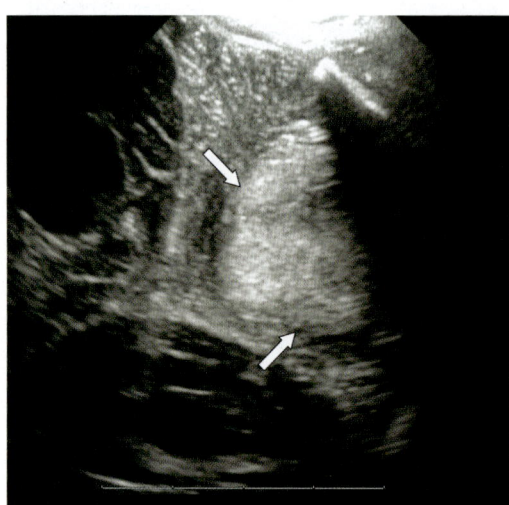

FIGURE 16-1

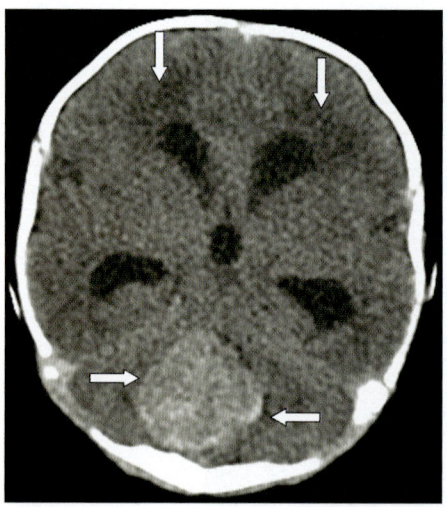

FIGURE 16-2

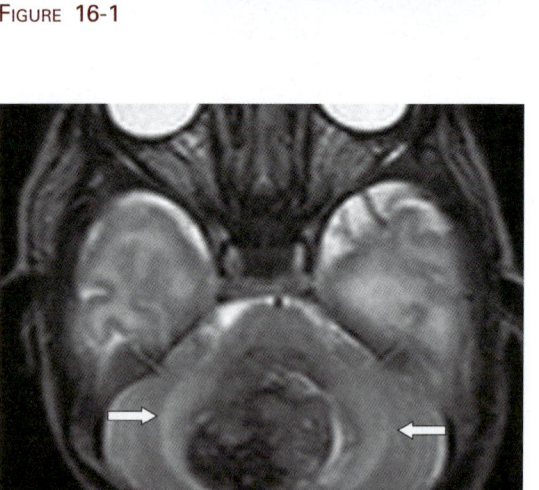

FIGURE 16-3

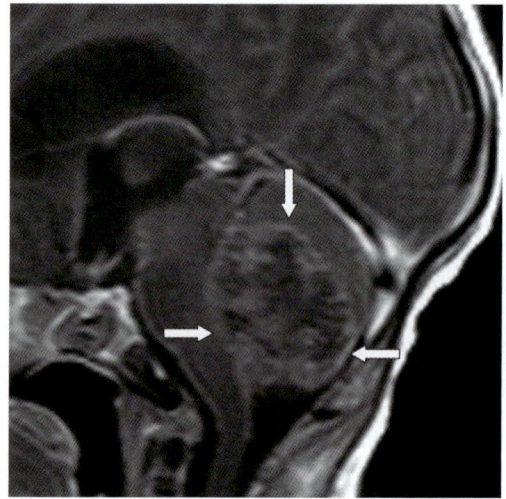

FIGURE 16-4

FINDINGS Figure 16-1. The initial imaging study was a head sonogram. This shows a large hyperechoic mass in the posterior fossa (arrows). Figure 16-2. Axial NCCT through the posterior fossa. The mass is hyperdense and well circumscribed (arrows). There is hydrocephalus with transependymal cerebrospinal fluid (CSF) flow (vertical arrows). Figure 16-3. Axial T2WI through the posterior fossa. The mass is heterogeneously hypointense with mild surrounding hyperintensity—edema (arrows). Figure 16-4. Sagittal post-contrast T1WI. The mass shows mild patchy enhancement (arrows). There is compression of the brainstem.

DIFFERENTIAL DIAGNOSIS Medulloblastoma, glioblastoma, atypical teratoid rhabdoid tumor (ATRT), ependymoma.

DIAGNOSIS ATRT.

DISCUSSION ATRT is an aggressive, WHO IV tumor most commonly found in infants and children under 3 years. The posterior fossa is the most common site of disease, but it can occur elsewhere. Up to 20% of patients present with leptomeningeal spread at diagnosis. Imaging features are similar to those of the more common medulloblastoma, with which ATRT shares quite a few features. On CT, the tumor is hyperdense reflecting both hemorrhage and a composition of densely packed small cells. Heterogeneous intensity is expected on T1WI and T2WI with evidence of cysts, hemorrhage, and enhancement. Leptomeningeal enhancement is indicative of CSF spread of the tumor.

Clinical presentation includes macrocrania because of hydrocephalus, vomiting, failure to thrive, and visual symptoms with headache in the older children. There is a male predominance. Evaluation of the entire neuroaxis is always necessary to exclude CSF seeding. The prognosis is poor. Longer survival is recorded in children older than 3 years presumably because of the use of intensive therapies.

Question for Further Thought

1. Can ATRT be differentiated from medulloblastoma by imaging?

Reporting Responsibilities

Direct reporting is essential in this obstructing tumor with hydrocephalus. Include ATRT in the differential for an aggressive-appearing tumor in young children under 3 years of age, particularly when medulloblastoma would also be appropriate. Look for evidence of leptomeningeal spread as this finding significantly impacts survival. If none is seen in the brain, suggest imaging of the remainder of the neuroaxis (also appropriate for medulloblastoma).

What the Treating Physician Needs to Know

- ATRT is an aggressive primitive tumor found in children mostly under 3 years of age
- Presence of leptomeningeal spread at diagnosis is not rare and significantly impacts survival
- Presence of complications such as hydrocephalus
- Spinal imaging is required to exclude CSF spread

Answer

1. No. By imaging, ATRT and medulloblastoma in the posterior fossa are identical. They are even to some degree similar histologically as they both contain small primitive-type cells. The age may be a helpful clue as ATRT is rare in children older than 3 years.

CLINICAL HISTORY *28-year-old female with gait abnormality and vision loss in right eye.*

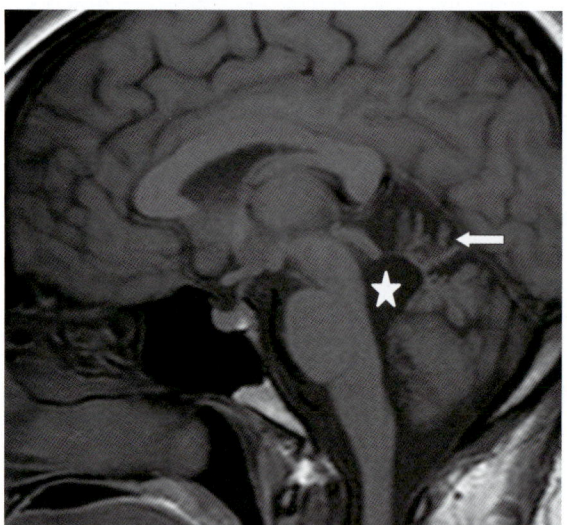

FIGURE 17-1

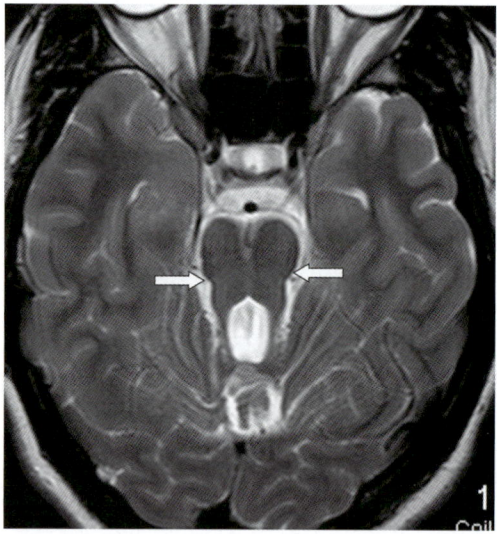

FIGURE 17-2

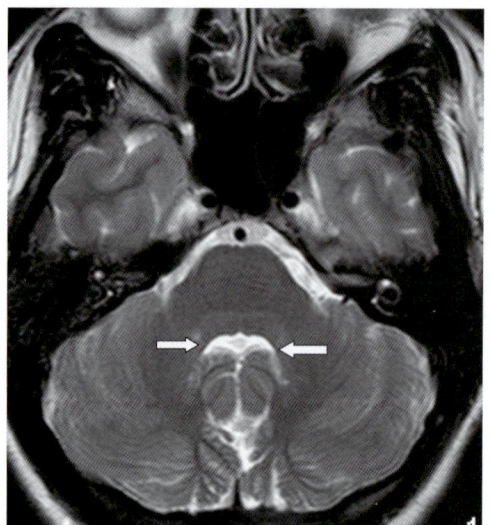

FIGURE 17-3

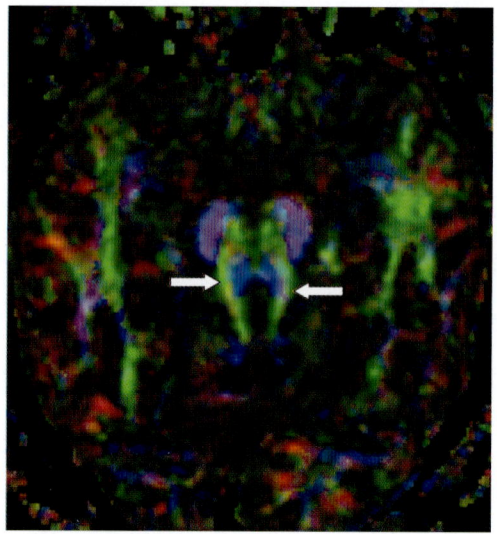

FIGURE 17-4

FINDINGS Figure 17-1. Sagittal MRI T1WI. There is a high-riding fourth ventricle (star) at the junction of the midbrain and the pons with obvious cerebellar vermis volume loss (arrow). The superior fourth ventricular velum is almost horizontal. Figure 17-2. Axial T2WI through the superior cerebellar peduncle demonstrates the molar tooth sign or malformation (MTS or MTM) (arrows). Figure 17-3. Axial T2WI inferior to the MTS. There is batwing appearance of the inferior fourth ventricle (arrows). Figure 17-4. DTI color directional map through MTS. There is thickening and horizontal disposition of the superior cerebellar peduncles (arrows).

DIFFERENTIAL DIAGNOSIS Joubert syndrome (JS), cerebellar vermian atrophy or hypoplasia, pontocerebellar atrophy.

DIAGNOSIS JS and Joubert syndrome-related disorder (JSRD).

DISCUSSION The hallmark of the diagnosis of JS or JSRD at imaging is the MTS or MTM. This is represented by large or thickened superior cerebellar peduncles projecting horizontally behind the pons/midbrain with deepening of the interpeduncular fossa resulting in a molar tooth configuration on CT or MRI as in Figure 17-2. The other findings include a high-riding fourth ventricle at the junction of the pons and midbrain. The velum of the fourth ventricle is almost horizontally directed. The nodulus and dentate nucleus could be heterotopic. There is a batwing or triangular appearance of the inferior fourth ventricle on the axial images as in Figure 17-3. The dentate nucleus has been shown to be laterally displaced. Interpeduncular heterotopia and hamartoma of the tuber cinerium have been reported in association with JSRD. DTI has been useful in demonstrating the underlying pathogenesis of the structural imaging findings. These include horizontally directed superior cerebellar peduncles with lack of decussation of the fibers, lack of decussation of the corticospinal tracts in the medulla, and laterally located deep cerebellar nuclei. Other abnormalities reported in this disorder include occipital cephaloceles, Dandy-Walker malformation, corpus callosal changes, and white matter (WM) T2 hyperintensities. MTS is absent in the other differential diagnoses.

JS is a rare complex malformation of the hind/midbrain inherited in an autosomal recessive mode with an estimated prevalence of 1 in 100,000. There are at least five identified chromosomal abnormalities associated with the JS spectrum responsible for about 50% of known JS population. The clinical presentations include irregular breathing in infancy, ocular apraxia, hypotonia, cognitive impairment, and ataxia. Imaging plays an important role in the diagnosis, and the MTS is the characteristic finding on axial CT or MRI. The underlying pathology is that of vermis aplasia or hypoplasia with thickening of the horizontally directed superior cerebellar peduncles associated with lack of decussation of its fibers. The corticospinal tracts in the caudal medulla also show lack of decussation. Other systemic changes include endocrine abnormalities, renal disease, ocular colobomas and retinal changes, occipital cephalocele, hepatic fibrosis, polydactyly, and oral hamartomas. The prognosis is generally poor as

there is no treatment. These patients are cognitively impaired and have problem coping.

Question for Further Thought

1. Is the MTS pathognomonic for JS?

Reporting Responsibilities

This is not an acute disorder, and as such routine reporting is sufficient. Recognizing the MTS is important in placing the patient in a definitive disease category that should lead to the necessary genetic testing to confirm which of the five mutations may be responsible for the disease.

What the Treating Physician Needs to Know

- Is there a definite MTS? This would exclude other differential diagnoses
- Are there other central nervous system (CNS) abnormalities outside the posterior fossa? These may suggest the degree of severity
- How can the other systemic changes be evaluated? US and/or CT may be useful for evaluation of the renal, hepatic, and skeletal abnormalities and neuroophthalmologic evaluation for the ocular changes

Answer

1. MTS is found throughout the spectrum of JS disorders known as JSRDs. JSRDs are classified into six phenotypic subgroups: pure JS, JS with ocular defect, JS with renal defect, JS with oculorenal defects, JS with hepatic defect, and JS with orofaciodigital defects. With the exception of rare X-linked recessive cases, JSRDs follow autosomal recessive inheritance and are genetically heterogeneous. Mutations in at least five genes (*TMEM216*, *CEP290*, *TMEM67*, *RPGRIP1L*, and *CC2D2A*) are known to be responsible for the anomalies in this spectrum.

CLINICAL HISTORY *35-year-old female with paraesthesia in bilateral upper extremities.*

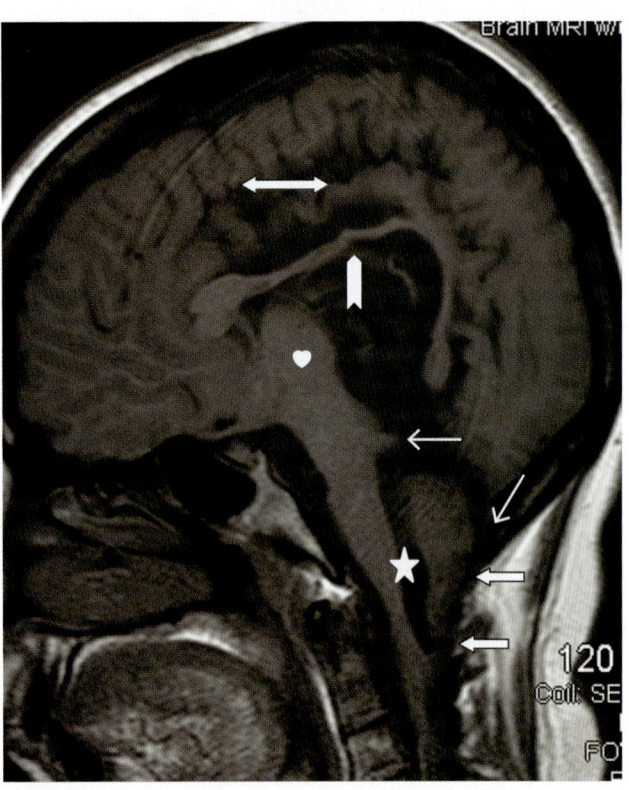

FIGURE 18-1

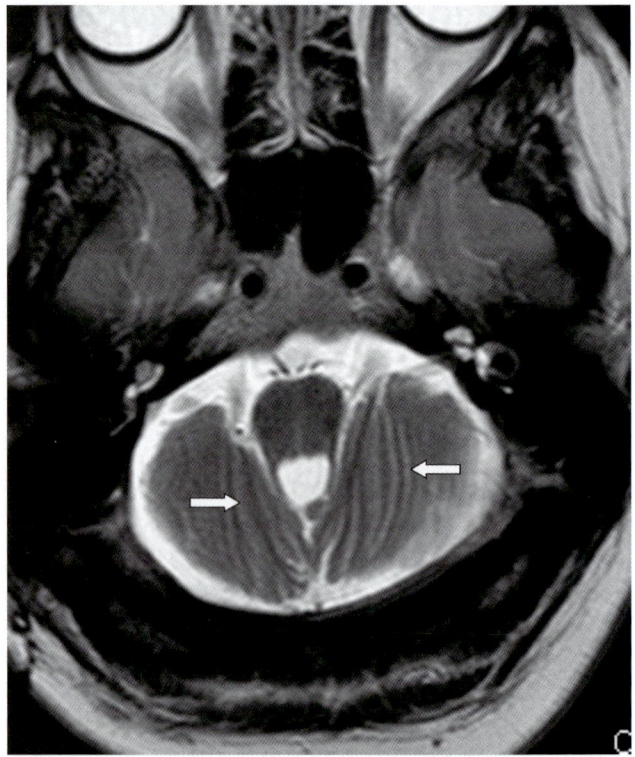

FIGURE 18-2

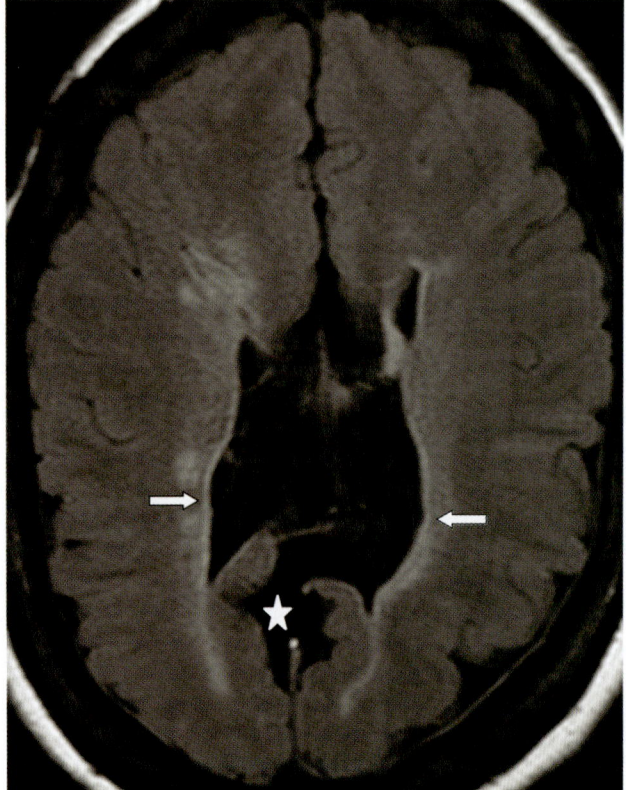

FIGURE 18-3

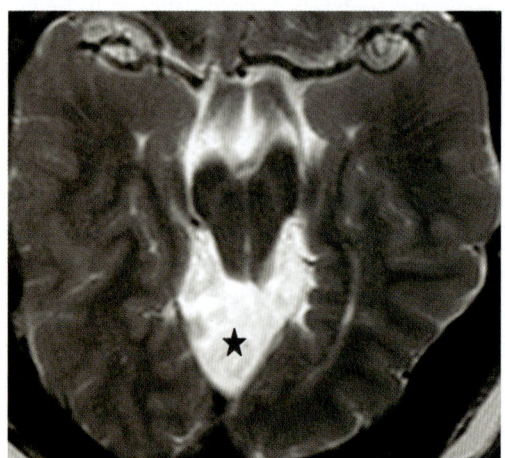

FIGURE 18-4

FINDINGS Figure 18-1. Sagittal MR T1WI. There is a very small posterior fossa with a very small cerebellum extending through wide foramen magnum into the upper cervical spinal canal (transverse thick arrows). The vertical thin arrow points to the low position of the torcula. There is a pointed (beaked) tectum (thin transverse arrow). The fourth ventricle is tubular and continuous inferiorly into the upper spinal canal with no visible fastigium (star).

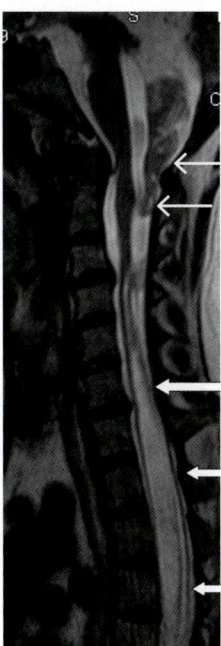

FIGURE 18-5

The body/splenium of the corpus callosum is severely atrophic (chevron). Parasagittal cerebral dysgenesis is present (right left arrow). The massa intermedia (heart) is large. Figure 18-2. Axial T2WI through the small posterior fossa. There is anteroposterior orientation of the cerebellar folia (transverse arrows). There is concavity of posterior petrosal surface. Figure 18-3. Axial FLAIR through the lateral ventricles. There is dysgenesis of the parasagittal occipital lobes and dilation of the posterior interhemispheric fissure (star). There is scalloping of the ventricular walls with periventricular hyperintensities due to leukomalacia (transverse arrows). There is bilateral cortical malformations, a mixture of pachygyria and polymicrogyria. Figure 18-4. Axial T2WI through midbrain. Beaked tectum protrudes into dilated quadrigeminal cistern (star). Figure 18-5. Sagittal cervical spine T2WI. There is inferior descent of the medulla, the fourth ventricle, and the cerebellum through the large foramen magnum into the upper cervical spine (thin arrows). There is a cervical thoracic syringomyelia from about C3–C4 disc level to the visualized upper thoracic spine (transverse thick arrows).

DIFFERENTIAL DIAGNOSIS Chiari II malformation (CIIM), CIM, occipital cephalocele (OC), rhombencephalosynapsis (RES).

DIAGNOSIS Chiari II malformation (CIIM).

DISCUSSION The focus of the malformation is in the posterior fossa and the changes include a small posterior fossa with low attachment of the torcula and transverse sinuses, descent of the medulla, fourth ventricle and the cerebellum into the upper cervical spinal canal, elongated tubular fourth ventricle without a visible fastigium, wrapping of the cerebellum around the brainstem resulting in anteroposterior orientation of cerebellar folia, beaking of the tectum with flattening of basis pontis, and bundling of the vermis as it pushes through the tentorial incisura. The posterior petrosal surface is concave. The sagittal and axial T1WI and T2WI demonstrate these abnormalities very well. The supratentorial abnormalities include hydrocephalus in over 90% and corpus callosum dysgenesis in over 60%. Deficient falx with interdigitation of cerebral hemispheres across the midline, sulcal, and cortical malformations such as hypoplasia, heterotopia, pachygyria, and polymicrogyria; colpocephaly; and large massa intermedia are common. Symptomatic hydrocephalus is considered a complication of repair of the associated myelomeningocele (MM). Once the hydrocephalus is shunted, there could be dilatation of midline subarachnoid spaces around the incisura. Lacunar skull is always a feature of CIIM in babies and is best demonstrated by CT. The spinal malformations are best evaluated by spinal MRI and include open dysraphism with MM in virtually 100% of patients, tethering of the spinal cord and syringohydromyelia in over 50%. Changes of CIIM are conveniently evaluated in utero by US and MRI. This may allow in utero intervention which has been shown to improve outcome in these children. CIM is not associated with the constellation of supratentorial changes and MM and usually, apart from cerebellar tonsillar ectopia, there is no significant cerebellar or brain stem abnormality. Lack of cerebellar fusion excludes RES, while occipital bone defect with protruding cerebellum is always present in OC.

These children are born with open spinal MM. It is more common in females than males. CIIM may present with lower limb paralysis, developmental delay, hindbrain symptoms of cranial nerve palsies, and respiratory problems. Spasticity and bladder dysfunction are subsequent problems. Incidence of CIIM is decreasing due to prophylactic folate therapy during pregnancy. Folate deficiency and use of anticonvulsants during pregnancy have been linked to open spinal dysraphism. It is suggested that constant leak of CSF from open MM result in lack of intracranial CSF space distention crucial to brain and cranial vault development. This lack of distention results in developmental domino effect leading to hypoplasia, maldevelopment, and malposition of various posterior fossa and supratentorial structures. In utero or early postnatal repair of the MM has been shown to improve outcome.

Questions for Further Thought

1. Is there a genetic basis for CIIM?
2. Is there a screening method for detection of fetal CIIM?

Reporting Responsibilities

Discovery of CIIM either on fetal US/MRI or in postnatal imaging requires direct reporting for prompt treatment which has been linked to improved outcome. Evaluation of CIIM is incomplete without evaluation of entire craniospinal axis, and this should be recommended.

What the Treating Physician Needs to Know

- Complete head and spine MRI is crucial for initial evaluation of CIIM and subsequent evaluation with any new symptoms
- CT may be enough for follow-up of shunted hydrocephalus
- Other associated anomalies as detailed above

Answers

1. Yes. Mutation of methylene-tetra-hydrofolate reductase (*MTHFR*) gene is common in neural tube closure anomaly. Prophylactic folate therapy during pregnancy is known to reduce this risk.
2. Yes. Maternal serum and amniocentesis testing for elevated α-fetoprotein and fetal US.

CLINICAL HISTORY *Young patient with hypotonia and developmental delay.*

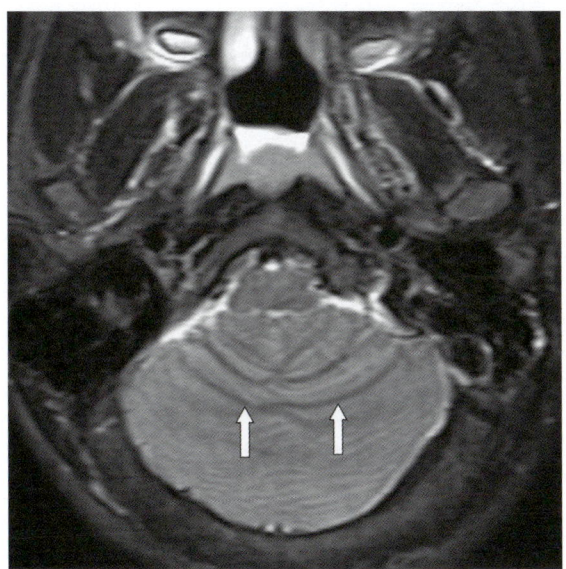

FIGURE **19-1**
Courtesy of M. Castillo MD.

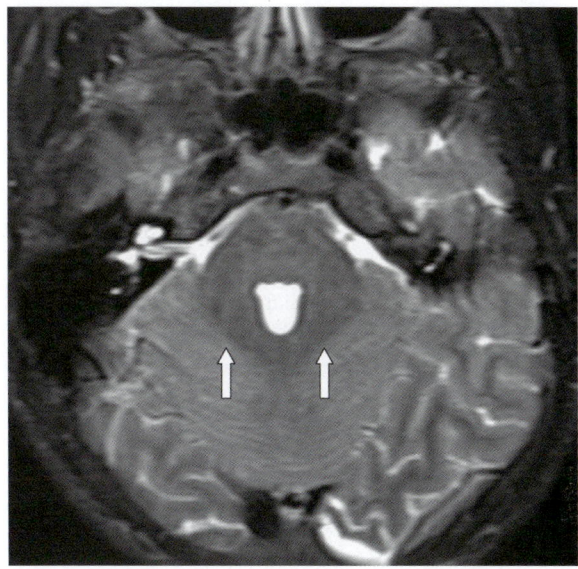

FIGURE **19-2**
Courtesy of M. Castillo MD.

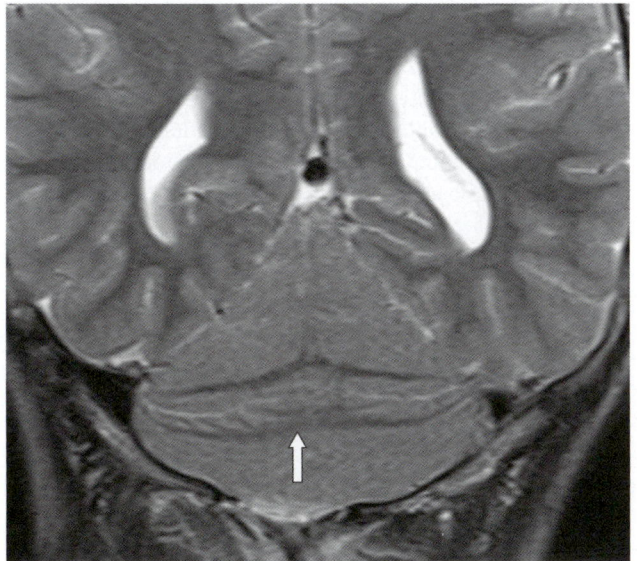

FIGURE **19-3**
Courtesy of M. Castillo MD.

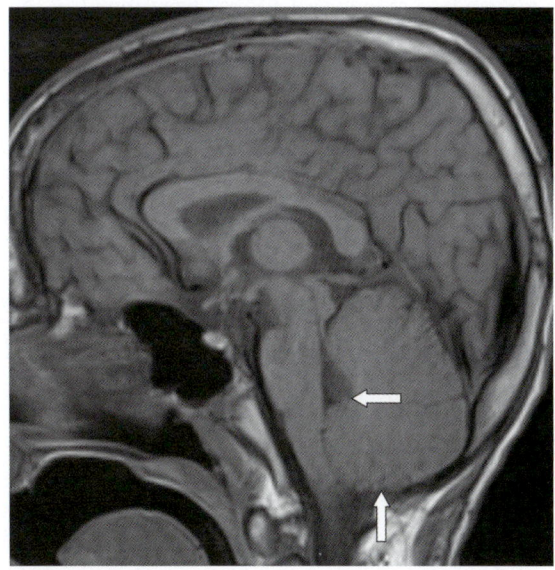

FIGURE **19-4**
Courtesy of M. Castillo MD.

FINDINGS Figure 19-1. Axial T2WI through the lower cerebellum. There is a single cerebellum without a midline fissure. The folia are oriented transversely, and there is continuity of the cerebellar white matter (WM) across the midline (arrows). There is no distinct vermis. Figure 19-2. Axial T2WI through the fourth ventricle. There is fusion of bilateral middle cerebellar peduncles and dentate nuclei around the deformed fourth ventricle (arrows). There is no obvious nodulus. There is lack of midline fissure in the single cerebellar hemisphere. Figure 19-3. Coronal T2WI through the cerebellum. There is transverse orientation of the folia and WM (arrow). The cerebellum is pear shaped. Figure 19-4. Sagittal T1WI demonstrates what appears to represent the fastigium (transverse arrow). The cerebellar hemisphere bulges inferiorly obliterating the cisterna magna (vertical arrow). The vermis is not visualized. There is normal appearance of supratentorial midline structures in this instance. There is no hydrocephalus. The aqueduct is thin but otherwise normal.

DIFFERENTIAL DIAGNOSIS N/A.

DIAGNOSIS Rhombencephalosynapsis (RES).

DISCUSSION The hallmarks of RES at imaging are a lack of central fissuring in the cerebellum with formation of a single cerebellum, transverse orientation of the folia with continuity of white matter across the midline, a diamond-shaped (deformed) fourth ventricle with fusion of the cerebellar peduncles and dentate nuclei around it. The vermis is not visualized except in mild cases. The single cerebellum is continuous at its base and bulges inferiorly to obliterate the cisterna magna. The cerebellar volume is preserved to slightly decreased. Fusion of the colliculi could be present. Some associated supratentorial anomalies may include hydrocephalus which occurs in about 50% usually due to aqueductal stenosis, deficiency or hypoplasia of the septum pellucidum, and dysgenesis of the corpus callosum and other midline anomalies, none of which is present in this case. MR rather than CT offers the complete way to evaluate this anomaly.

RES is a rare congenital anomaly of the hindbrain. It is usually sporadic, but syndromic forms exist. Clinically, these patients are generally hypotonic with developmental delay. There is no gender preference. RES has been found in the context of two other syndromes; Gomez-Lopez-Hernandez (GLH) syndrome where there is temporal parietal alopecia, dysmorphic features, trigeminal anesthesia and turricephaly, and the VACTERL anomaly which consists of vertebral anomalies, anal atresia, cardiovascular anomalies, trachea–esophageal fistula, renal anomalies, and limb defects. The etiology is unknown and is generally ascribed to dorsoventral patterning defect between the 8 and 16 weeks of gestation. The clinical outcome varies depending on the severity and could be compatible with long life and incidentally discovered in adulthood.

Question for Further Thought

1. Is RES strictly a hindbrain malformation?

Reporting Responsibilities

Routine reporting is sufficient unless there is unexpected hydrocephalus. RES could easily be missed on CT evaluation of congenital hydrocephalus. These patients should at least have the benefit of MR evaluation, and this should be recommended. Detailed scrutiny of supratentorial structures should be undertaken in any situation where the imaging is positive for RES.

What the Treating Physician Needs to Know

- Babies with congenital hydrocephalus should be evaluated for the presence of RES
- RES cannot be adequately evaluated by CT. CT is therefore not sufficient for evaluation of congenital hydrocephalus. MR is the examination of choice
- In utero diagnosis of RES can be made by fetal MR

Answer

1. No. There is associated mid- and forebrain malformations that suggest that there is a domino effect of some form. These malformations include tectal fusion, mammillary body, corpus callosal, septum pellucidum and anterior commissural anomalies, absence of olfactory bulb, holoprosencephaly, and septooptic dysplasia to mention a few.

CLINICAL HISTORY *70-year-old female, healthy otherwise, presenting with rapidly progressive dementia for the last 2 to 3 months and language difficulties. Upon admission to the hospital, she was nonverbal, became progressively ataxic, and elicited myoclonus.*

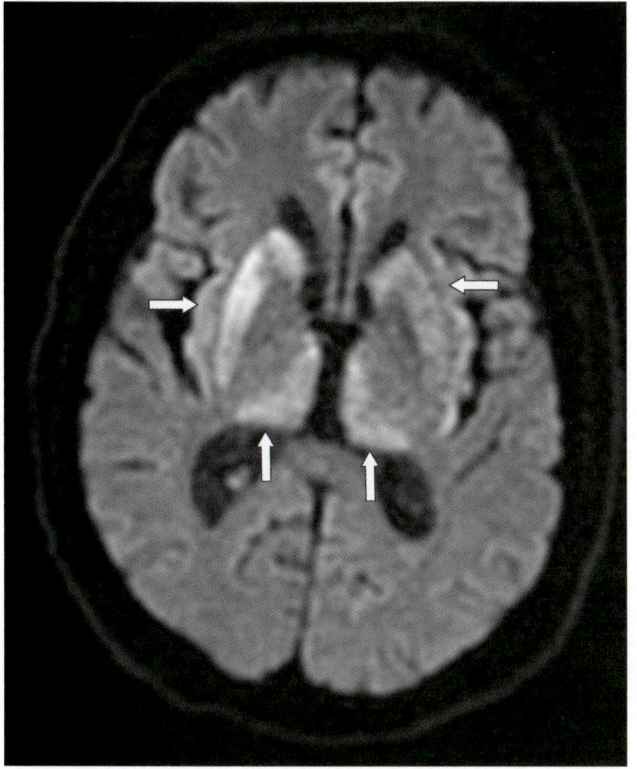

FIGURE 20-1

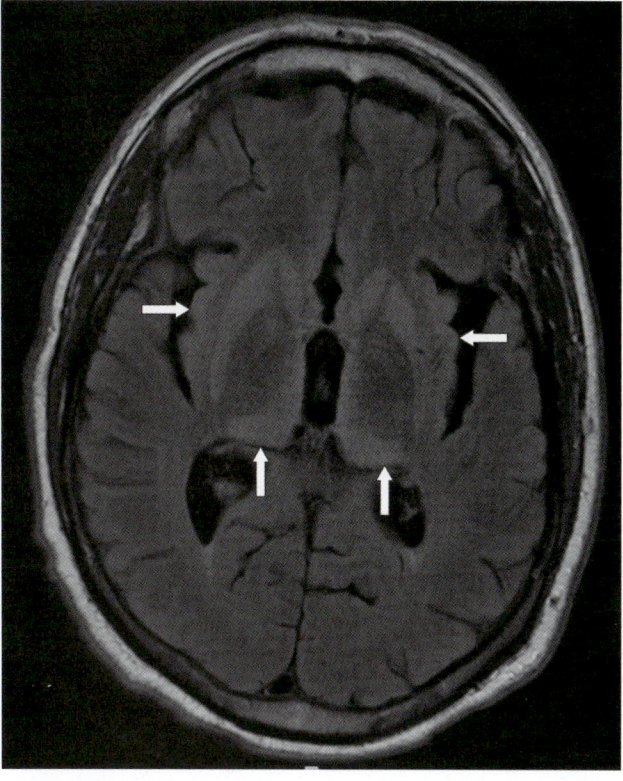

FIGURE 20-2

FINDINGS Figures 20-1 and 20-2. Axial DWI, and corresponding FLAIR at the level of basal ganglia. Diffusion restriction and increased FLAIR signal are noted in the bilateral corpus striatum (transverse arrows) and thalamus (vertical arrows). Two characteristic signs—pulvinar sign (symmetric involvement of pulvinar, the posterior nuclei of thalamus) and "hockey stick" sign (symmetric involvement of pulvinar and dorsomedial thalamus)—are present (vertical arrows). There is also involvement of the insula cortex.

DIFFERENTIAL DIAGNOSIS Acute hypoxic ischemic encephalopathy (HIE), encephalitis, other causes of dementia (Alzheimer disease, frontotemporal dementia, multi-infarct dementia, corticobasal degeneration), Leigh syndrome, Wilson disease, Creutzfeldt-Jakob disease.

DIAGNOSIS Creutzfeldt-Jakob disease (CJD), variant form.

DISCUSSION Typical MRI findings of variant form are DWI-ADC abnormality and T2/FLAIR hyperintensity of the striatum (caudate and/or putamen), thalamus, and cortex (cerebral and/or cerebellar). Cerebral cortex is involved in the descending order of frontal, parietal, and temporal lobes. The involved areas do not show enhancement. Sporadic CJD dominates in the cerebral cortex. It predominantly involves the gray matter (GM) (cortex), basal ganglia (striatum, caudate and putamen more than globus pallidus), and thalamus in the descending order. Primary sensorimotor cortex is relatively spared until late stage and cortical involvement is asymmetric. PET and SPECT are nonspecific but adjunctive for diagnosis of early stages, with demonstration of regional glucose hypometabolism and decreased uptake of tracer and absolute values on rCBV.

CJD is a fatal, rapidly progressive neurodegenerative disorder caused by prions. The clinical presentation is nonspecific and is assessed under the umbrella of dementia syndromes. The definite diagnosis is obtained via brain biopsy. Three subtypes exist as sporadic (85%), familial (15%), and iatrogenic/infectious (<1%, includes variant form). The sporadic form is the most common and, as suggested by WHO in 2009, the diagnosis comprises combinations of myoclonus, visual or cerebellar signs, pyramidal/extrapyramidal signs, akinetic mutism, and diagnostic tests such as typical electroencephalography (EEG) (periodic sharp wave complexes), positive 14-3-3 or tau protein cerebrospinal fluid (CSF) assay and MRI findings. NECT is usually normal, besides brain atrophy on successive imaging.

Question for Further Thought

1. What is the most challenging differential diagnosis in CJD?

Reporting Responsibility

Direct reporting is essential in this transmissible disease. MRI findings can be subtle, but given high fatality of the disease, early diagnosis is essential to salvage the residual functional brain parenchyma with newly developed potential therapeutic agents as well as prompt offer of adequate palliative care.

What the Treating Physician Needs to Know

• The differential diagnosis of CJD is varied, with each of the diseases having diverse treatment options. Early and accurate diagnosis is crucial for best treatment options
• NECT of the head is often nonspecific, when there is clinical concern, brain MRI should promptly be obtained if there is no contraindication

Answer

1. Differentiation from acute HIE may sometimes be difficult given the specific cerebral/cerebellar cortical involvement in the variant form. Subacute symptom onset, lack of edema, and mass effect should steer away from HIE.

CLINICAL HISTORY   *61-year-old male presenting with memory problems.*

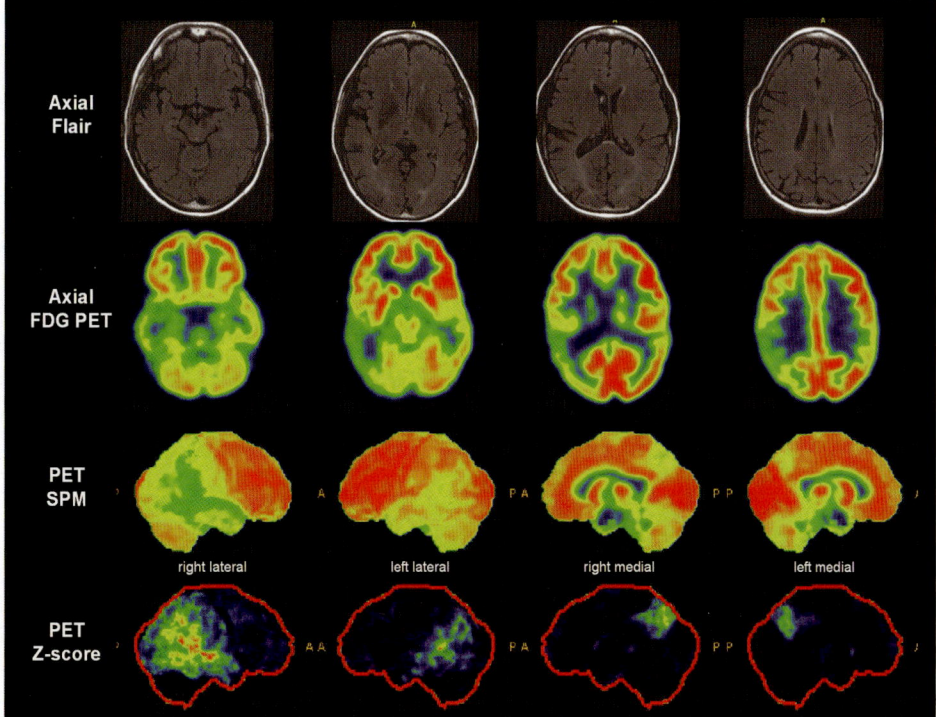

FIGURE 21-1

FINDINGS Figure 21-1. Top row: Axial FLAIR MRI. There is mild bilateral temporoparietal volume loss. Second, third, and fourth rows: Axial and surface projection maps F-18 FDG PET. There is bilateral posterior temporal and parietal hypometabolism (right greater than left). Posterior temporal and parietal hypometabolism with preservation of precentral gyrus metabolism is a characteristic feature of Alzheimer disease (AD).

DIFFERENTIAL DIAGNOSIS Vascular dementia, frontotemporal dementia, Lewy body dementia, corticobasal degeneration, normal pressure hydrocephalus.

DIAGNOSIS AD.

DISCUSSION AD is a progressive neurodegenerative disorder that manifests with gradual deterioration in cognition, behavior, and motor function. It is the most common dementia in the elderly followed by vascular and frontotemporal dementias. The definitive diagnosis is obtained through brain biopsy showing accumulation of extracellular senile β-amyloid plaques and intracellular neurofibrillary tangles formed by tau proteins.

The conventional CT and MRI are a part of the dementia workup primarily to rule out vascular dementia, normal pressure hydrocephalus, or secondary causes such as intracranial mass. Another common use of imaging is following up the degree of brain atrophy. There are no early CT or MRI findings of AD. Functional MRI shows diminished intensity and/or delayed activation in the prefrontal cortex and medial temporal lobe, which are primary circuits of learning and memory. The magnitude of FDG temporoparietal metabolic deficits on FDG-PET correlate well with cognitive impairment. Basal ganglia, thalamus, cerebellum, and primary sensorimotor cortex are usually spared. A normal β-amyloid PET imaging with preserved gray–white differentiation excludes the possibility of dementia due to AD. Patients with mild cognitive impairment and a positive β-amyloid PET imaging have greater chance of progressing to AD (50% to 60%) than those with a negative amyloid PET study (less than 4% to 7%). However, amyloid PET study can be positive even in elderly patients without cognitive difficulties.

AD insidiously starts at the temporal lobe entorhinal cortex and gradually progresses to hippocampus and neocortex followed by association areas. Therefore, the earliest affected abilities are learning and short-term memory. Then cognitive loss is enhanced with loss of orientation, long-term memory, and personality. The inevitable outcome is behavioral changes (e.g., hallucinations), loss of language, visuospatial skills, and eventually motor function. There is no cure available, but slowing the disease progression or prevention in case of early diagnosis is extensively investigated. Thus, early diagnosis is crucial as atrophy translates into irreversible neuronal death. The functional imaging techniques β-amyloid PET imaging sought to offer early recognition of the disease, potentially to slow devastating outcomes with antiamyloid therapies.

Question for Further Thought

1. What is the best follow-up imaging study for evaluating AD progression?

Reporting Responsibilities

Routine reporting is sufficient unless there are acute findings. The diagnosis of AD is clinical. Primary benefit of structural imaging (CT and MRI) is to rule out intracranial mass or acute infarct in an elderly patient. Secondary benefits are adjunctive providing areas of focal cerebral atrophy to support the diagnosis.

What the Treating Physician Needs to Know

- A negative β-amyloid PET imaging study is valuable to exclude AD
- A positive study in patients with mild cognitive impairment has prognostic implications
- The FDG PET is valuable in disease monitoring of AD and in the diagnosis of frontotemporal dementia and Lewy body dementia as the spatial pattern of FDG hypometabolism is characteristic

Answer

1. β-amyloid PET imaging is valuable in the early diagnosis or exclusion of AD. FDG PET/CT and MRI changes correlate best with disease progression and can be used for evaluating patients with AD in follow-up.

CLINICAL HISTORY *77-year-old male with a 2-year history of progressive dementia, urinary incontinence, gait instability, and increased frequency of falls.*

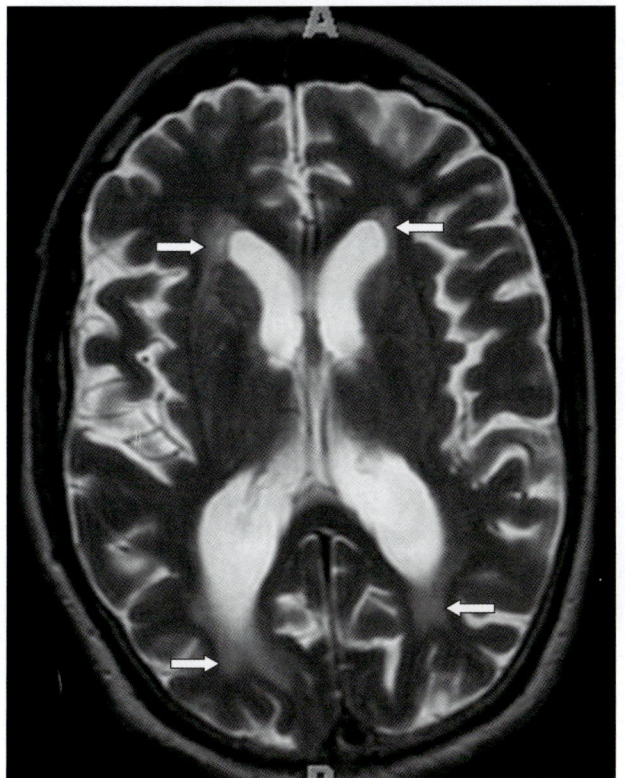

FIGURE 22-1

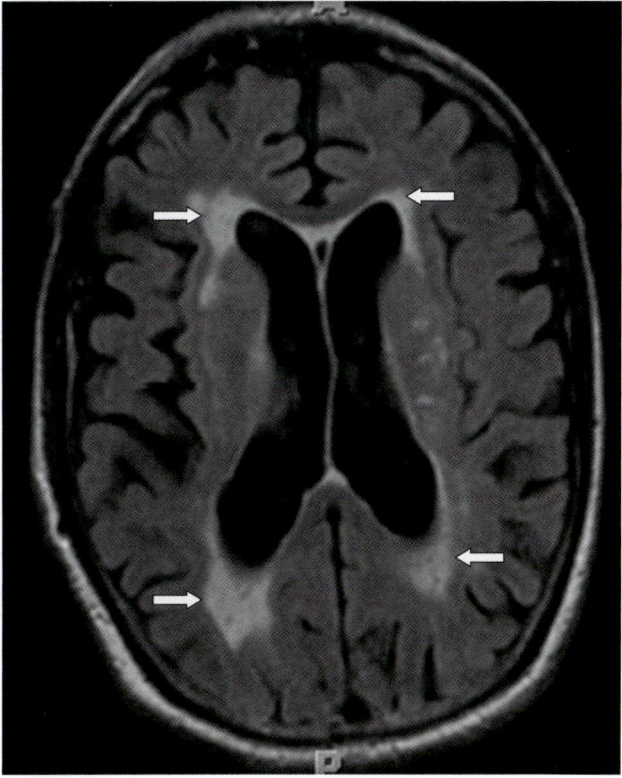

FIGURE 22-2

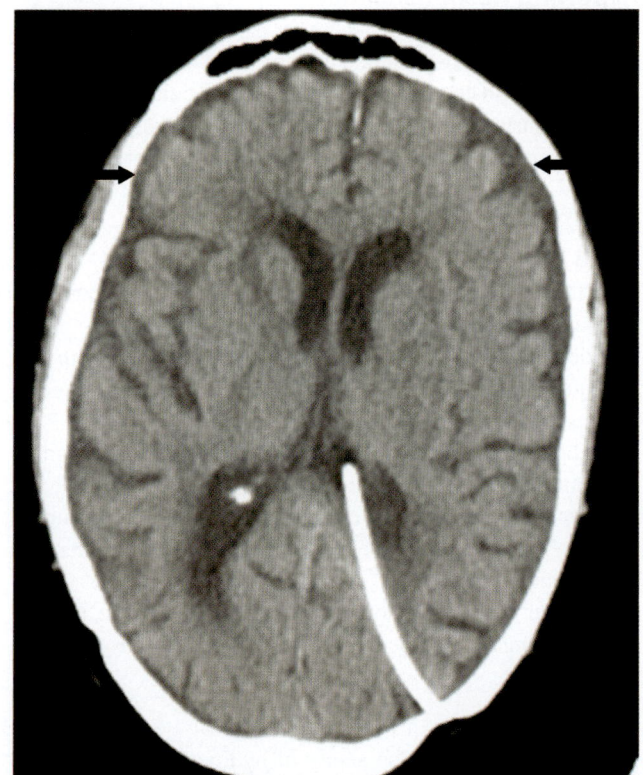

FIGURE 22-3

FINDINGS Figure 22-1. Axial T2WI through lateral ventricles. There is ventricular enlargement out of proportion to sulcal dilation. There is bilateral frontal and occipital periventricular caps (arrows). Figure 22-2. Axial FLAIR through the body of the lateral ventricle. There is confluent periventricular hyperintensity over the frontal and occipital regions suggestive of transependymal cerebrospinal fluid (CSF) flow (arrows). Figure 22-3. Axial NCCT through the lateral ventricles following ventriculoperitoneal (VP) shunting. There is normalized caliber of the ventricles with resolution of periventricular caps and interval appearance of thin subdural collections (arrows). Figure 22-4. Pre-operative In-111 diethylene triamine pentaacetic acid (DTPA) cisternography. There is persistent radiotracer uptake in the lateral ventricles (star) at 24 hours.

DIFFERENTIAL DIAGNOSIS Normal aging brain, Alzheimer disease, vascular dementia, sporadic subcortical arteriosclerotic encephalopathy, Parkinson disease, normal pressure hydrocephalus (NPH).

DIAGNOSIS NPH.

DISCUSSION NPH is defined as idiopathic communicating hydrocephalus where the degree of the triventricular dilatation is out of proportion to degree of cortical sulcal dilation

41

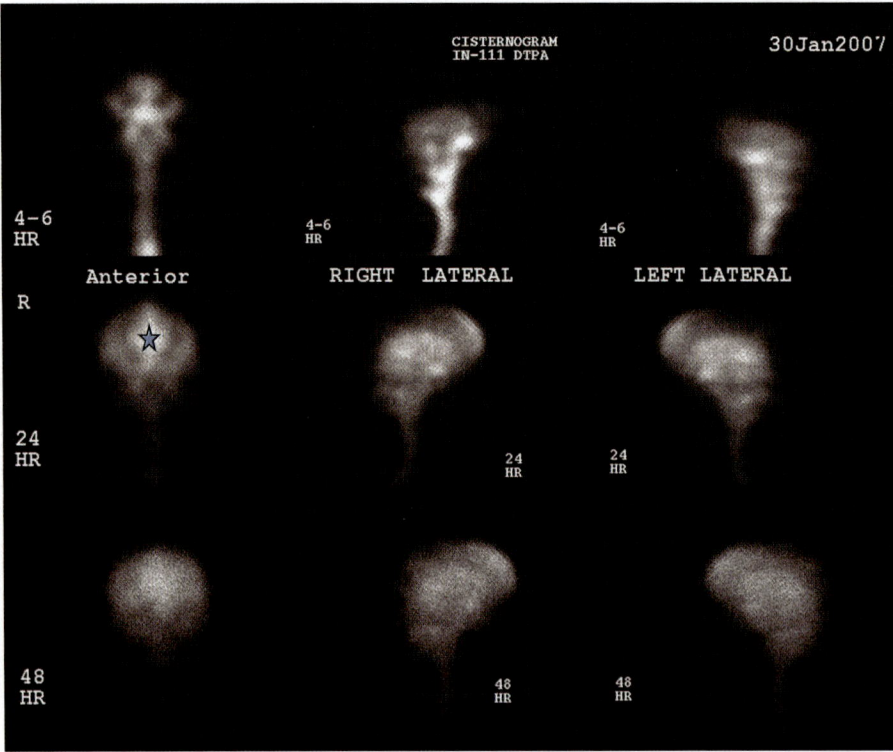

CISTERNOGRAM
IN-111 DTPA

30Jan2007

4-6
HR

Anterior

R

24
HR

48
HR

4-6
HR

RIGHT   LATERAL

24
HR

48
HR

4-6
HR

LEFT LATERAL

24
HR

48
HR

FIGURE 22-4

under normal CSF pressure. The fourth ventricle is usually spared. Conventional MRI demonstrates disproportional ventricular enlargement compared with sulcal dilatation. There may be confluent periventricular T2 hyperintensity, indicating transependymal CSF flow and/or edema secondary to impaired venous flow and/or periventricular arterial ischemia. Biphasic flow at the cerebral aqueduct on cine phase–contrast MRI is well correlated with good response to shunting. Periventricular and deep white matter (WM) T2 hyperintense lesions which may be due to small vessel ischemic changes are signs of poor outcome after ventricular shunting. The diagnostic indicators of NPH are flow void in cerebral aqueduct on MRI and prominent ventricular activity at 24 hours on In-111 DTPA cisternography. Aqueductal flow void sign reflects increased uncompensated CSF flow. Thinning of the corpus callosum is always present.

Presence of significant WM infarctions could point in the direction of vascular dementia as centrally predominant atrophy may produce similar disproportionate enlargement of the ventricles. The disproportionate ventricular enlargement rules out normal aging process and Parkinson disease.

NPH is a treatable cause of dementia, and imaging is adjunctive to determine the candidates who will benefit from ventricular decompression. The typical presentation is the Hakim triad of gait apraxia, urinary incontinence, and dementia. Lumbar puncture (LP) was performed in this patient with the CSF opening pressure at 18 cm H_2O. LP may be used as a therapeutic trial of VP shunting. Patients who respond to large-volume tap are generally supposed to benefit from VP shunting.

Question for Further Thought

1. Does the degree of ventricular enlargement correlate with symptoms?

Reporting Responsibilities

Direct reporting may be necessary particularly if this entity is not clinically suspected. The lack of WM T2 hyperintensities in a mild-to-moderate triventricular enlargement may be secondary to normal aging. If that is the case and diagnosis is indeterminate, radionuclide cisternography with In-111 DTPA should be performed.

What the Treating Physician Needs to Know

- NPH is a surgically treatable condition, whereas Alzheimer disease or vascular dementia is not
- If dementia is the preceding symptom compared with gait disturbance or lack of urinary incontinence, other dementing syndromes should be suspected
- Alzheimer disease should be favored where hippocampal or medial temporal volume loss is the most significant finding. Disproportional dilatation of the parahippocampal fissure is characteristic for atrophy seen in Alzheimer disease but not in NPH
- Vascular dementia should be favored if multiple infarcts are striking especially in the deep WM and the basal ganglia

Answer

1. To our knowledge the acuity of hydrocephalus correlates with symptoms instead of degree of hydrocephalus. The degree of hydrocephalus is a better sign of cortical atrophy.

CLINICAL HISTORY *48-year-old female with metastatic infiltrating ductal breast carcinoma to the T12 vertebral body, staging examination.*

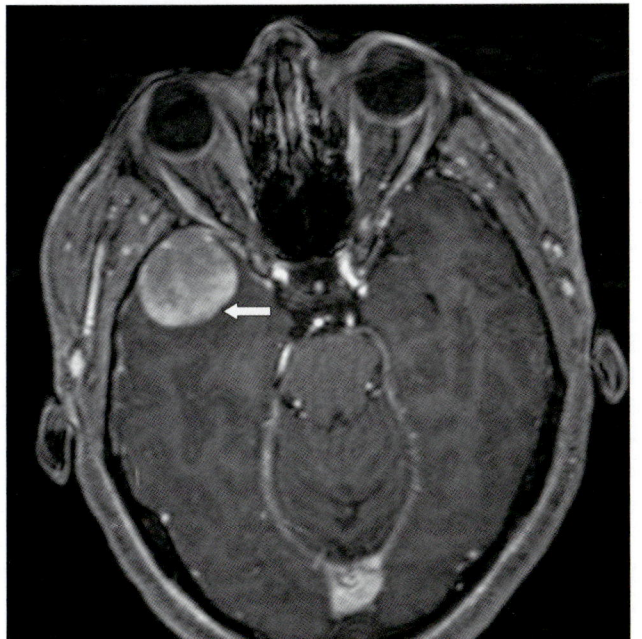

FIGURE 23-1

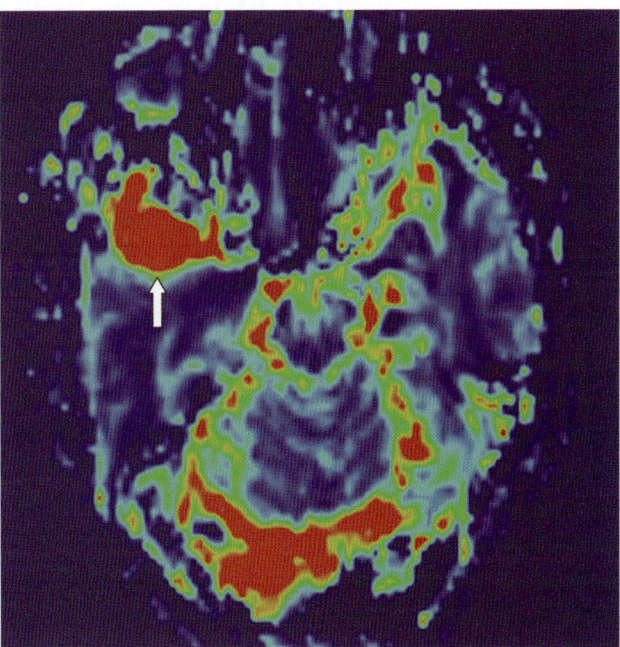

FIGURE 23-2

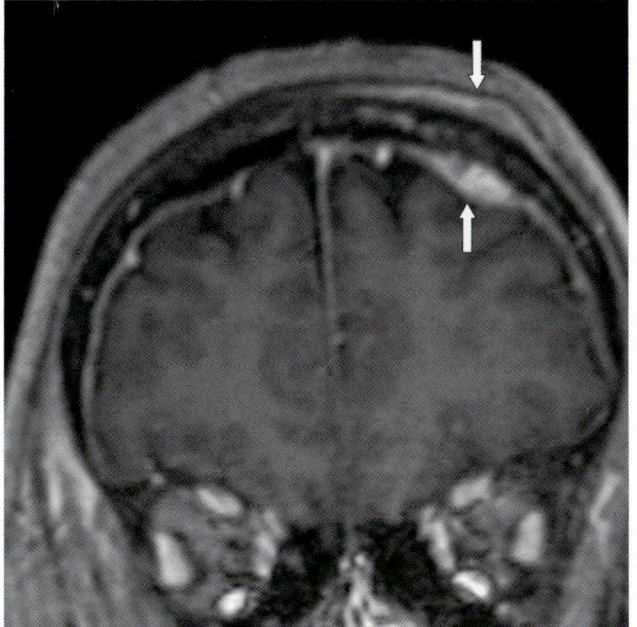

FIGURE 23-3

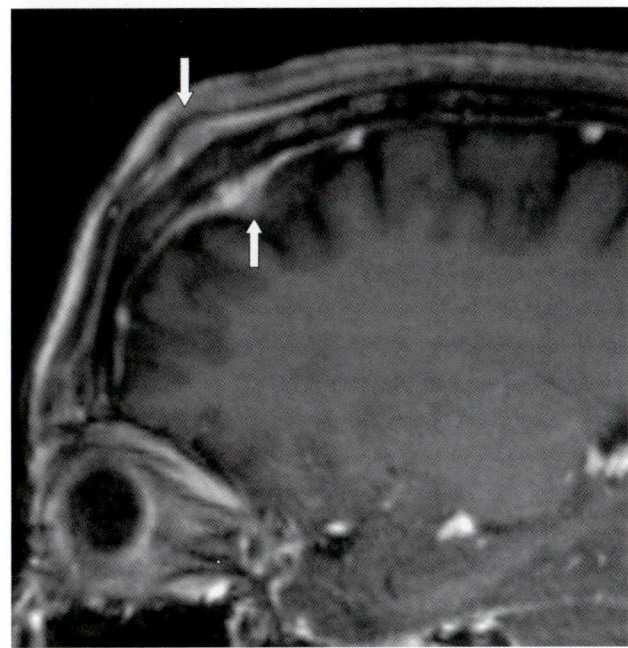

FIGURE 23-4

FINDINGS Figure 23-1. Axial post-contrast T1WI through the temporal lobes. There is a homogenously enhancing extraaxial mass within the right middle cranial fossa (arrow). Figure 23-2. Cerebral blood volume (CBV) map from dynamic susceptibility contrast MR perfusion. There is markedly elevated relative Cerebral Blood Volume (rCBV) within the right middle cranial fossa mass (arrow). Figures 23-3 and 23-4. Coronal and sagittal reformatted post-contrast 3D T1WI through the frontal lobes, respectively. There is a concurrent dural-based enhancing mass with dural tails at the left frontal convexity with contiguous osseous and extracranial components (arrows).

DIFFERENTIAL DIAGNOSIS Meningioma, lymphoma, hemangiopericytoma, metastases.

DIAGNOSIS   Dural metastatic breast cancer.

DISCUSSION   Dural metastasis shares the same features with most dural-based extraaxial aggressive lesions; extra-axial compression of the brain, avid contrast enhancement, dural tail, and overlying bone destruction and in this case transcalvarial subgaleal extension of the tumor in the frontal component. Hemorrhagic masses most likely will present with GRE blooming. There may or may not be infiltration of the underlying brain. Meningioma is the most common extraaxial homogenously enhancing mass in an adult patient and statistically would be the likely diagnosis for a right middle cranial fossa extraaxial mass in this patient age group. The key to this case is the patient's history of metastatic breast cancer and previous brain imaging (4 months prior) which did not depict a right middle cranial fossa mass. Meningiomas are slowly growing extraaxial lesions, unless they degenerate into a higher grade, which typically occurs with a preexisting meningioma. MR perfusion imaging has been suggested to help differentiate between dural-based metastasis and meningioma, whereby meningioma showed significantly more elevated rCBV compared to dural-based metastases. Interestingly, our case demonstrates markedly elevated rCBV. Therefore, MR perfusion was not helpful in excluding the possibility of a meningioma in our case.

Additional imaging with CT would likely have demonstrated permeative change in the right greater sphenoid wing with dural-based metastatic disease, rather than the hyperostosis typically seen with meningioma. Certainly more aggressive neoplasms such as lymphoma and hemangiopericytoma could have arisen within the short time frame of less than 4 months. However, the concurrent left frontal dural-based lesion with contiguous osseous and extracranial components overwhelmingly confirms that the right middle cranial fossa lesion is a metastasis rather than a meningioma, in this patient with known metastatic breast cancer.

Questions for Further Thought

1. What are the four most common dural-based metastatic lesions in adults?
2. What is the single most common dural-based metastatic lesion in children?

Reporting Responsibilities

Direct reporting is essential in every metastatic disease. Presence of an additional enhancing dural-based lesion with osseous and extracranial extension confirms metastatic disease and effectively excludes meningioma from the differential diagnosis.

What the Treating Physician Needs to Know

- Location, number, and size
- Comparison to prior imaging

Answers

1. Breast, prostate, lung, and melanoma.
2. Neuroblastoma.

CLINICAL HISTORY *50-year-old female with subacute headache and acute onset of bilateral lower extremity weakness (right greater than left).*

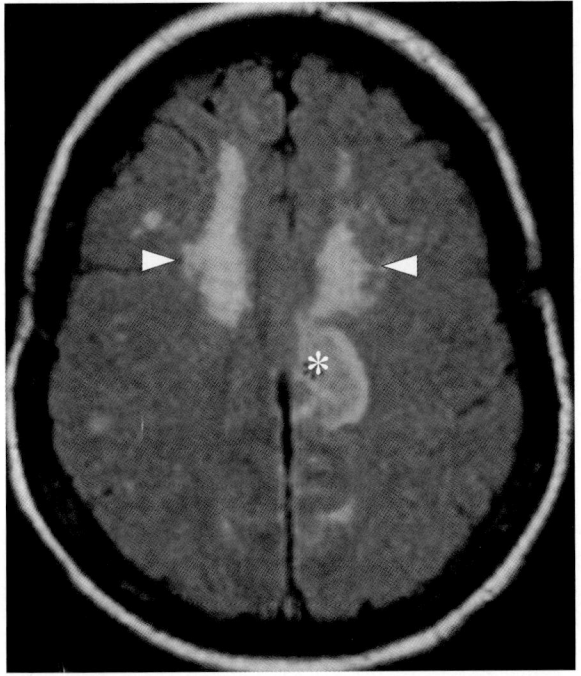

FIGURE 24-1

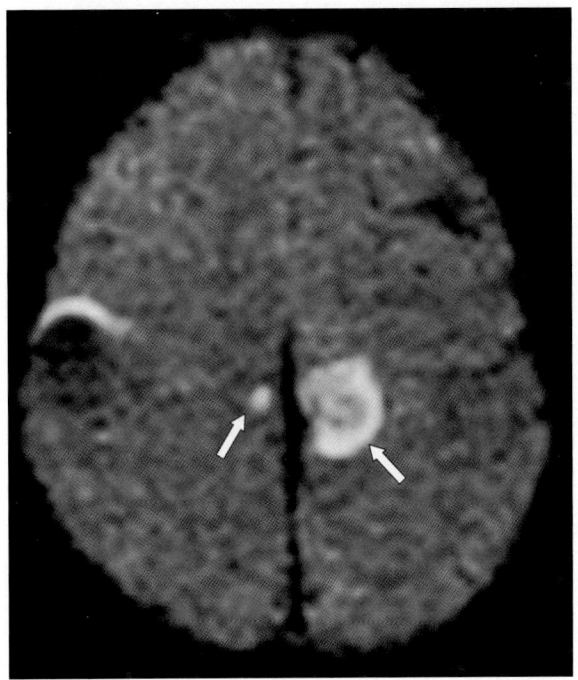

FIGURE 24-2

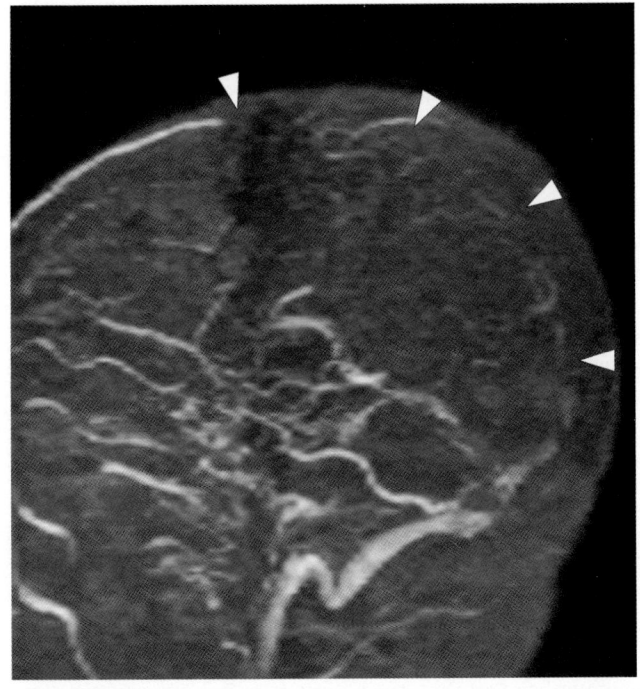

FIGURE 24-3

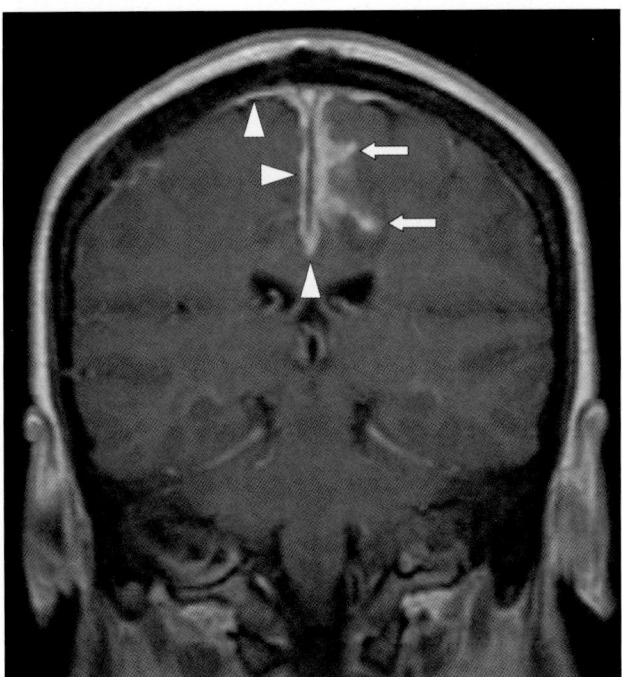

FIGURE 24-4

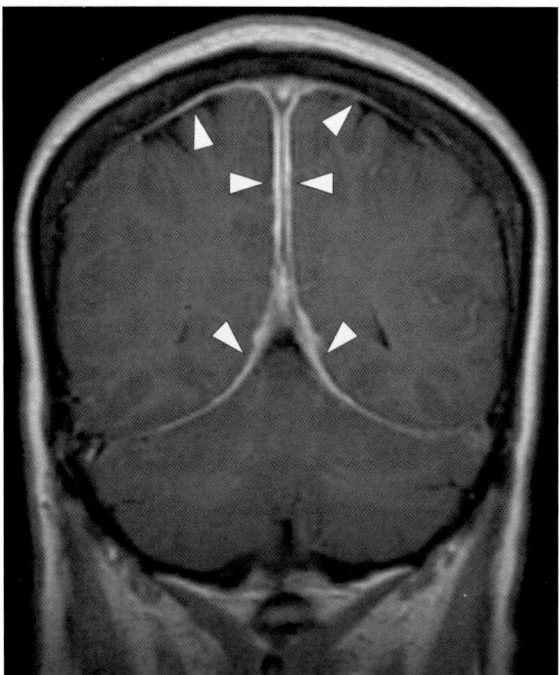

FIGURE **24-5**

FINDINGS Figure 24-1. Axial FLAIR image through the centrum semiovale. There is bilateral subcortical white matter signal hyperintensity within the centrum semiovale (arrowheads). There is a suggestion of increased signal intensity in the posterior aspect of the sagittal sinus. There is also focally hyperintense FLAIR signal involving the cortex of the medial surface of the left hemisphere (paracentral lobule*) that shows corresponding diffusion restriction on axial DWI in Figure 24-2 (arrows). Note the small, medial contralateral focus of diffusion restriction (Note: the DWI signal hyperintensity along the right convexity is artifactual). Figure 24-3. Sagittal 2D TOF MR venography MIP image shows absence of flow-related enhancement along the mid and posterior aspect of the superior sagittal sinus (arrowheads). Figures 24-4 and 24-5. Coronal post-contrast T1WI anteriorly and posteriorly, respectively. There is abnormal pachymeningeal thickening and enhancement (small arrowheads) in addition to sulcal leptomeningeal (pia-arachnoid) enhancement along the medial surface of the left cerebral hemisphere (small arrows).

DIFFERENTIAL DIAGNOSIS Dural and leptomeningeal metastatasis (breast, lymphoma), leukemia, en plaque and lymphoplasmacyte-rich meningiomas (LRM), neurosarcoidosis, Wegener granulomatosis, tuberculous meningitis, noninfectious inflammatory meningitis (i.e., rheumatoid pachymeningitis), bacterial and fungal meningitis, hypertrophic pachymeningitis, idiopathic granulomatous meningitis, intracranial hypotension.

DIAGNOSIS Idiopathic granulomatous pachymeningitis complicated by secondary sagittal sinus thrombosis, venous congestion, and venous infarction.

DISCUSSION MRI is the examination of choice for evaluation of pachymeningitis which primarily affects the dura arachnoid. There is usually dural thickening which could be focal or extend over a sizable portion particularly of the falx and tentorium. The thickened dura is isointense on pre-contrast T1WI. Post-contrast T1WI shows enhancement of the convexity dura. Where the meningeal dura (as opposed to the periosteal dura) folds on itself to form the falx and the tentorium, there is usually a central hypointensity separating the enhancing dura, forming a triple-layered structure with dural enhancement enclosing the hypointensity as seen in Figures 24-4 and 24-5. At other times there is apparent fusion of the two leaves of dura. There may be associated nodularity or focal thickening or leptomeningeal thick enhancement as seen in Figure 24-4. On T2WI, the dura is hypointense with peripheral hyperintensity. CT is not as sensitive as MRI, but it generally replicates the MRI findings of enhancing triple-layered falx and tentorium. Convexity dural enhancement may blend with overlying bone density on CT. The thickened dura is hyperdense without contrast. Imaging is much better in the detection of complications or sequelae of extensive pachymeningeal deposits, such as hydrocephalus, venous sinus thrombosis, and venous infarction as demonstrated in this case.

The thrombosis of the superior sagittal sinus and bilateral cerebral venous infarction are secondary to the extensive dural inflammation. The dura may normally enhance, most notably over the upper convexities. This physiologic phenomenon is most conspicuous at 3T MR, particularly with isovolumetric post-contrast gradient T1 techniques. It is smooth and usually no thicker than a couple of millimeters. Reactive, diffuse dural thickening and enhancement may be observed following intracranial surgery. Most of the differentials tend to present nodular characteristics or mass-like lesions that tend to separate them from the idiopathic hypertrophic pachymeningitis but not from each other. Intracranial hypotension on the other hand presents a rather diffuse smooth pachymeningeal enhancement with sagging of the mid- and hindbrain.

Pachymeningitis is a rare disorder with diverse etiology. Two major forms are identified: the primary or idiopathic hypertrophic pachymeningitis when the cause cannot be found as in our case and the secondary pachymeningitis when a definable association can be made. Early reports of pachymeningitis were in association with tuberculosis and syphilis, but there are several other associations. Its pathogenesis remains speculative but presumed to be due to autoimmune phenomenon or a result of direct infiltrative process. Imaging has very low specificity regarding the cause or etiology of pachymeningitis. It has multiple clinical presentations with headache and craniopathies being some of them. An extensive clinical workup including cerebrospinal fluid

(CSF) analysis, dural, leptomeningeal, and brain biopsy may be required, and a specific cause is not always identified. In this case, the pathologic specimens showed nonspecific inflammatory process with granulomatous features.

Questions for Further Thought

1. How does the anatomy of the dura contribute to the changes seen on imaging?
2. What is the nature of the relationship between lumbar puncture and diffuse intracranial dural thickening/enhancement on MRI?

Reporting Responsibilities

The finding of dural venous sinus thrombosis, with or without venous congestion, venous infarction, or parenchymal hemorrhage is a clinical emergency requiring prompt reporting and urgent treatment to prevent life-threatening consequences. Secondary hydrocephalus and any focal mass effect or brain edema should also be reported emergently.

What the Treating Physician Needs to Know

- Extent/distribution of disease
- Complications of pachymeningitis (venous sinus involvement, venous congestion/edema/infarction), mass effect, leptomeningeal component, hydrocephalus
- The cause of the thrombosis is usually not evident on imaging. Additional workup including expeditious lumbar puncture and blood work is required to exclude infection and malignancy

Answers

1. The dura or pachymeninges is the thick, fibrous outer layer of the meninges that consists of two layers (outer periosteal and inner meningeal) in the intracranial compartment, unlike the single layer in the spinal canal. The two intracranial dural layers are closely applied along the inner table of the skull, separating to form the dural venous sinuses. Hence inflammation of the dura can lead to inflammation of the venous sinuses resulting in sinus thrombosis. The inner layer is redundant and folds into the interhemispheric fissure as the falx cerebri and similarly forms the roof of the posterior fossa as the tentorium cerebelli. It also forms the small falx cerebelli along the midline of the posterior fossa, between the cerebellar hemispheres. The two layers of this fold enclose a loose layer which forms the nonenhancing portion of the triple layer on contrast-enhanced T1WI.

2. Diffuse intracranial dural enhancement is rare following uncomplicated lumbar puncture. Intracranial hypotension either spontaneous or following a lumbar puncture or "wet tap" (inadvertent subarachnoid needle placement during epidural anesthesia) shows characteristically smooth, thin, and diffuse dural enhancement which resolves once the leak is treated.

CLINICAL HISTORY *40-year-old female with no past medical history presenting with headaches.*

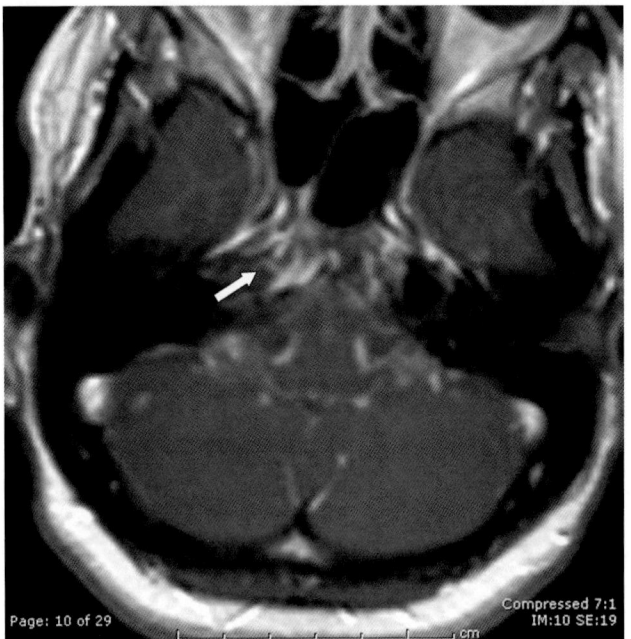

FIGURE 25-1

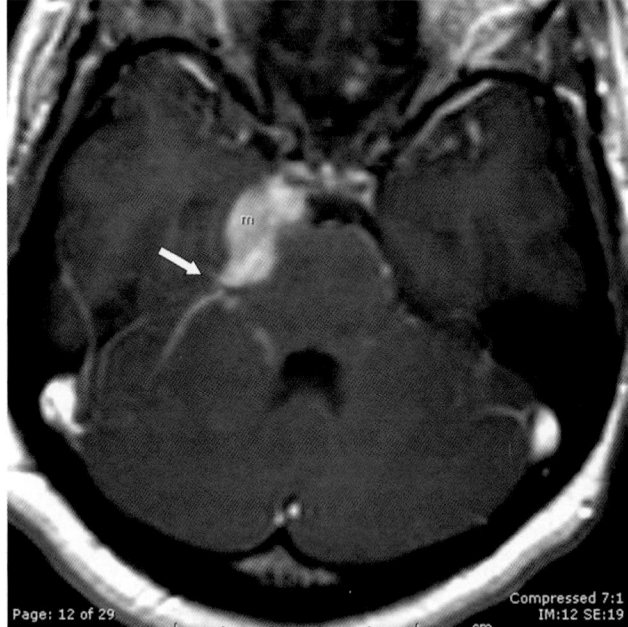

FIGURE 25-2

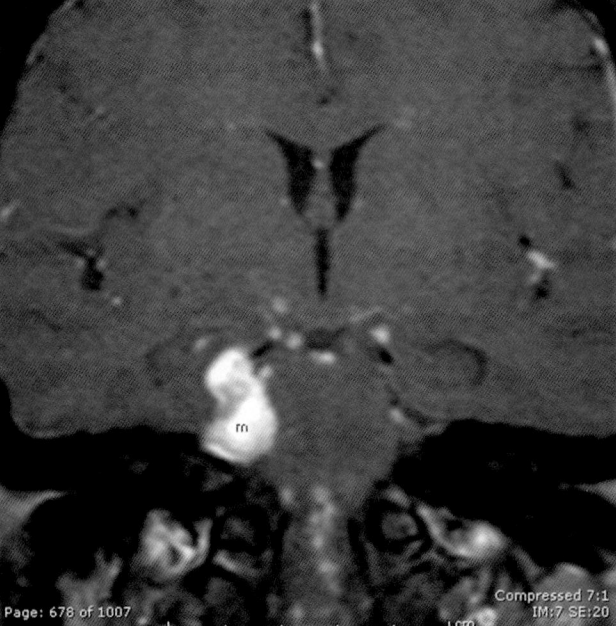

FIGURE 25-3

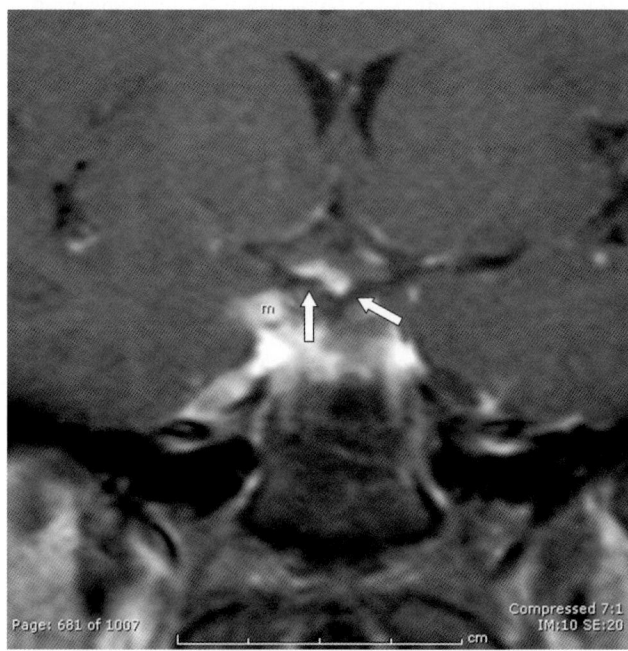

FIGURE 25-4

FINDINGS Figure 25-1. Axial post-contrast T1WI through the inferior posterior fossa. There are multifocal meningeal enhancements bilaterally along the cerebellum and brainstem with irregular enhancement in the right near the Meckel cave (arrow). Figure 25-2. Axial post-contrast T1WI through the pons. There is a lobulated, enhancing dural-based mass (m) extending from the region of the right Meckel cave posterolaterally along the right tentorial edge (arrow). Figure 25-3. Coronal post-contrast T1WI through the mass. The mass (m) extends from the Meckel cave to the cerebellopontine angle (CPA), as well as scattered leptomeningeal enhancing foci predominantly around the brainstem and upper cervical cord. Figure 25-4. Post-contrast coronal T1WI through the pituitary fossa. There is enhancement and thickening of the infundibulum and undersurface of the optic chiasm (arrows) in addition to the mass (m) extension into the right cavernous sinus.

DIFFERENTIAL DIAGNOSIS Neurosarcoidosis, lymphoma, leptomeningeal carcinomatosis, metastatic disease, and infectious etiologies.

DIAGNOSIS Neurosarcoidosis.

DISCUSSION Sarcoidosis is a multisystem inflammatory disease characterized by noncaseating granulomas. Neurosarcoidosis has been reported in up to 5% of patients with sarcoidosis (with higher percentages seen in postmortem series). Imaging findings typically consist of pachymeningeal/dural masses, leptomeningeal involvement, enhancing brain parenchymal lesions, and cranial nerves thickening and enhancement. Approximately 1/3 to 1/2 of the lesions tend to involve the dura. Approximately 1/3 of the lesions tend to involve the leptomeninges, with the cranial nerves, optic nerves, and brain parenchyma (hypothalamus/infundibulum) the next most common location. The remaining occur in the spine, most commonly dural-based. The dural-based and parenchymal lesions of neurosarcoid typically enhance homogeneously on post-contrast T1WI and have a predilection for involvement of the skull base. Contrast-enhanced MRI including multiplanar sequences and fat saturation is the best imaging tool for diagnosis of neurosarcoidosis.

Question for Further Thought

1. What other imaging would help in confirming your suspicion of neurosarcoidosis?

Reporting Responsibilities

As with most intracranial lesions, location and acuity of the lesion(s) and potential complications generally dictate the urgency of relaying findings. Dural-based neurosarcoid lesions may obstruct the arachnoid granulation or ventricular outlets causing hydrocephalus. Other lesions may cause significant mass effect on vital structures warranting urgent communication of findings. While in many cases routine reporting is sufficient, a phone call to the referring clinician with an unexpected finding is usually helpful and appreciated.

What the Treating Physician Needs to Know

- Diagnosis of neurosarcoidosis is based on documentation of systemic sarcoidosis in the absence of other neurologic disease
- Neurologic manifestations are frequently the presenting symptoms but may be nonspecific
- Neurosarcoidosis is usually included in the differential diagnosis when an abnormality involving the leptomeninges and/or dura is detected particularly in the setting of systemic sarcoidosis
- Imaging is important in the clinical evaluation of sarcoidosis for both diagnosis and follow-up to assess response to treatment and to guide the next best course of action
- Early diagnosis of neurosarcoidosis is important because of its associated high morbidity and mortality. Recognition of the constellation of findings of neurosarcoidosis in association with systemic sarcoidosis may help to avoid additional invasive testing and biopsy

Answer

1. Look for a recent prior chest X-ray or chest CT if one has been performed. Chest abnormalities, predominantly hilar adenopathy, can be seen in greater than 90% of patients with systemic sarcoidosis and neurosarcoidosis.

CLINICAL HISTORY *Motor vehicle accident with anterior and central skull base fractures 1 year ago. Patient is presenting with persistent headaches now.*

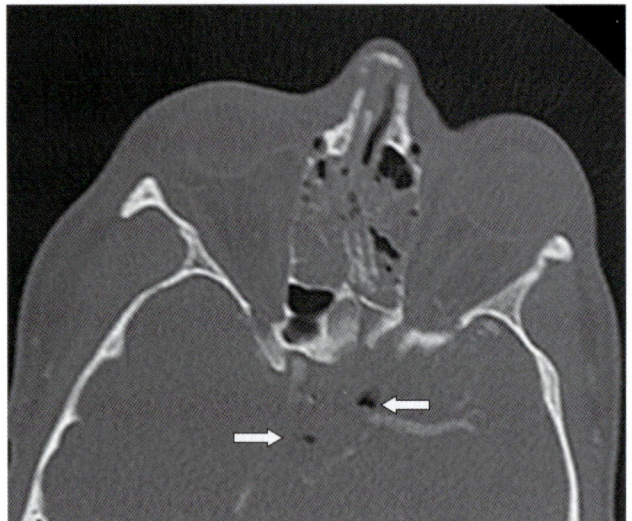

FIGURE 26-1

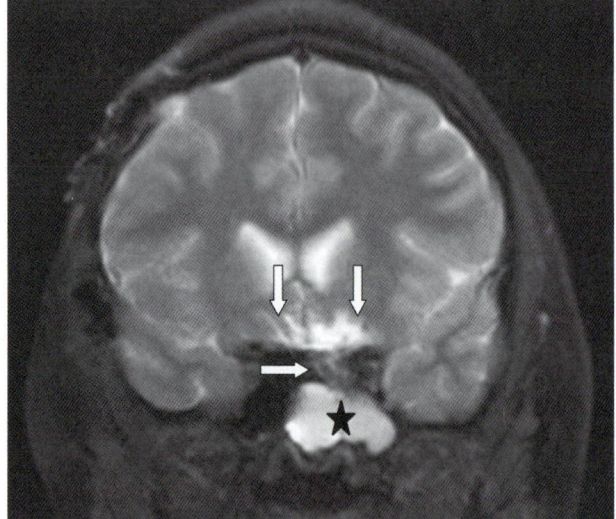

FIGURE 26-2

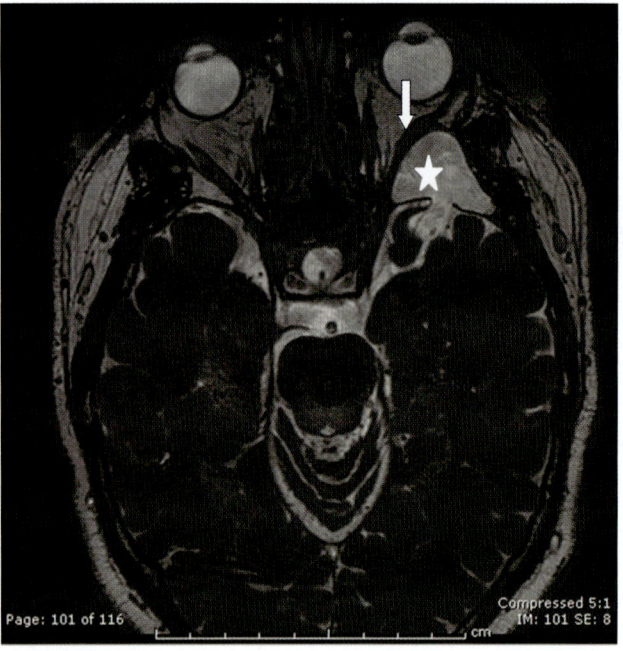

FIGURE 26-3

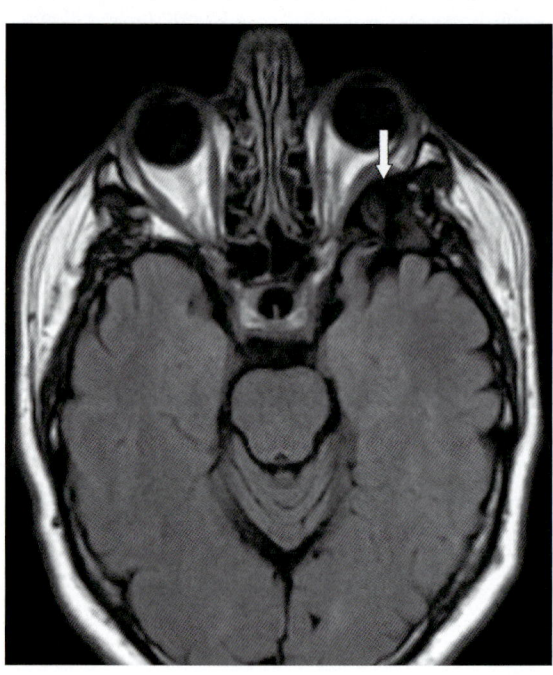

FIGURE 26-4

FINDINGS Figure 26-1. Axial CTA image, bone window through the ethmoid. There is comminuted ethmoidal fracture. Additionally, there is a fracture through the sphenoid roof at the skull base with pneumocephalus in the region of the suprasellar cistern (arrows). Figure 26-2. Coronal T2WI through the planum sphenoidale 1 year later. There is encephalomalacia and gliosis of the bilateral subfrontal lobes (vertical arrows). Additionally, there is hyperintense opacification in the region of the posterior ethmoid and sphenoid sinuses (star). There appears to be a tenuous tract through the planum on the left (transverse arrow). Figures 26-3 and 26-4. Axial heavily T2WI fast imaging employing steady state acquisition (FIESTA) and FLAIR, respectively, in a companion case. There is hyperintense collection anterior to the left middle cranial fossa (star) through a defect in the dura and the left greater wing of sphenoid. Fluid collection abuts and compresses the left lateral rectus (arrows). The fluid suppresses on FLAIR in Figure 26-4.

DIFFERENTIAL DIAGNOSIS Growing skull fractures, pseudomeningocele, leptomeningeal cyst, sinus retention cyst and infection.

DIAGNOSIS Posttraumatic cerebrospinal fluid (CSF) collection (pseudomeningocele).

DISCUSSION High-resolution CT at the level of skull base is highly sensitive for demonstrating skull base fractures acutely, and the lack of healing, bony resorption or "growing fractures" may be identified on follow-up imaging.

Advanced MR techniques such as T2 FIESTA, FLAIR, T1, and T2 sequences can be extremely helpful in determining the extent of posttraumatic fluid collections and oftentimes permit identification of the direct communication with the subarachnoid space (as shown in our companion case). The fluid collection in pseudomeningoceles should be the same as the CSF within the ventricles and the subarachnoid space on all MRI sequences.

For definitive documentation of communication of the fluid collection with the subarachnoid space and identification of the exact point of communication, radionuclide cisternography or CT cisternography is required. For radionuclide cisternography, indium is instilled into the thecal sac via lumbar puncture and the patient tipped head down on the fluoroscopy table in order to advance the radionuclide into the intracranial subarachnoid space. Imaging is obtained immediately and delayed in order to define the location of the communication. Nasal and external auditory canal pledgets may be employed and counted for radioactivity when active CSF leak is suspected. For CT cisternography, myelographic nonionic iodinated contrast is instilled into the thecal sac via lumbar puncture and the patient tipped head down on the fluoroscopy table in order to advance the contrast into the intracranial subarachnoid space. Direct coronal CT imaging is extremely useful in the depiction of contrast leaking into the dependent fluid collection in the setting of a skull base fracture.

Asymptomatic or minimally symptomatic cases of posttraumatic fluid collection without active CSF leak may be identified and subacutely treated surgically. When active leak is present, the increased risk of meningitis, empyema, or infectious complications warrants emergent surgical treatment.

A growing skull fracture (leptomeningeal cyst) is a rare but well-documented complication of craniofacial trauma less commonly seen following fractures of the skull base. A well-defined fracture of the skull base in association with traumatic dural injury results in exposure of the fracture to the pulsations of the cerebrospinal fluid within the subarachnoid space. Pulsatile pressure begins to gradually widen the fracture line permitting the dura/meninges to prolapse through the defect. The content may be slightly hyperintense on T1WI reflecting slightly more proteinaceous contents within the leptomeningeal cyst as compared with a pseudomeningocele.

With infection, abscess will present with single or multiple fluid pockets with poorly defined margins associated with overlying soft tissue swelling and edema. The exact constellation of findings is related to the path of spread of the infection. The fluid collections associated with infection do not follow the imaging characteristics of CSF.

Questions for Further Thought

1. What is the natural history of this disease?
2. What treatment options are there?

Reporting Responsibilities

Direct reporting is essential in view of the possible complications. Location and density or signal intensity of the fluid collections and their proximity to the location of the skull base fracture and the presence of complications such as pneumocephalus, empyema, or other infection must be urgently reported.

What the Treating Physician Needs to Know

- Location, size, and relationship to adjacent structures
- Presence/absence of complications as assessed by imaging
- Usefulness of cisternography for identification of the tract

Answers

1. Increasing fracture diastasis over time may lead to prolapse of meninges and meningocele formation. Progressive neurologic deficits may develop from low CSF pressure states and from infection in cases of active CSF leak.
2. All of these complications of skull base fractures are treated surgically with the addition of antibiotic therapy in those patients with active CSF leak and/or meningitis.

CLINICAL HISTORY *70-year-old male with smoldering multiple myeloma developed mental status changes. Rule out meningitis.*

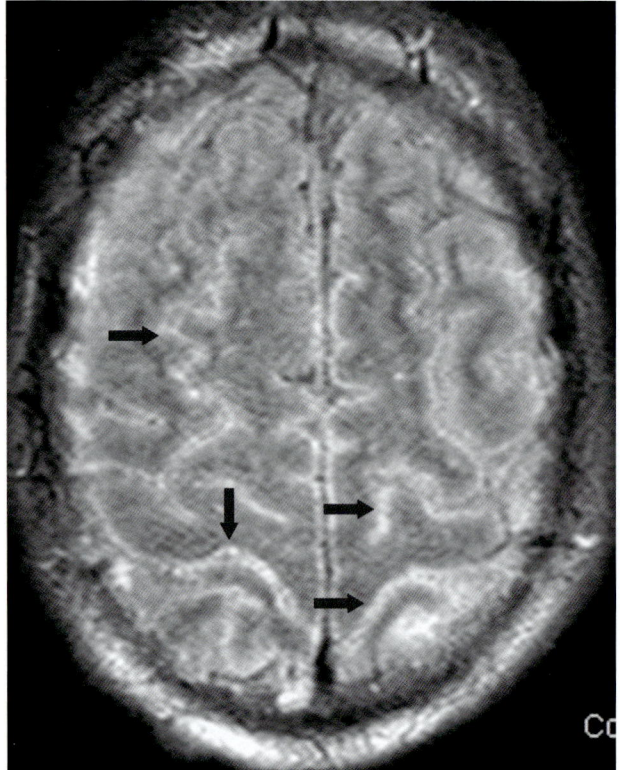

FIGURE 27-1

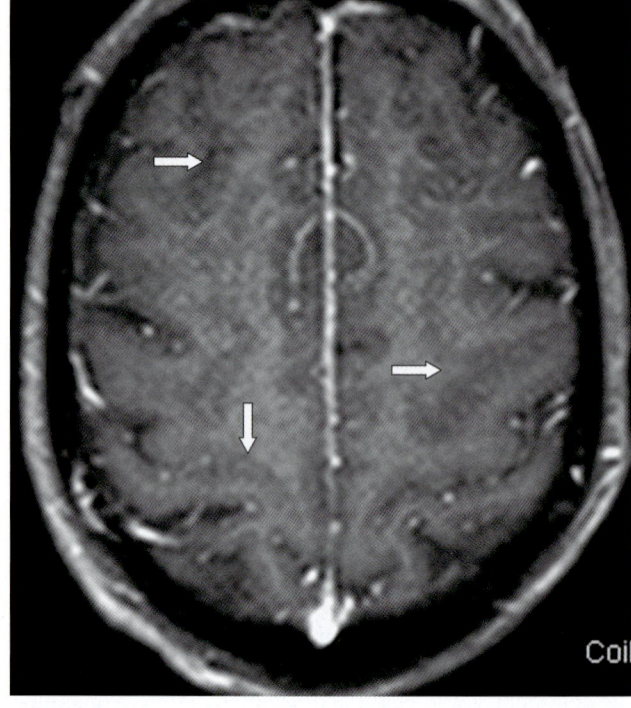

FIGURE 27-2

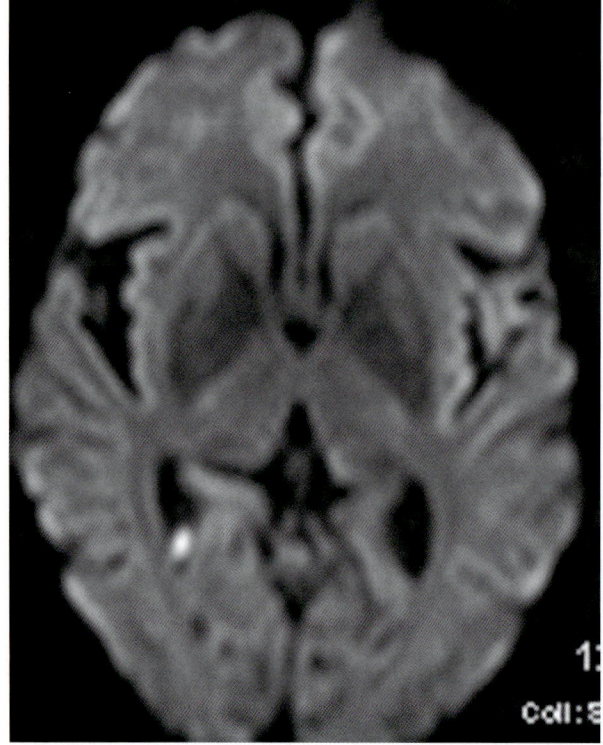

FIGURE 27-3

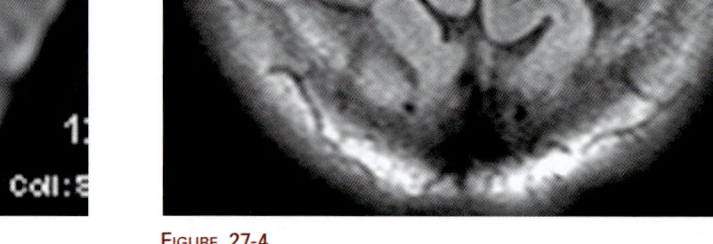

FIGURE 27-4

FINDINGS Figure 27-1. Axial FLAIR through the vertex. There is diffuse sulcal hyperintensity over bilateral cerebral hemispheres (arrows point to some of the hyperintense sulci). The sulci appear prominent on T2WI (not shown). Figure 27-2. Axial post-contrast T1WI through same levels as Figure 27-1. There is bilateral sulcal effacement with very little or no leptomeningeal enhancement (arrows). Figure 27-3. Axial DWI through the trigone 2 weeks following antimicrobial treatment. There is a tiny right trigonal restricted diffusion (arrow) compatible with ventricular debris and ventriculitis. Figure 27-4. Axial FLAIR at the same time as Figure 27-3. There is residual right frontal superior sulcus hyperintensity (arrow) with resolution of sulcal hyperintensity and effacement elsewhere.

DIFFERENTIAL DIAGNOSIS Meningitis, subarachnoid hemorrhage (SAH),ventriculitis.

DIAGNOSIS Bacterial meningitis (BM).

DISCUSSION MRI is the most sensitive imaging modality for evaluation of BM. Contrast-enhanced MRI is normal in about 50%. It should therefore be emphasized that normal imaging does not exclude BM. In those with positive imaging, findings include sulcal FLAIR hyperintensity as in this patient, generally believed to be due to the high protein content of the cerebrospinal fluid (CSF) in BM, leptomeningeal enhancement due to inflammation, subcortical edema, and brain swelling. Complications such as hydrocephalus, vasculopathy, cerebritis, abscess, ischemic infarcts, venous sinus thrombosis, ventriculitis, and subdural collections either empyema or hygroma could easily be detected by imaging. FLAIR sulcal hyperintensity is not unique to BM and may be seen in SAH, supplemental oxygen administration, propofol administration, and leptomeningeal metastases. The history may be useful in excluding these situations. The pattern of leptomeningeal enhancement in BM may not be distinguishable from some normal physiologic situations. CT is capable of showing the complications but not as effective as MRI. Neuroimaging can identify conditions that may predispose to BM such as skull base fractures, paranasal sinus or mastoid infections, and congenital anomalies and monitor response of the complications to treatment. MRA and MRV are useful in evaluation of the vascular complications such as vasculopathy, infarctions, and venous sinus thrombosis.

BM is a severe and often lethal neurologic illness with about 30% to 50% of survivors having permanent neurologic disability. BM can occur in all ages and both genders. The diagnosis of BM is based on clinical and CSF findings. However, imaging particularly CT may be requested before lumbar puncture (LP) to exclude raised intracranial pressure (RIP) and mimics of meningitis. Unfortunately, while RIP is considered a contraindication to LP, normal CT scan does not completely exclude RIP in patients with BM. Imaging is not needed in most patients with meningitis as it is often normal. It may, however, be necessary in patients not responding to treatment as expected or in those suspected to have complications. The causative organisms reach the central nervous system (CNS) by inhalation, via the bloodstream, by direct extension from surrounding paranasal sinuses and mastoid infections or by direct inoculation during intervention. The common organisms in the immunocompetent are *Streptococcus pneumoniae* and *Neisseria meningitidis* accounting for about 80% of cases, while *S. pneumoniae*, *Listeria monocytogenes*, and gram-negative bacilli are common in the immunosuppressed. Group B *streptococci* and coliform bacilli are responsible for most cases in neonates. The CSF is this patient was described as very cloudy with evidence of acute inflammation. *S. pneumoniae* was isolated from the blood, and he responded to a combination of antimicrobials. The follow-up MRI showed resolving sulcal hyperintensity and evidence of complicating ventriculitis.

Question for Further Thought

1. In what ways could DWI be useful in evaluation of meningitis?

Reporting Responsibilities

Findings compatible with meningitis or its complications should be directly reported.

What the Treating Physician Needs to Know

• Is there RIP? Is it safe to perform LP?
• Are there complications? If so what are they?
• On follow-up studies, is there response to treatment or are there new findings or progression of complications?

Answer

1. The most common complication of meningitis is hydrocephalus. This could easily be established by CT or routine MRI. However abscess, subdural empyema, and ventriculitis require DWI for characterization. These three complications usually show restricted diffusion (hyperintense on DWI and hypointense on ADC map) due to cellular debris, thus making it possible to distinguish subdural empyema from subdural hygroma, abscess from tumors, and ventriculitis from hemorrhage. Hemorrhage may sometimes produce heterogeneous restricted diffusion. DWI can also be used to monitor response of these complications to treatment.

CLINICAL HISTORY *37-year-old male with seizures.*

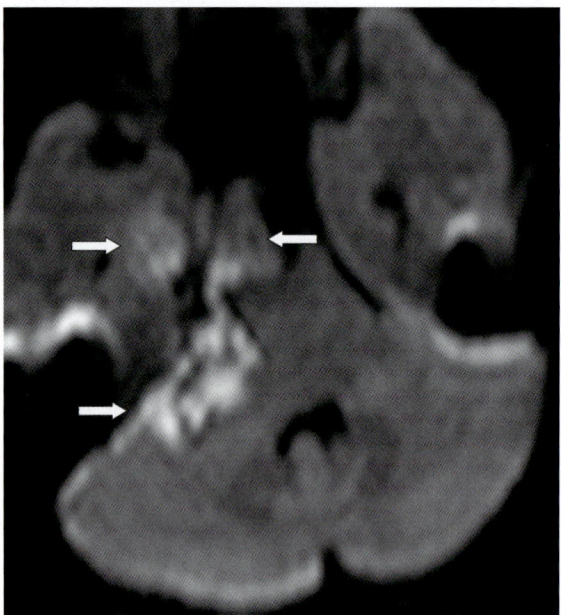

FIGURE 28-1

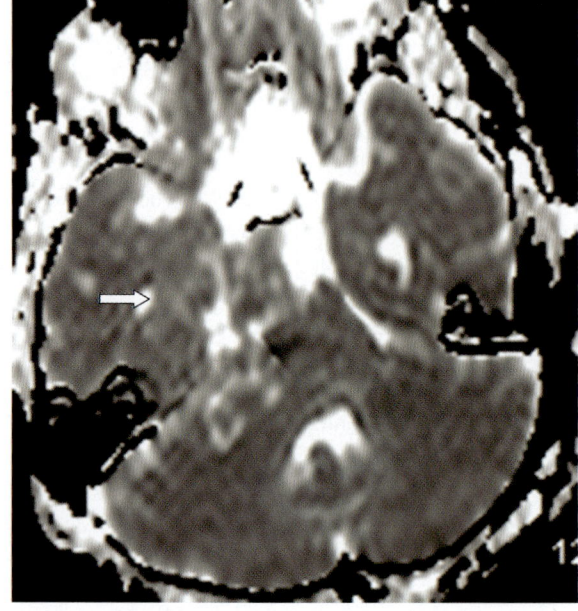

FIGURE 28-2

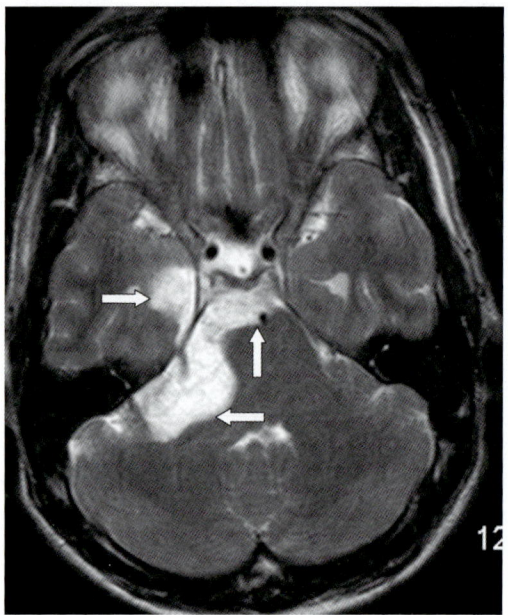

FIGURE 28-3

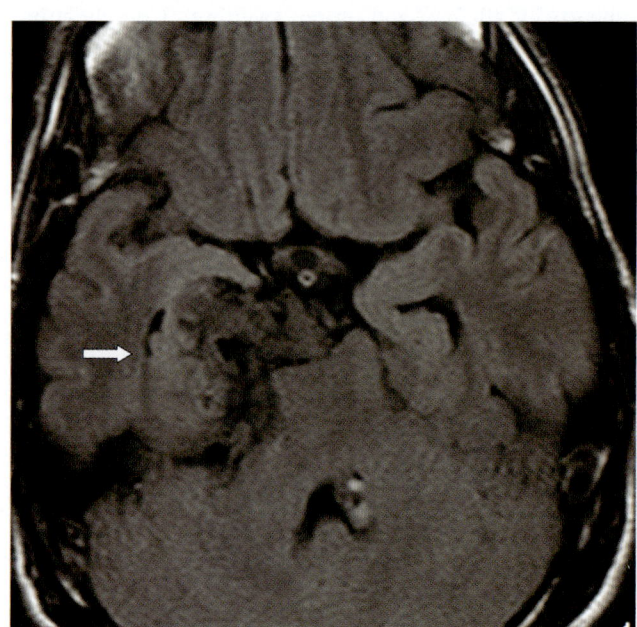

FIGURE 28-4

FINDINGS Figures 28-1 and 28-2. Axial DWI with corresponding ADC map through the posterior fossa. There is a heterogeneous DWI hyperintense mass which is isointense (to brain) on ADC map in the right cerebellopontine angle (CPA). The mass extends into the right middle cranial fossa and suprasellar region (arrows). Figure 28-3. Axial T2WI through the posterior fossa. There is a right CPA, prepontine cistern, suprasellar and adjacent right mesiotemporal hyperintense mass with mass effect on surrounding structures (arrows). The intensity is that of

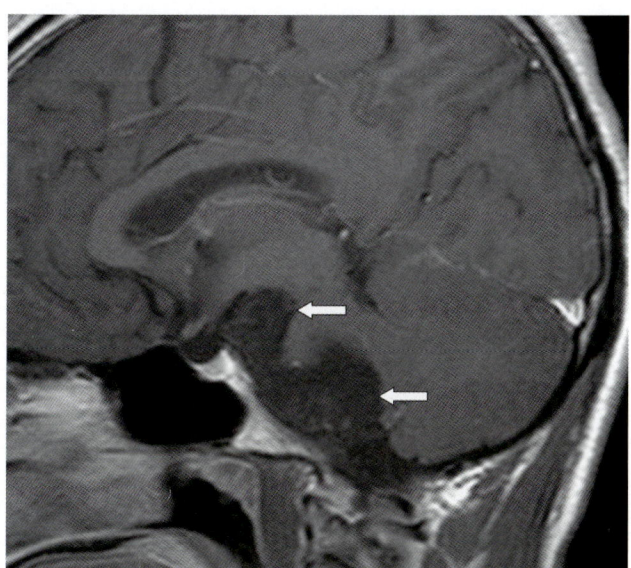

FIGURE **28-5**

reach a large size with significant mass effect on surrounding structures but absolutely no parenchymal edema or contrast enhancement. White epidermoid which is a rarer form of epidermoid cyst has unique imaging characteristics appearing hyperintense on T1WI and hypointense on T2WI, thus resembling dermoid.

Epidermoid cyst is usually a well-circumscribed lobulated non-contrast-enhancing hypodense (CSF density) mass on CT. However, minimal rim enhancement along the periphery has been demonstrated in approximately 25% to 35% of cases. Just as in the MRI, there is no surrounding edema. Secondary dystrophic calcification is a rare occurrence in about 10% and is thought to be caused by peritumoral leakage of cyst contents. Hyperdense cyst, the so-called white epidermoid, is uncommon.

Epidermoid cyst is rare and typically asymptomatic until the third to fifth decades of life with presentation at a mean age of 40 years. Clinical presentation depends on the location of the lesion, extension, and mass effect on adjacent vital structures. Presentation may include mild headaches, seizures, and rare fatal events. Trigeminal neuralgia, hemifacial spasm, tinnitus, gait ataxia, diplopia, and dysphagia are some of the presenting symptoms of posterior fossa epidermoid. Pineal region lesions may cause hydrocephalus and Parinaud syndrome. Epidermoid cyst is a congenital anomaly thought to arise from misplaced inclusions of ectodermal squamous epithelial remnants trapped during neural tube closure and separated from the ectoderm between the third and fifth weeks of intrauterine development. During this same period of embryogenesis, the otic and optic vesicles are also being formed, and it is believed that migration along these or other developing neurovascular structures accounts for the lateral placement seen in most epidermoid cysts. It is speculated that inclusions occurring prior to the third week of embryologic development may result in intraventricular and intracerebral lesions, as this coincides with formation of the primary cerebral vesicle. The cyst is lined with keratinizing stratified squamous epithelium. As desquamation occurs, the cystic cavity fills with epithelial cells consisting predominantly of keratin in concentric layers, water, and cholesterol from cell membrane degradation, giving the tumor its pearly appearance.

Treatment is gross total surgical resection which generally carries a good prognosis. The potential for damage to cranial nerves and adjacent critical structures during aggressive resection exists. Aseptic meningitis due to remnant cyst material is a known complication of surgery.

CSF. Figure 28-4. Axial FLAIR through the suprasellar cistern. There is a right mesiotemporal/prepontine/upper right CPA somewhat heterogeneous hypointense mass. There is deformity of and mass effect on the brainstem and right temporal lobe with compression of the right temporal horn (arrow). Figure 28-5. Right parasagittal post-contrast T1WI. There is a non-contrast-enhancing lobulated hypointense right CPA and suprasellar mass (arrows) compressing the right cerebellum, brachium pontis, and midbrain.

DIFFERENTIAL DIAGNOSIS Arachnoid cyst, epidermoid cyst, dermoid cyst.

DIAGNOSIS Epidermoid cyst.

DISCUSSION Epidermoid cyst or pearl tumor is best imaged by MRI. This tumor is subarachnoid in location. It is most frequently located in the CPA. Location in or extension into the prepontine and suprasellar cisterns and the middle cranial fossa is not uncommon. It could be found in the pineal region or within the ventricles and anywhere intracranially. It generally follows CSF intensity on spin echo sequences appearing hypointense on T1WI and hyperintense on T2WI. However, this presentation has been shown to be somewhat variable depending on the cyst contents with some degree of signal heterogeneity. It could be slightly hyperintense on FLAIR. Epidermoid cyst is usually heterogeneously hyperintense on DWI with ADC map approaching that of the brain parenchyma. This distinguishes it from arachnoid cyst which has CSF intensity pattern on DWI/ADC map. Dermoid on the other hand is well circumscribed mainly midline to parasagittal in location with T1 hyperintensity and heterogeneous T2 hypointensity. Epidermoid cyst could

Question for Further Thought

1. Why is white epidermoid different from the regular epidermoid cyst?

Reporting Responsibilities

Although this is a benign process, the significant mass effect requires direct reporting. Presence of hydrocephalus makes direct reporting more urgent. The location and extent of the mass should be described in detail.

What the Treating Physician Needs to Know

- Location and extent of the mass
- Presence of significant mass effect or hydrocephalus

Answer

1. White epidermoid is hyperdense on CT and hyperintense on T1WI; changes thought to be due to a relatively high protein concentration and large fraction of albumin. It is hypointense on T2WI probably on the basis of the higher viscosity of the cyst content. Its lipid content is also believed to be different from typical epidermoid cyst.

CLINICAL HISTORY *61-year-old male with headache. He was an outpatient at the time of the CT!*

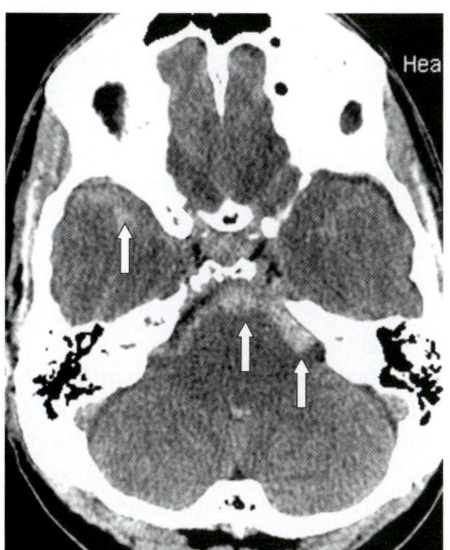

FIGURE 29-1

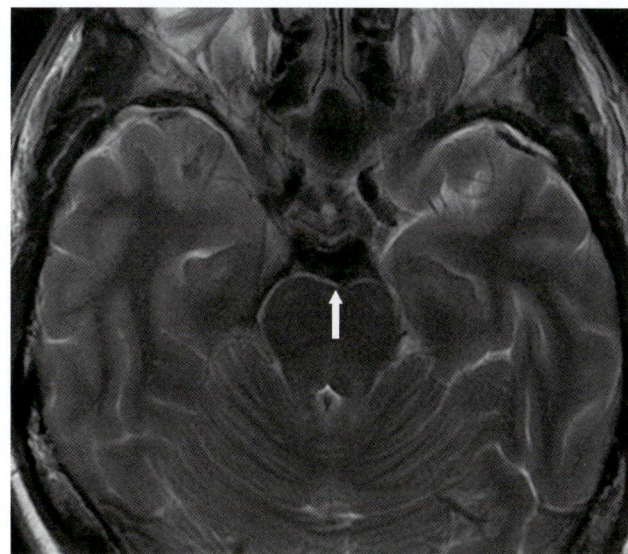

FIGURE 29-2

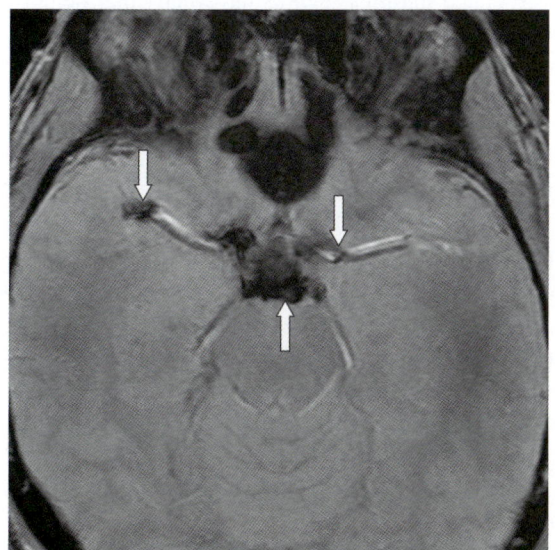

FIGURE 29-3

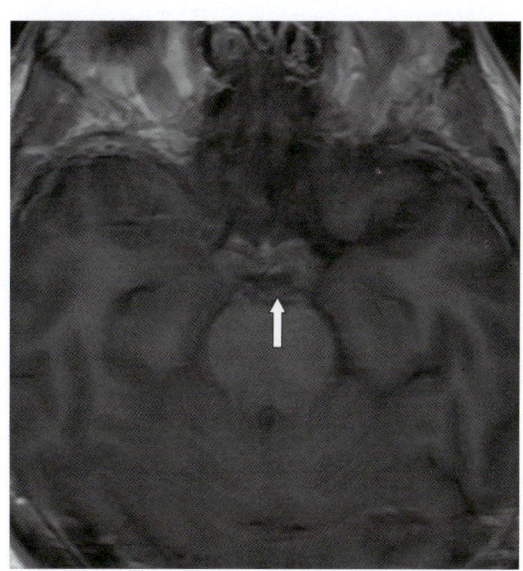

FIGURE 29-4

FINDINGS Figure 29-1. Axial NCCT through the posterior fossa. There is subarachnoid space (SAS) hyperdensity in the posterior and middle cranial fossae (arrow). Figure 29-2. Axial T2WI through the suprasellar cistern. There is diffuse hypointensity in the SAS (arrow). Figure 29-3. Axial GRE through the suprasellar cistern. There is diffuse hypointensity/signal void in the suprasellar cistern and lateral fissures (arrows). Figure 29-4. Axial non-contrast T1WI through the suprasellar cistern. There is diffuse isointensity in the suprasellar cistern (arrow). Figure 29-5. Axial FLAIR through the

lateral ventricles in a companion patient with SAH. There is bilateral scattered sulcal hyperintensity (arrows).

DIFFERENTIAL DIAGNOSIS N/A.

DIAGNOSIS Acute subarachnoid hemorrhage (ASAH).

DISCUSSION The classical NCCT sign of ASAH is subarachnoid space hyperdensity. NCCT is the gold standard for the diagnosis of ASAH with a sensitivity of up to 100%

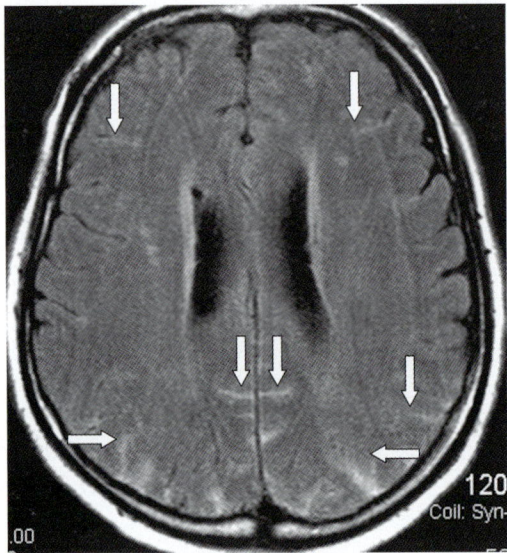

FIGURE 29-5

within the first 6 hours. The location and size of the hemorrhage may influence the sensitivity of CT. About 10% of SAH may not be visible on CT after 24 hours. There has been an emphasis on FLAIR MRI sulcal hyperintensity for demonstrating this group of CT-negative SAH. As seen in this case, acute SAH could be visible on other MRI sequences. There is SAS isointensity on T1WI, hypointensity on T2WI, and hyperintensity on FLAIR. The location of the SAH is predominantly posterior fossa in this case with some diffusion into the convexity sulci. The logical follow-up evaluation of SAH is either CTA or MRA, both of which are equally effective in uncovering the aneurysmal origins of most nontraumatic SAH. If either of this fails to show the cause, DSA is the next logical examination.

Initial CTA and DSA were negative for aneurysm in this patient. A follow-up CTA showed extensive vasospasm but no aneurysm. MRI showed multifocal infarcts. A follow-up DSA did not reveal any aneurysm. This therefore is one form of nonaneurysmal subarachnoid hemorrhage (NASAH). NASAH forms about 15% of all nontraumatic SAH. The location of the hemorrhage is predominantly posterior fossa and around the midbrain into the suprasellar region in this case with some convexity diffusion in the companion patient

(Figure 29-5). The thinking used to be that NASAH is a benign process compared to aneurysmal SAH. Complications in a recent cohort of NASAH include early hydrocephalus 25%, late hydrocephalus 13%, vasospasm 4%, infarction 2%, and death 3%. Follow-up angiograms usually show aneurysm in about 24%. It is therefore essential that a repeat angiogram, CTA, MRA, or DSA be performed. There is controversy as to how soon the follow-up angiogram should be performed but usually within 4 weeks. If that is negative, then another follow-up between 2 and 6 months may be desirable.

Question for Further Thought

1. What is the cause of NASAH?

Reporting Responsibilities

This is an acute situation requiring direct reporting. The extent of the hemorrhage and recommendation for angiogram should be mentioned. Visible cause such as venous thrombosis, arteriovenous malformation (AVM), cerebral cavernous malformation (CCM), or dural arteriovenous fistula (DAVF) on the MRI should be mentioned.

What the Treating Physician Needs to Know

- Location of hemorrhage
- Other associated findings such as intraventricular hemorrhage (IVH), hydrocephalus, parenchymal hemorrhage, or focal clot that may suggest location of aneurysm, parenchymal changes that may point in the direction of a cause of the hemorrhage
- Recommendation for finding out the cause of the SAH: CTA or MRA

Answer

1. Repeat angiograms show aneurysm in about 24% of NASAH. These aneurysms may not be visible initially because of their size, presence of spasm, or complex anatomy of their locations. Other possible causes may include occult AVM, CCM, telangiectasia, coagulopathy, venous thrombosis, pituitary apoplexy, arterial dissections, spinal AVM, and DAVF. DSA in NASAH should always include external carotid injections to exclude DAVF. However, the cause of the hemorrhage is never found in the majority of NASAH.

CLINICAL HISTORY *62-year-old female for stroke evaluation.*

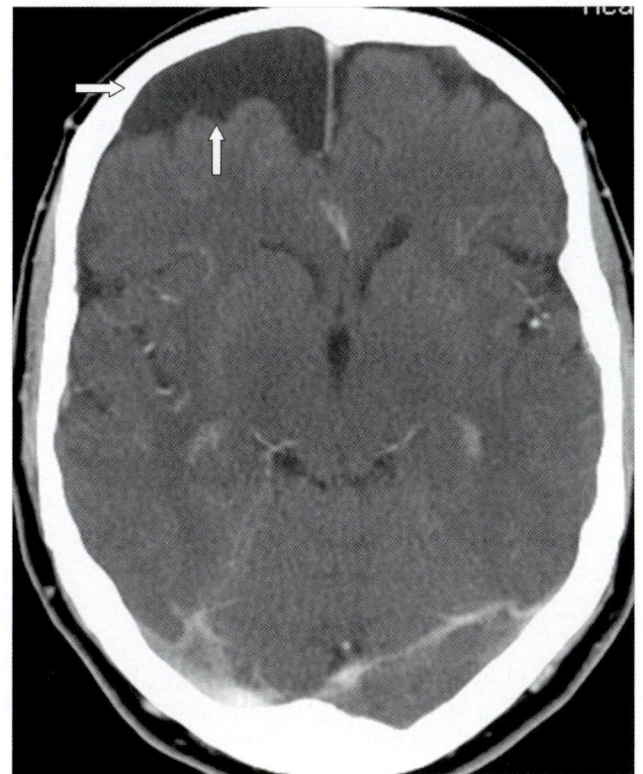

FIGURE 30-1

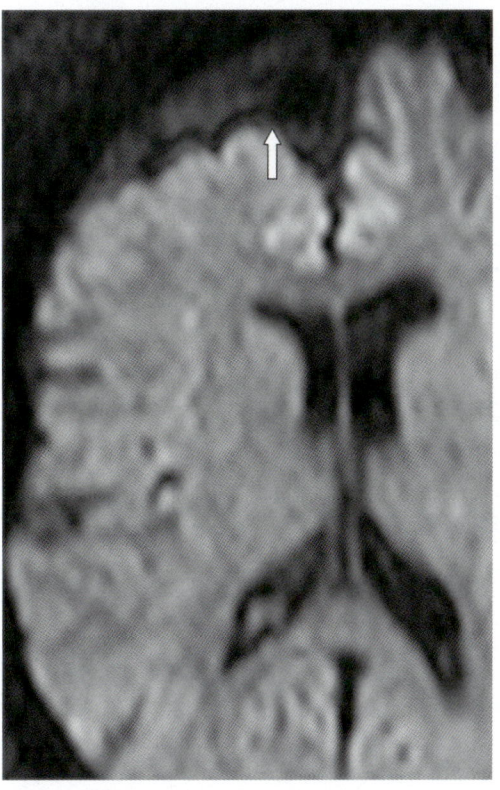

FIGURE 30-2

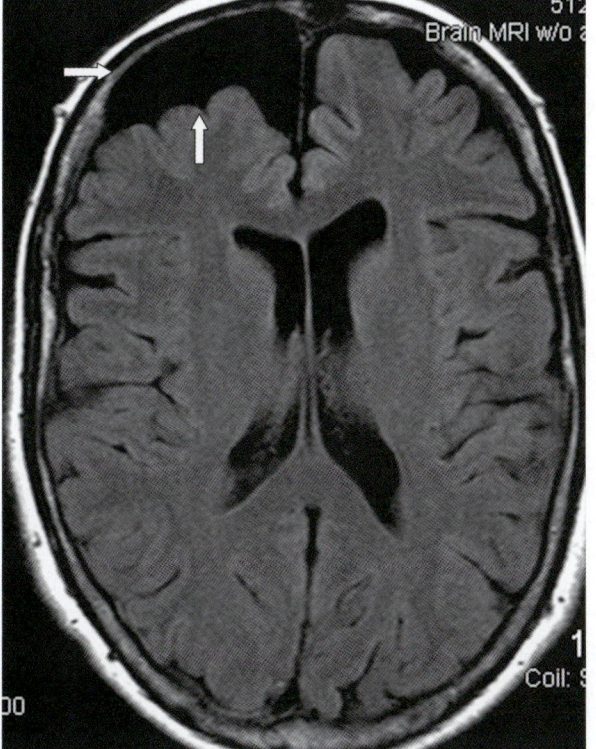

FIGURE 30-3

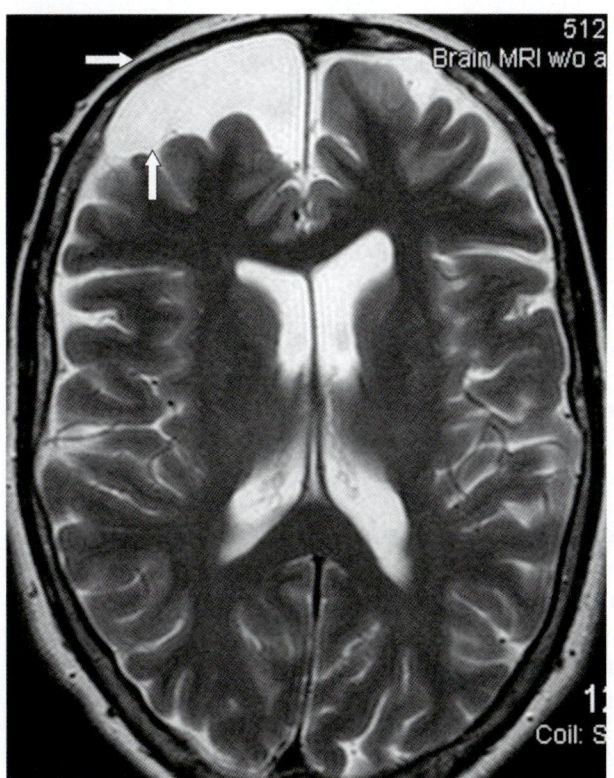

FIGURE 30-4

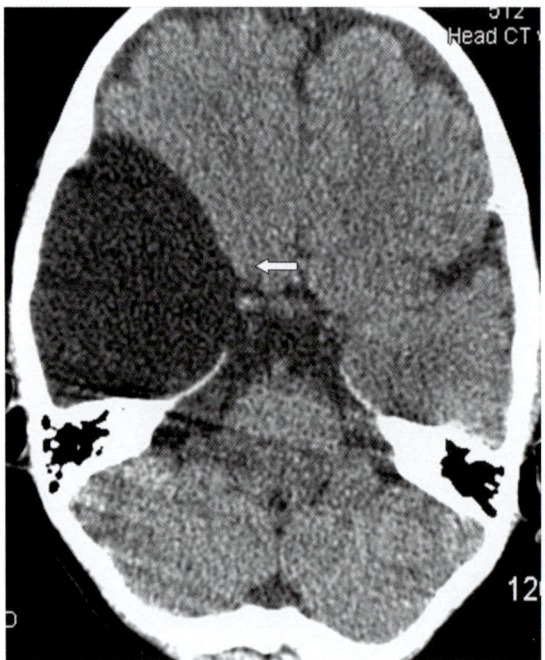

FIGURE 30-5

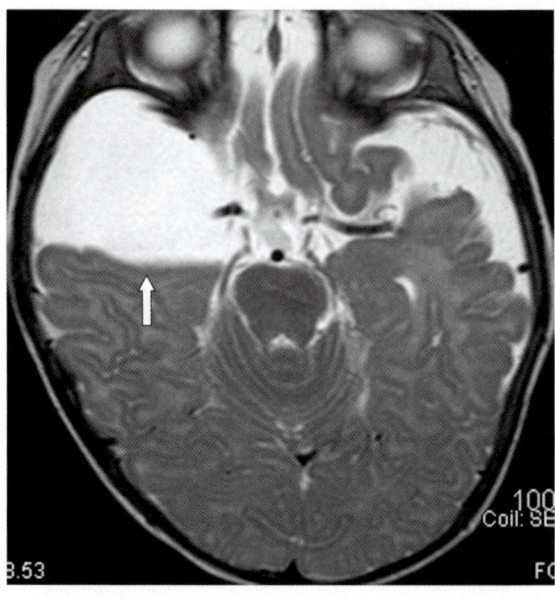

FIGURE 30-6

FINDINGS Figure 30-1 Axial post-contrast CT. There is a right frontal extraaxial cerebrospinal fluid (CSF) density collection with compression of the right frontal lobe (vertical arrow). There is mild thinning and remodeling of the overlying right frontal bone (transverse arrow). Figures 30-2 to 30-4. Axial DWI, FLAIR, and T2WI, respectively, through the lesion. The collection follows CSF intensity on all sequences. There is compression of the frontal lobe (vertical arrows). Thinning of the right frontal bone is again demonstrated (transverse arrows). Figures 30-5 and 30-6. Axial NCCT and axial T2W MRI, respectively, through the right middle cranial fossa in a 3-year-old boy. These demonstrate an arachnoid cyst (AC) in a more typical location in the right middle cranial fossa. There is smooth compression of the frontal and temporal lobes (arrows) with overlying right temporal bone remodeling and thinning seen on the CT. In these two cases like in all cases, the mass is extraaxial to cortical gray matter (GM).

DIFFERENTIAL DIAGNOSIS AC, epidermoid cyst, neurocysticercosis, porencephalic cyst (PC), pilocytic astrocytoma, hemangioblastoma.

DIAGNOSIS Arachnoid cyst (AC).

DISCUSSION Both CT and MRI are capable of demonstrating the changes of AC, but MRI is the preferred method of choice. AC is an extra axial CSF containing mass located in the subarachnoid space compressing the underlying brain with remodeling and thinning of the overlying calvarium. It is homogeneously CSF hypodense on CT and follows CSF intensity on all MRI sequences. There is usually no vascular structure within it, and the wall can rarely be identified being composed of a very thin arachnoid membrane. The immediate surrounding brain is usually cortical GM which could be slightly thickened and flattened due to mass effect. PC on the other hand is surrounded by gliotic tissue since it is a result of parenchymal destruction. PC also communicates freely with the CSF space. The majority of ACs are noncommunicating, while a small percentage may communicate via a ball valve mechanism which could be demonstrated by CT cisternogram or phase contrast cine MR. Epidermoid tumor follows CSF intensity on all spin echo sequences but restricts diffusion which distinguishes it from AC. However, some ACs may contain proteinaceous fluid or become hemorrhagic making differentiation difficult. Hemorrhage into ACs could be spontaneous, traumatic, or due to a ruptured aneurysm. Racemose neurocysticercosis is usually multiloculated with septations. Pilocytic astrocytoma and hemangioblastoma are parenchymal lesions with solid mostly contrast-enhancing components.

AC accounts for less than 1% of all intracranial masses and is widely accepted as developmental anomalies in which splitting or duplication of the primitive arachnoid membrane allows subarachnoid fluid collection. It is a common benign lesion occurring in the CNS both within the intracranial compartment (most common) and within the spinal canal. Common intracranial locations include the middle cranial fossa/sylvian fissure (50% to 60%), suprasellar (10%), quadrigeminal plate cistern (10%), cerebellopontine angle (5% to 10%), supracerebellar cistern (<5%), and cisterna magna (<5%).

Most cases begin during infancy; however, onset may be delayed until adolescence. Although the vast majority is sporadic, they are seen with increased frequency in mucopolysaccharidoses. The majority of ACs is small and asymptomatic. Headache and seizures are the most common symptoms. When symptoms occur, they are usually the result of gradual enlargement resulting in mass effect. This results in either direct neurologic dysfunction, or distortion of normal CSF pathways resulting in obstructive hydrocephalus. Surgical treatment when necessary includes surgical excision, surgical fenestration, or cyst shunting into the CSF space or peritoneum.

Questions for Further Thought

1. Does AC cause seizure?
2. Is there any difference between communicating and noncommunicating AC?

Reporting Responsibilities

This is a benign usually incidental finding and requires routine reporting. It is important to report the size, presence of bone remodeling, and associated hydrocephalus if any.

What the Treating Physician Needs to Know

- Size and location
- Presence of adjacent compressed or dysplastic tissue
- Communicating or noncommunicating in symptomatic lesions at CT cisternogram or phase contrast cine MR

Answers

1. No. Most ACs are incidental, asymptomatic, and do not cause seizures. However, since ACs are more common in the middle cranial fossa than elsewhere, there is the suggestion that underlying temporal lobe compression, dysplasia, or hypogenesis could lead to seizures.
2. It has been suggested that symptomatic ACs are usually the growing or enlarging ACs and that these symptomatic ACs tend to communicate with the arachnoid space via a ball valve mechanism that allows CSF to enter but not exit. CT cisternography and/or phase contrast cine MR have been used to demonstrate presence of such communication. There is a consensus that symptomatic cysts causing seizures, hydrocephalus, focal neurologic deficits, or raised intracranial pressure may benefit from surgical management and demonstration of communication between the ACs and the subarachnoid space is important in the preoperative evaluation.

CLINICAL HISTORY *2-year-old with increasing ataxia, irritability, and new onset vomiting.*

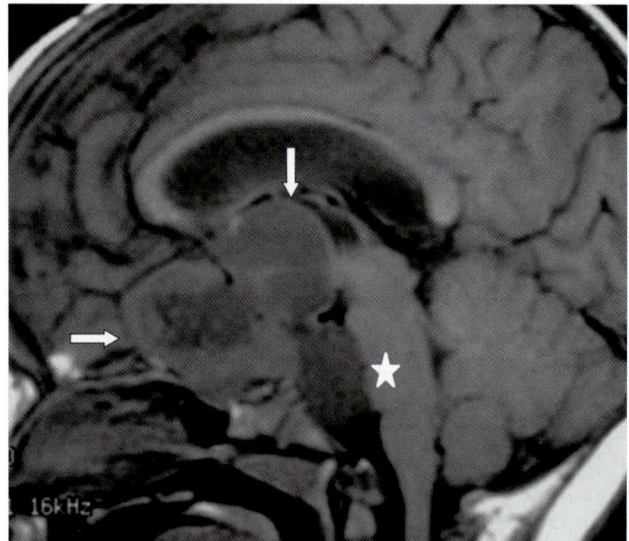

FIGURE 31-1

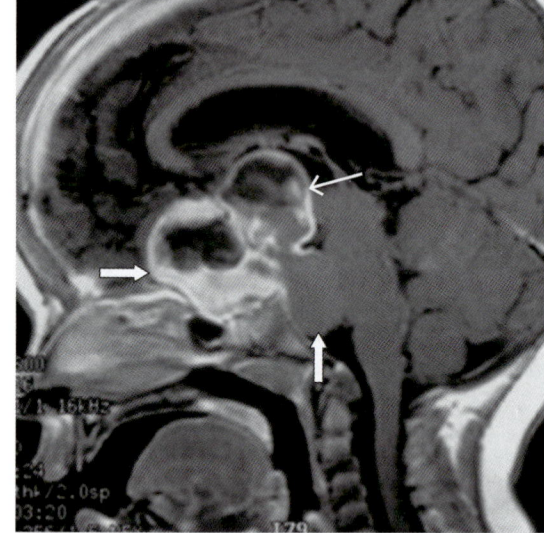

FIGURE 31-2

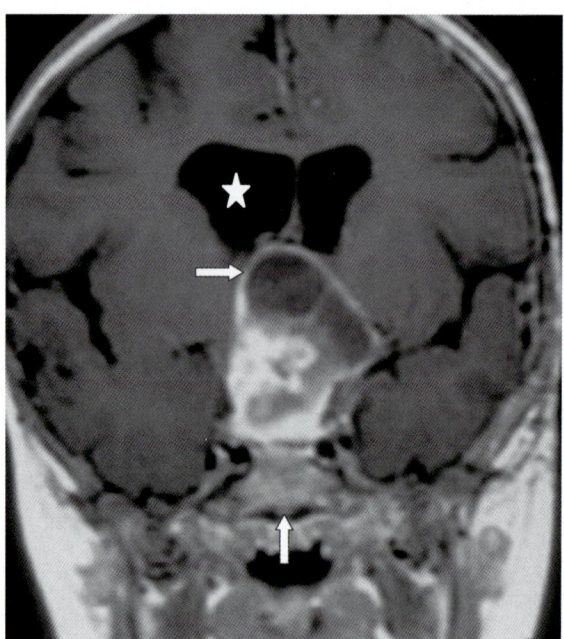

FIGURE 31-3

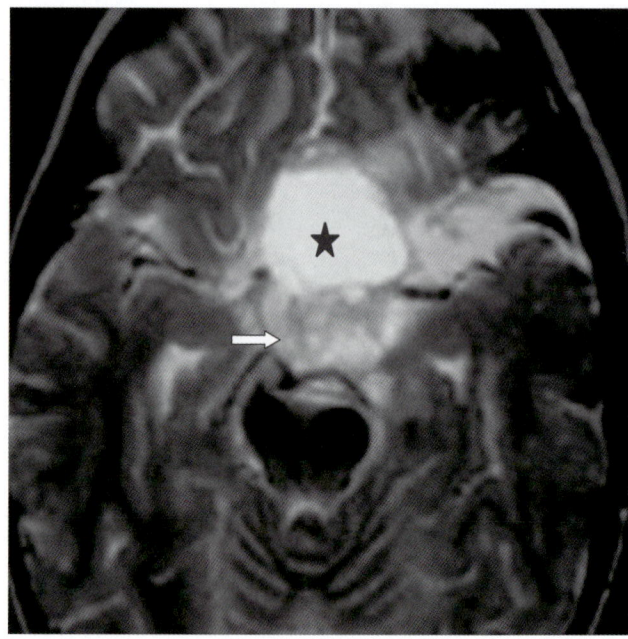

FIGURE 31-4

FINDINGS Figure 31-1. Sagittal non-contrast T1WI. There is a large multilobulated solid cystic mass in the suprasellar cistern. There is marked mass effect and displacement of the floor of the third ventricle (vertical arrow), posterior inferior frontal lobes (transverse arrow), midbrain and pons (star). The lesion is heterogeneous hypo- to isointense. Figure 31-2. Sagittal post-contrast T1WI. Thin (thin arrow) and thick (thick anterior arrow) walls of enhancement are present. The

component in front of the pons (vertical arrow) is not enhancing. Figure 31-3. Coronal post-contrast T1WI. The superior extension of the lesion to the foramina of Monro (transverse arrow) and the dilation of the lateral ventricles (star) are demonstrated. The sella turcica is compressed (vertical arrow). Figure 31-4. Axial T2WI. The cystic component is noted to be hyperintense to cerebrospinal fluid (CSF) (star), and the more solid component is only mildly hyperintense (arrow). There is mild surrounding edema. No evidence of calcifications was found on the MRI.

DIFFERENTIAL DIAGNOSIS Optic nerve glioma, craniopharyngioma, meningioma, metastatic tumor, macroadenoma, aneurysm, sarcoid, tuberculoma, pilocytic astrocytoma (PA).

DIAGNOSIS PA of optic pathway.

DISCUSSION PA has a strong propensity to present as a complex cystic and solid mass but can be mainly cystic or solid. Calcification and hemorrhage can occur (24% and 31%, respectively), but some series have yielded no calcifications. The cystic component is iso- to slightly hyperintense to CSF on T1WI, incompletely suppressed on FLAIR, and hyperintense to CSF on T2WI. The solid component is iso- to hypointense on T1WI and iso- to hyperintense on T2WI. The solid component and cyst wall have variable contrast enhancement from none to avid enhancement. Mass effect is usual with very little or no surrounding edema. PA in the optic pathway such as this may not always be well-defined like elsewhere but can be infiltrating, spreading along the optic tracts and nerves. MRS may show a high choline and creatine peak with reduced *N*-acetyl aspartate (NAA) in the solid component. Perfusion MRI usually shows reduced relative cerebral blood volume (rCBV) and cerebral blood flow (CBF) in the solid portion. The CT findings follow the MR morphology. PA is isodense to hypodense without contrast. It may show hyperdense calcification or hemorrhage and variable contrast enhancement of a mural nodule or solid component within a nonenhancing cyst. Cyst wall may enhance. The majority of PA occur in the posterior fossa with a reported incidence of 75% with the remainder split between the supra/parasellar region as in this case and supratentorial lobar regions. The supratentorial lobar location is more common in adults and occurs more in the temporal and parietal lobes.

The absence of calcifications makes craniopharyngioma unlikely. The lack of skull base thickening, marrow infiltration, dural tail, and overall complex morphology excludes meningioma. This lesion or any lesion is unlikely to be a pituitary adenoma if the sella is unremarkable. The lack of flow artifact, lack of blood clot, and presence of solid and cystic areas rule out a giant aneurysm. Sarcoid is excluded by the complex solid enhancing and nonenhancing components. One may expect associated leptomeningeal and cranial nerve enhancement (especially CN V and VII) in sarcoidosis. Metastatic disease or glioblastoma presents in this location rarely, and the features could be similar, but more associated edema would be expected. With metastatic disease solid nonenhancing tumor would not be present.

Patients with neurofibromatosis type 1 have a propensity for developing PA. If stigmata of neurofibromatosis type 1

(NF1) are identified, then the diagnosis of a PA becomes very likely. PAs occur mostly in the first two decades of life although the age of presentation can extend to late adulthood. PA occurs equally in males and females. PAs often present with symptoms of hydrocephalus due to CSF pathway obstruction but can also present with symptoms related to local mass effect or invasion. These symptoms include loss of vision, pituitary hypofunction, diencephalic syndrome, cranial nerve dysfunction with cavernous sinus involvement, and/or proptosis. PA is the most benign of all astrocytic tumors and the most common glioma in children 1 to 19 years forming about 5% to 6% of all gliomas. PA is a relatively circumscribed tumor composed of compact cellular areas consisting of elongated and fibrillated cells that alternate with loose myxoid, microcyst-rich areas. Nuclei contain bland chromatin. Mitoses are none to rare. Brightly eosinophilic Rosenthal fibers are common in compact areas, whereas eosinophilic granular bodies (EGBs) can be seen in either region. Necrosis and glomeruloid vascular hyperplasia can be seen and should not be confused with high-grade glioma. It is a WHO I tumor with a good chance of cure following complete removal.

Question for Further Thought

1. What are the factors associated with event-free survival?

Reporting Responsibilities

Presence of hydrocephalus or herniation deserves direct reporting to the referring physician. Although PA is a WHO I tumor, presence of leptomeningial enhancement may suggest the occasional but rare tumor dissemination, and evaluation of the craniospinal axis may be warranted. A vascular mass such as aneurysm should not be confused with a tumor. If in doubt suggest MRA or CTA.

What the Treating Physician Needs to Know

- There is a strong association of PA with NF1. If this has not already been established, it may be necessary to look for this association
- Is the tumor well circumscribed or infiltrating? Any complications?
- Location and size on both initial and follow-up recording any tumor growth

Answer

1. Four pathologic features (necrosis, oligodendroglioma-like features, vascular hyalinization, and calcification) show a significant correlation with decreased event-free survival. Also, PAs involving the optic pathway are associated with worse event-free survival compared with those arising in other locations.

CLINICAL HISTORY   *75-year-old male with new onset left-sided leg and foot weakness.*

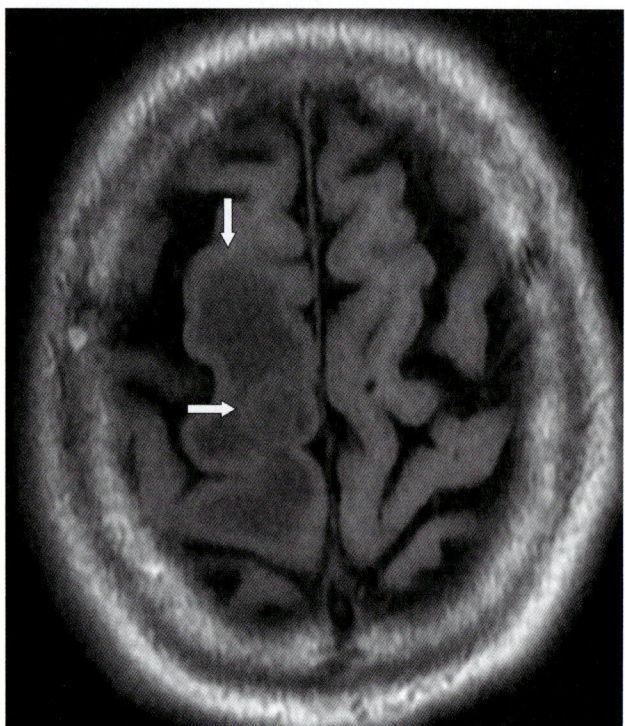

FIGURE 32-1

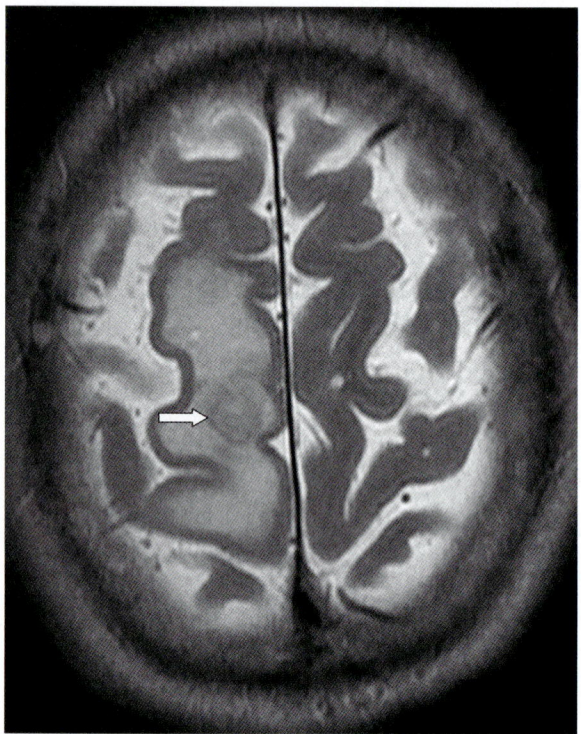

FIGURE 32-2

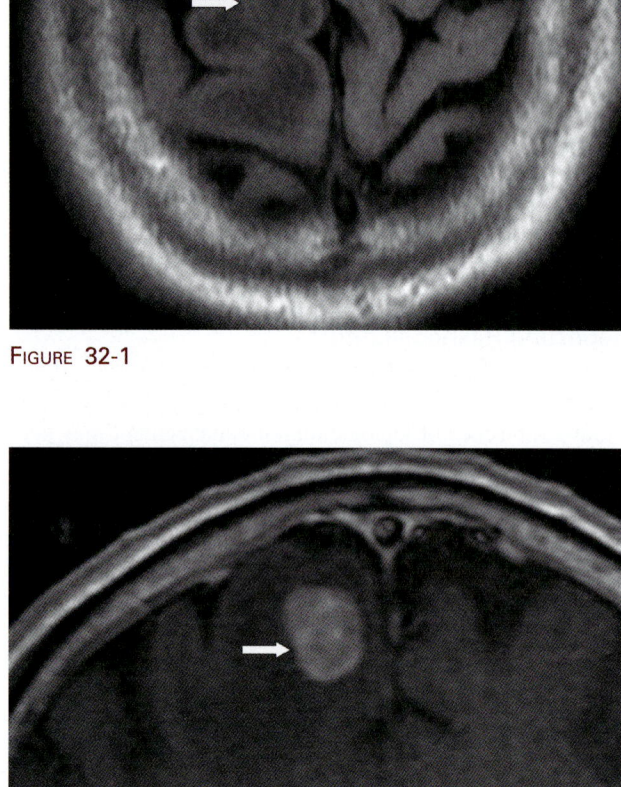

FIGURE 32-3

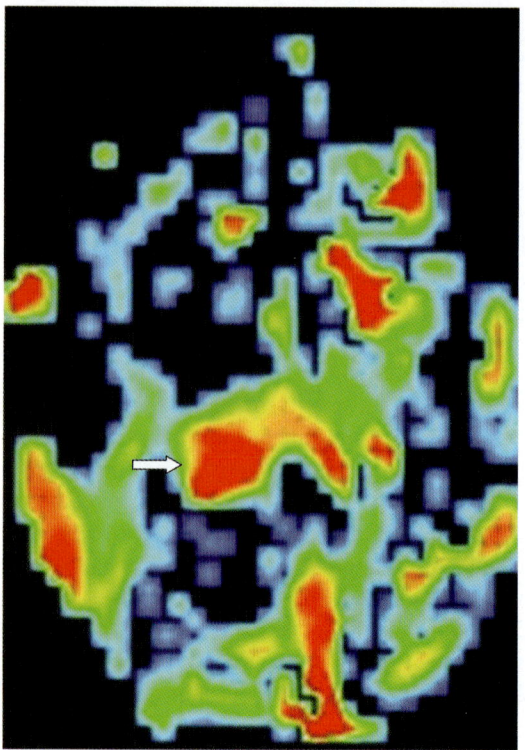

FIGURE 32-4

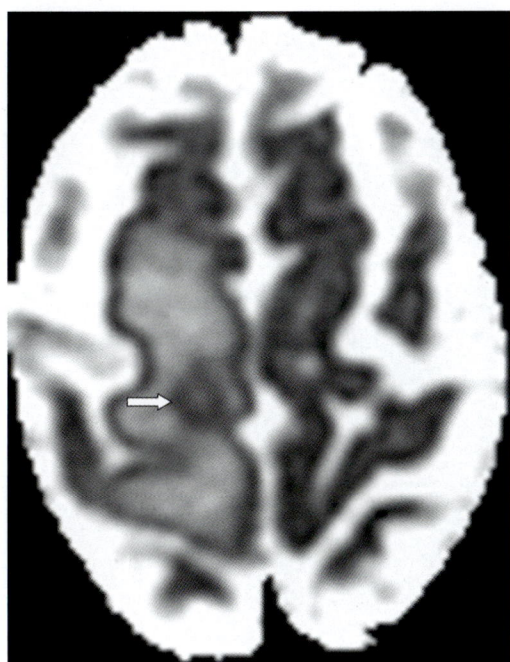

FIGURE 32-5

FINDINGS Figure 32-1. Axial non-contrast T1WI through the cerebral convexities. There is a round right posterior frontal lobe parasagittal small well-circumscribed mass (transverse arrow) in the premotor area, mildly heterogeneous but isointense compared to surrounding expanded hypointense white matter (WM) that is consistent with edema (vertical arrow). Figure 32-2. Corresponding axial T2WI. The mass is mildly heterogeneous and slightly hypointense (arrow) compared to the surrounding hyperintense edema. The right superior frontal gyrus is expanded, and adjacent sulci are partially effaced. Figure 32-3. Coronal post-contrast T1WI. There is a single mildly heterogeneous contrast-enhancing, sharply marginated, subcortical mass in the posterior parasagittal right frontal lobe. There is surrounding hypointensity consistent with edema or infiltrating tumor. Figure 32-4. Axial blood volume perfusion map through the mass. There is significant increase in the relative Cerebral Blood Volume (rCBV) (arrow). Figure 32-5. ADC map through the mass. The mass has relative restricted diffusion peripherally compared to the adjacent brain. This likely indicates hypercellularity in the mass and the surrounding elevated ADC values indicate that most of the surrounding abnormality is likely vasogenic edema.

DIFFERENTIAL DIAGNOSIS Metastasis, anaplastic astrocytoma, anaplastic oligodendroglioma, ganglioglioma (GG), pilocytic astrocytoma (PA), pleomorphic xanthoastrocytoma (PXA), lobar ependymoma.

DIAGNOSIS Granular cell astrocytoma (GCA).

DISCUSSION GCA is a rare WHO IV astrocytoma. The tumors almost all occur in the cerebral hemispheres. More tend to occur in the parietal or frontal lobes than in the temporal lobe or occipital lobe. CT demonstrates a well-defined hypodense mass. Mass is usually hypointense on T1WI and hyperintense on T2WI and FLAIR. There is a solid or irregular rim enhancement and extensive surrounding edema. The lesion in this instance demonstrates relative restricted diffusion with elevated rCBV consistent with a cellular high-grade tumor. Anatomic imaging features are similar to a solitary metastasis from which it could be difficult to differentiate. GG, cortical ependymoma, lobar PA, and PXA could have a similar appearance since all of these lesions can present as a solidly enhancing mass rather than the more standard cystic and nodular mass. However, these other cortical/subcortical masses tend to have less surrounding edema. Enhancement is more unusual in dysembryoplastic neuroepithelial tumor (DNET) which is often multicystic/bubbly in nature. Low-grade astrocytomas and oligodendrogliomas would in general not enhance, and surrounding edema is usually absent. Higher-grade anaplastic astrocytomas and oligodendrogliomas may have surrounding edema. Glioblastoma could present as a solid mass with microscopic necrosis that is not visible at imaging but will usually present with a thick irregular rim of enhancement.

GCA occurs over a broad age range but in general occur in adults older than 50 years with a male predominance. Presentation depends on location with seizures and focal neurologic deficits as common presentations. GCA at pathology can be confused with reactive conditions such as multiple sclerosis, progressive multifocal leukoencephalopathy, and infarction secondary to the granular cells resembling macrophages. Most patients with GCA die within 1 year. The aggressive behavior is opposite of the benign nature of granular cell tumors in other locations in the body. Follow-up after excision in this patient revealed a new anterior right frontal lobe mass with similar characteristics.

Questions for Further Thought
1. What is the choice of therapy?
2. Are there any common genetic alterations?

Reporting Responsibilities
Direct reporting is essential. Presence of significant edema and mass effect makes reporting more urgent. Presence of tumors or enhancement elsewhere may suggest multifocal lesions or cerebrospinal fluid (CSF) seeding.

What the Treating Physician Needs to Know
- Location and size
- Presence of significant mass effect or herniation
- Place of advanced imaging to further characterize the mass

Answers
1. Surgical excision plus postoperative chemotherapy or radiotherapy is the treatment of choice for most patients with GCA.
2. Loss of 9p and 10q are present in almost all cases and may help explain the aggressive behavior.

CLINICAL HISTORY *25-year-old male with seizure activity on Sunday morning following a Saturday night out of heavy drinking.*

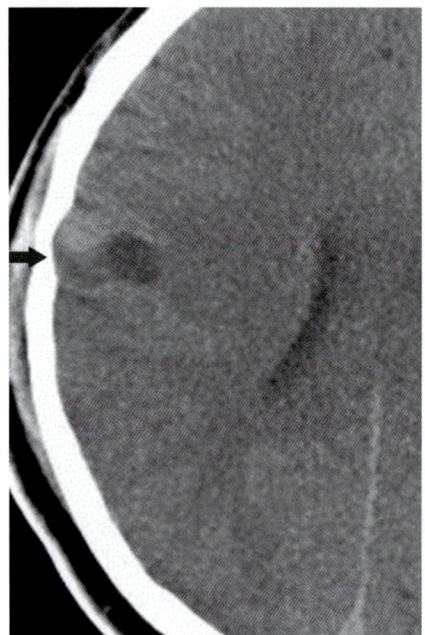

FIGURE 33-1

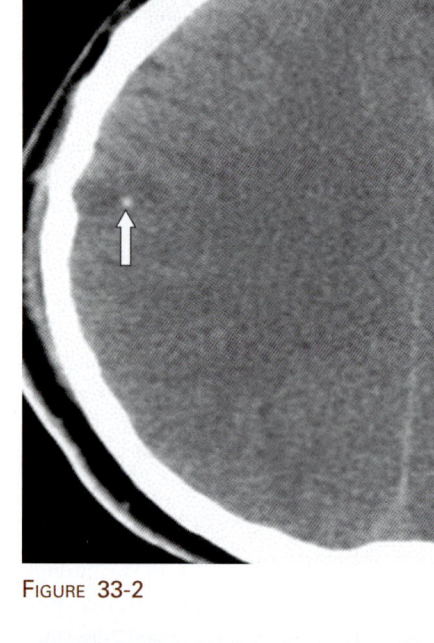

FIGURE 33-2

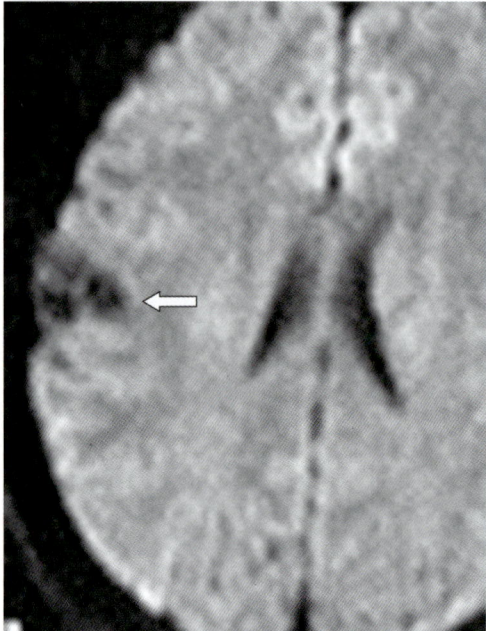

FIGURE 33-3

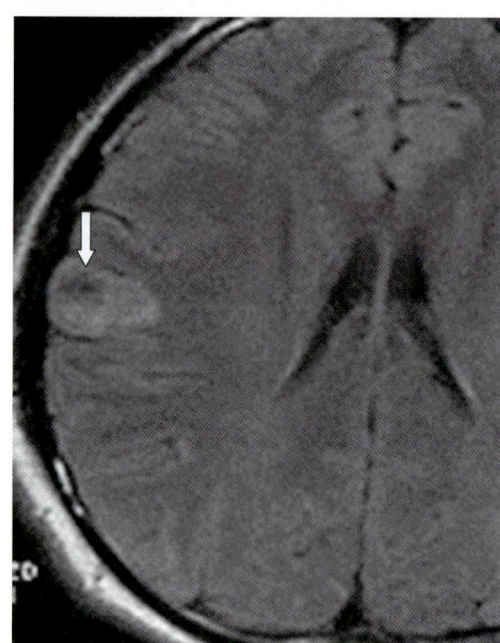

FIGURE 33-4

FINDINGS Figures 33-1 and 33-2. Axial contiguous NCCT through the level of the corona radiata. There is a cortical-based suprasylvian right frontal lobe mass with a hyperdense lateral component and a hypodense medial component. There is scalloping of the adjacent inner table (arrow in Figure 33-1) and a medial peripheral focal calcification (arrow in Figure 33-2). Figure 33-3. Axial DWI through the mass. There are three areas of increased diffusion within the mass. Figure 33-4. Axial T2 FLAIR. The mass is well circumscribed and hyperintense with a small area of profound hypointensity anterolaterally (arrow). There is no surrounding edema. Figure 33-5. Axial GRE. There is an area of

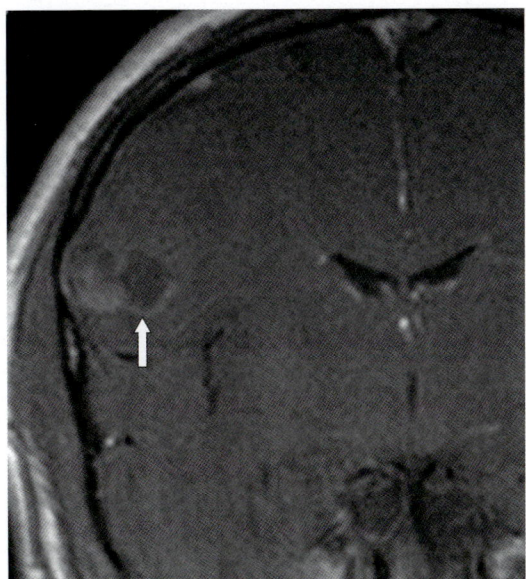

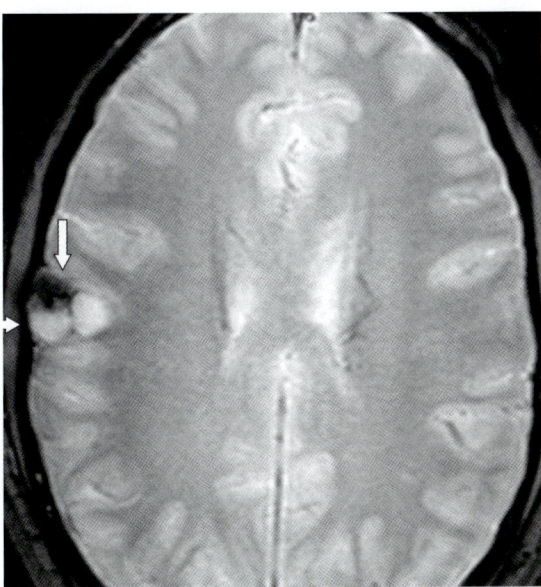

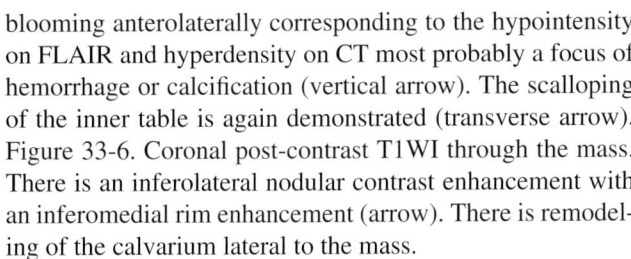

FIGURE 33-5

FIGURE 33-6

blooming anterolaterally corresponding to the hypointensity on FLAIR and hyperdensity on CT most probably a focus of hemorrhage or calcification (vertical arrow). The scalloping of the inner table is again demonstrated (transverse arrow). Figure 33-6. Coronal post-contrast T1WI through the mass. There is an inferolateral nodular contrast enhancement with an inferomedial rim enhancement (arrow). There is remodeling of the calvarium lateral to the mass.

DIFFERENTIAL DIAGNOSIS Ganglioglioma, pilocytic astrocytomas (PAs), dysembryoplastic neuroepithelial tumor (DNET), meningioma, oligodendroglioma, astrocytoma, pleomorphic xanthoastrocytoma (PXA).

DIAGNOSIS PXA.

DISCUSSION PXA is usually a cortical-based supratentorial well-circumscribed solid/cystic lesion with variable surrounding edema abutting the meninges and scalloping the adjacent calvarium. Deep-seated PXA does occur. PXA is more common in the temporal lobes but does occur in the frontal and parietal lobes. Posterior fossa and spinal PXA are rare. The solid part or mural nodule is hypodense to isodense on CT with hypointensity to isointensity on T1WI and mild hyperintensity on T2WI/FLAIR. The cystic component shows cerebrospinal fluid (CSF) intensity on MRI and CSF density on CT. It may contain calcification which is hyperdense on CT in over a third of the cases. It may also contain areas of hemorrhage which is hyperdense on CT and hypointense on T2WI/FLAIR and GRE. There is heterogeneous contrast enhancement with a nodular solid portion and the cystic portion showing rim or ring enhancement. Meningeal enhancement and the presence of a dural tail are not uncommon. Calcification or hemorrhage in PXA obscures analysis

of the perfusion and diffusion data. PXA can be nonenhancing and may not have elevated perfusion. The diffusion and perfusion data for PXA are very limited. Differential diagnosis usually includes other cortical- or dural-based tumors such as ganglioglioma, oligodendroglioma, DNET, lobar PA, and meningioma. A cystic component is unusual in a meningioma which generally occurs in the older population. Meningeal enhancement and bone remodeling are uncommon in the other differentials. DNET generally shows a bubbly pattern.

PXA is a rare WHO II neoplasm constituting less than 1% of all astrocytic tumors. It usually occurs in the second and third decades of life but could be seen in younger population and in older adults. PXA occurs approximately equally in men and women. It is a slow-growing tumor with the patients presenting with a long history of seizures or symptoms of raised intracranial pressure (such as headaches or nausea and vomiting). PXA usually demonstrates a superficial compact component and an infiltrating component resembling diffuse astrocytoma. The typical histologic features include cellular pleomorphism, xanthomatous change (vacuolization of tumor cells), thick sclerotic vessels, eosinophilic granular bodies (EGB), perivascular lymphocytes, and abundant reticulin. Mitoses are usually absent or rare if detected at all. It has a favorable prognosis following gross total resection.

Question for Further Thought

1. What is the preferred treatment and how successful is treatment?

Reporting Responsibilities

Like any other tumor, PXA deserves direct reporting. PXAs can present with hydrocephalus and mass effect, and these factors should be immediately communicated. Location is important for treatment purposes.

What the Treating Physician Needs to Know

- Location and size. These will affect surgical planning
- Presence of CSF obstruction particularly by deep-seated tumor

Answer

1. Surgical resection results in a high cure rate of 70% to 80% at 5 years. These tumors do have a higher recurrence rate and higher transformation to anaplastic grade than other low-grade astrocytomas. Acting swiftly likely helps to avoid anaplastic transformation.

CASE 34

CLINICAL HISTORY *6-year-old female has symptoms (phantosmia and paraosmia; stomachache subsequently followed by an angry outburst, followed by a headache) that correlate with possible seizures. Subsequently she "looks out of it," is drowsy, and sleeps for approximately 12 to 14 hours. This has become progressively worse over the past year.*

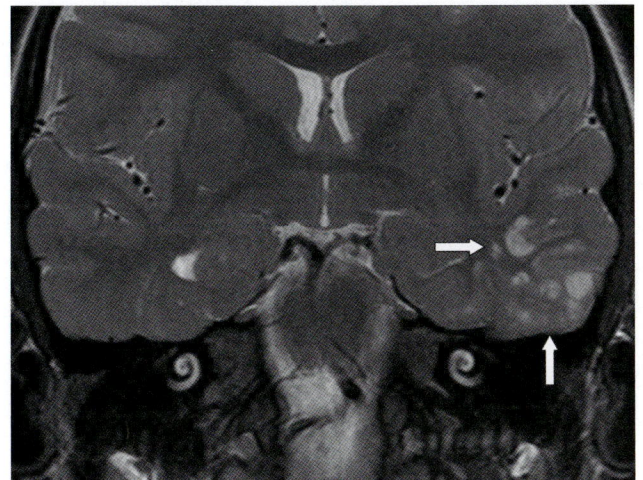

FIGURE 34-1

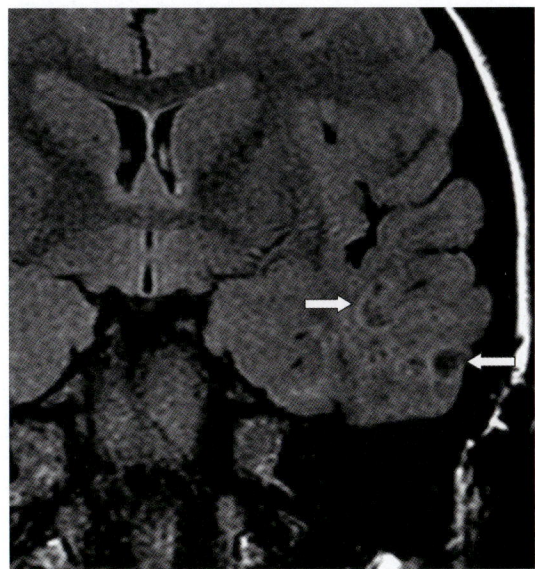

FIGURE 34-2

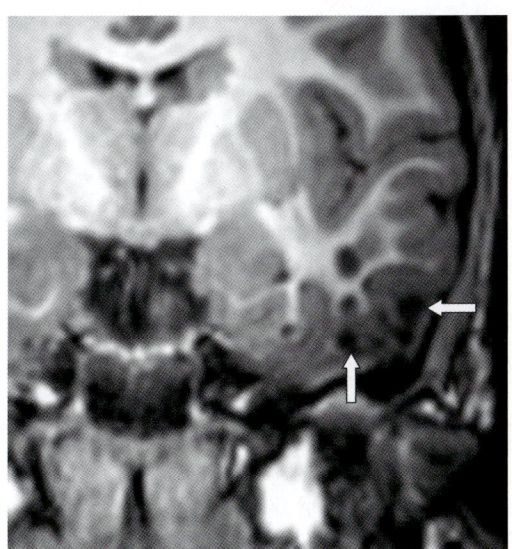
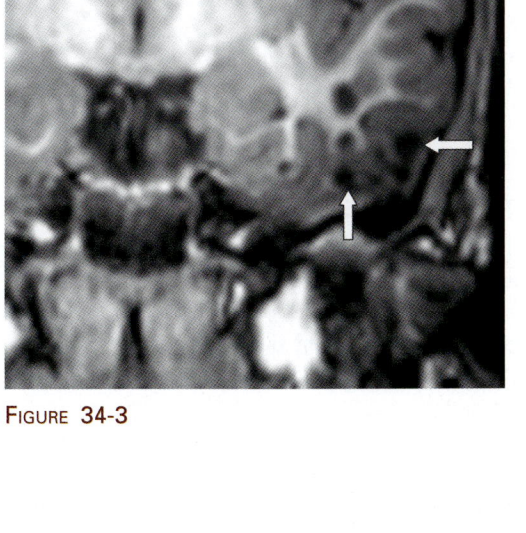

FIGURE 34-3

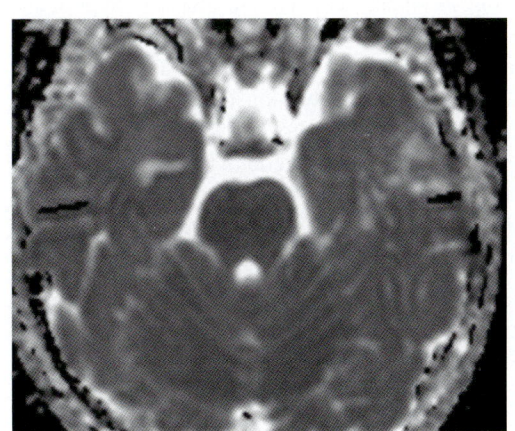

FIGURE 34-4

FINDINGS Figure 34-1. Coronal T2WI through the temporal lobes. There is a collection of hyperintense foci (cysts) (arrows) scattered inferolaterally in the left temporal lobe. Figure 34-2. Coronal T2-FLAIR through same region. The hyperintense foci (cysts) show cerebrospinal fluid (CSF) hypointensity with surrounding hyperintense rims within a poorly defined area of low-level hyperintensity (arrows) that is not adequately appreciated on the coronal T2WI. Figure 34-3. Coronal T1WI. The cysts are markedly hypointense (arrow). No enhancement was present with gadolinium. Figure 34-4. ADC map demonstrates high values throughout the region. No evidence of calcification

or hemorrhage on the MRI. Figure 34-5. Photomicrograph shows characteristic mucinous pools containing ganglion cells (floating neurons). The other component is composed of monomorphic cells with round nuclei and pericellular clearing artifact (H&E stain).

DIFFERENTIAL DIAGNOSIS Dysembryoplastic neuroepithelial tumor (DNET), astrocytoma or other glioma, neurocysticercosis, hydatid cysts, enlarged perivascular spaces, dysplastic brain, multiple bacterial abscesses, herpes encephalitis, ganglioglioma (GG), pilocytic astrocytoma (PA), pleomorphic xanthoastrocytoma (PXA).

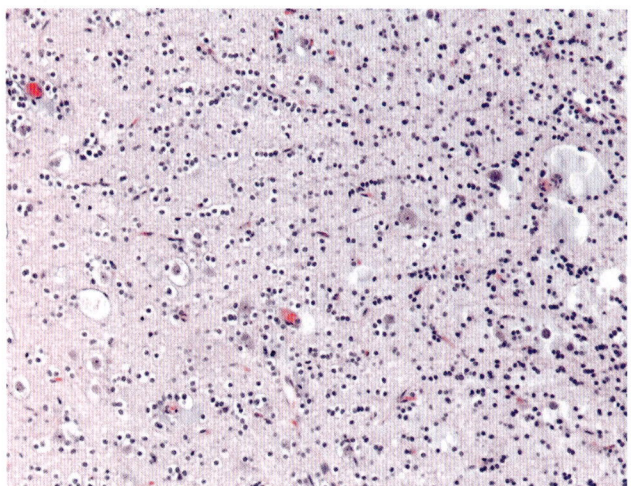

FIGURE 34-5

DIAGNOSIS Dysembryoplastic neuroepithelial tumor (DNET).

DISCUSSION DNET is most commonly seen in the temporal lobe followed by the frontal lobe. MRI and CT show a sharply demarcated mass, ranging greatly is size (1 mm to 5 cm), cortical and subcortical in location with or without surrounding vasogenic edema. The mass is hypodense on CT, hypointense on T1WI, and hyperintense on T2WI. Common radiologic features include cystic or microcystic pattern, remodeling of the overlying calvarium with focal enhancement in a minority (19% to 21.6%) and rarely calcification (11% to 15.2%). The cysts tend to have a hyperintense rim on FLAIR as seen in Figure 34-2. The enhancement has been described as focal, nodular, ring like, or heterogeneous. DNETs are often described as having a multicystic or bubbly appearance, but great variation exists on the reported rate of cyst/pseudocysts ranging from being present in a minority to 100% of the lesions. Hemorrhage has been noted very rarely in less than 5%. Another pattern described is the wedge-shaped pattern with the tumor wider at the cortex with overlying deformation of the skull and extension into the white matter (WM). MRS of DNET shows preservation or suppression of N-acetyl aspartate (NAA) with nonelevated choline. DNETs generally have lower relative Cerebral Blood Volume (rCBV) compared to normal brain, but some tumors may have mildly elevated rCBV. The ADC is elevated in DNET.

DNET has to be differentiated from other cortical tumors/lesions such as oligodendroglioma, PXA, cortical dysplasia, and enlarged perivascular spaces. The surrounding gliosis of T2 hyperintensity on FLAIR excludes perivascular spaces.

The bubbly pattern is almost pathognomonic excluding oligodendroglioma, PXA, PA, cortical dysplasia, abscess, and neurocysticercosis. Abscess, PXA, and PA have much greater rates of enhancement. An abscess should have restricted diffusion centrally. The rarity of calcification in DNET helps to exclude consideration of neurocysticercosis. GG can be quite similar but tends to enhance more, commonly have calcifications, and have a single or a few cysts rather than a multicystic bubbly appearance. The spectral pattern of DNET helps to exclude other tumors.

DNETs are WHO I tumors found usually in young adults in the second decade but can be seen in younger and older patients with a 1:1 male–female ratio. A protracted history of seizure is usually the presenting symptom. DNETs are largely intracortical and lack diffuse infiltration as seen in diffuse gliomas. They are composed of multiple intracortical nodules and an internodular "glioneuronal element," which shows microcystic change and axons ensheathed by oligodendroglia-like cells (OLCs), extending to the pial surface. Large cortical neurons floating in small pools of mucin is a characteristic finding. Extranodular diffuse hypercellular areas composed of OLCs are usually seen.

Questions for Further Thought

1. What is the surgical outcome for treating DNET?
2. Can DNET have malignant transformation?

Reporting Responsibilities

Direct reporting is important for all tumors to enable early treatment. Tumors located in eloquent areas may benefit from functional imaging. Significant changes on follow-up should be reported.

What the Treating Physician Needs to Know

- Location is important for treatment planning.
- Will advanced imaging be useful in further characterization to exclude higher-grade lesion, malignant transformation, or infiltration of eloquent sites?
- Any significant changes on follow-up to suggest malignant transformation?

Answers

1. Surgery alone for DNET is very successful for controlling seizures.
2. Malignant transformation of DNET has rarely been reported. Given this regular follow-up imaging is suggested to identify progression at an early stage for tumors located in eloquent areas. It is possible that the discovery of a higher-grade glioma within a histologically proven DNET is a coincidence.

CLINICAL HISTORY *70-year-old female with cough and shortness of breath. She lost 30 pounds over the last 3 months.*

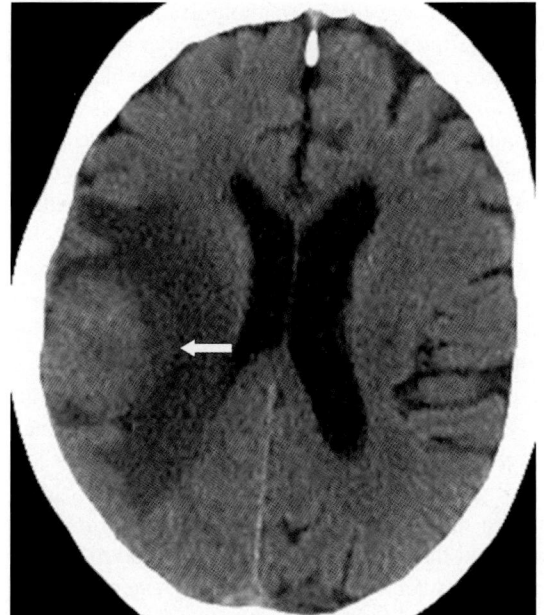

FIGURE 35-1

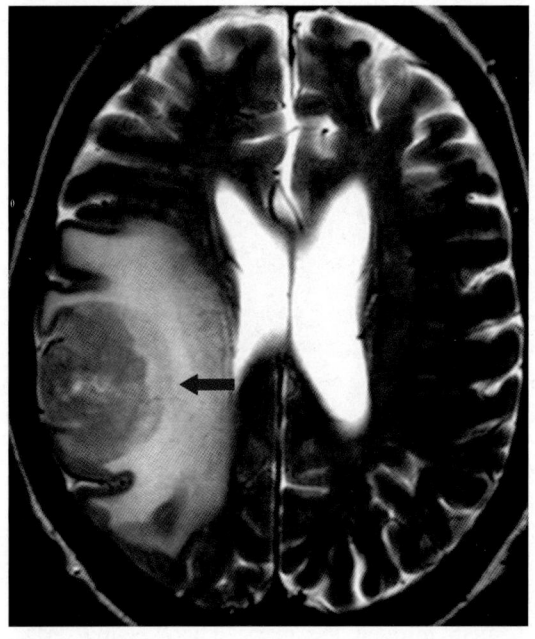

FIGURE 35-2

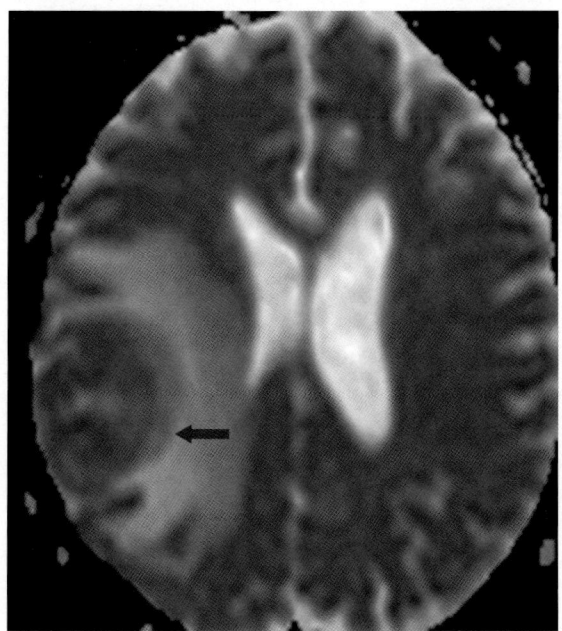

FIGURE 35-3

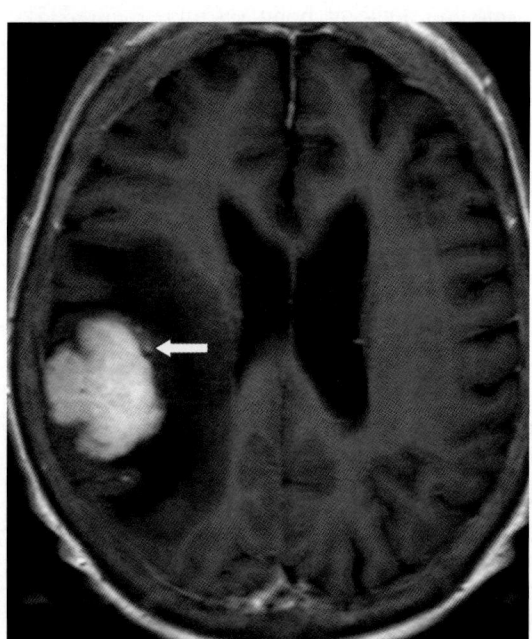

FIGURE 35-4

FINDINGS Figure 35-1. Axial NCCT through the lateral ventricles. There is a mildly hyperdense mass in the right frontoparietal lobe with extensive surrounding hypodensity consistent with vasogenic edema. There is local mass effect but no midline shift. There is a crescentic medial component that is less hyperdense (arrow) suggesting infiltration of surrounding edema. Figure 35-2. Axial T2WI through the mass. There is a heterogeneous minimally

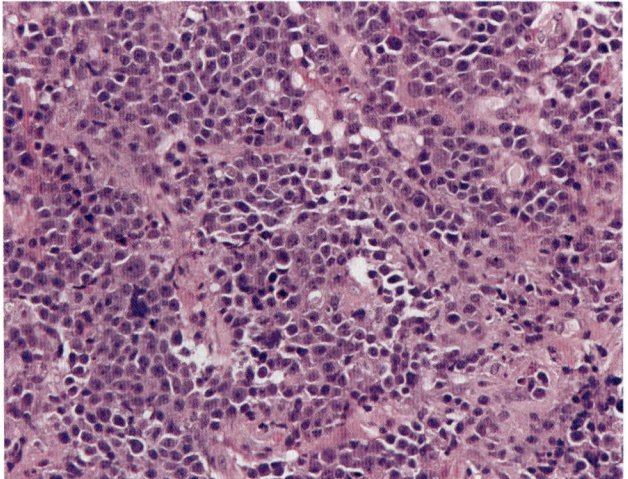

FIGURE 35-5

hyperintense mass in the right frontoparietal junction with surrounding marked hyperintensity consistent with vasogenic edema. The medial crescent is of intermediate hyperintensity (arrow). There is mild mass effect on the right lateral ventricle with effacement of overlying sulci. Figure 35-3. ADC map through the mass. There is low ADC within the mass (arrow) consistent with restricted diffusion. Figure 35-4. The mass demonstrates marked homogeneous enhancement. Abutment of the cortex is clearly identified. Anteriorly and medially there is mild infiltration seen into the adjacent brain (arrow). Figure 35-5. Photomicrograph shows discohesive population of large lymphoid cells with atypical hyperchromatic nuclei; some with one or more nucleoli (H&E stain).

DIFFERENTIAL DIAGNOSIS Lymphoma, hypercellular metastatic disease, hypercellular glioma.

DIAGNOSIS

Lymphoma (primary central nervous system lymphoma [PCNSL]).

DISCUSSION Hyperdensity on CT is a key feature of lymphoma (PCNSL) and is due to its hypercellularity. This imaging feature is very useful since a head CT without contrast is often obtained initially when a patient presents with neurologic complaints. PCNSL could also be hypo- to isodense. The tumor has a great propensity to present adjacent to the cerebrospinal fluid (CSF) either cortical or periventricular including in the corpus callosum. When lymphoma presents as a mass abutting the dura, it can mimic a meningioma in appearance. However, MRI remains indispensable since even large lymphoma masses might present as isodense to brain on a CT without contrast and be difficult to detect. The hypercellularity of a lymphoma mass results in lower ADC values and relatively hypointense masses on T2WIs. The enhancement of PCNSL is more homogeneous than what is seen in the majority of gliomas. However, the enhancement pattern in any particular case can be quite heterogeneous and in unusual cases there may be infiltration into the brain without enhancement. These tumors pathologically could present a very infiltrating pattern along perivascular spaces with a minimal degree of nodularity or mass. Ring enhancement is more typically seen in immunosuppressed patients associated with transplantation or HIV. PCNSL may have many appearances but necrosis, peripheral enhancement, hemorrhage, or calcifications are unusual in an immunocompetent patient.

PCNSLs tend to present as large masses. Edema is present in 90% of patients. PCNSL has a preference for the cerebral hemispheres (38.2%), basal ganglia (27%), and masses involving the ventricular borders account for 11.8% of cases. Imaging is poor at detecting leptomeningeal disease in lymphoma and CSF analysis is required. Glioblastoma (GB) may show heterogeneous high diffusion and low ADC values in areas of hypercellularity. Perfusion imaging demonstrates a leakage pattern more commonly in lymphoma than in high-grade glioma and the perfusion is usually low due to lack of angiogenesis. Massively elevated lipid and greater elevation of the Cho/Cr level in PCNSL may help differentiate lymphoma from glioma.

PCNSL occurs predominantly in older immunocompetent adults with a mean age of 59.8 years with a range of 27 to 82 years in one series. It occurs equally in both male and female. More than 90% of PCNSL are B-cell non-Hodgkin lymphomas. They more often demonstrate an angiocentric proliferation of large malignant lymphocytes from where they diffusely infiltrate the brain parenchyma. Mitoses are frequent, and necrosis is common. Intervening parenchyma shows an astrocytic and microglial response, macrophages, and reactive lymphocytic infiltrates. T-cell phenotype is very rare and anaplastic large cell lymphoma is exceptional. Low-grade B-cell tumors occur, but a precise definition is lacking, and less than 5% of CNS lymphoma cases are considered low grade.

Question for Further Thought

1. What type of CNS lymphoma presents with ischemia?

Reporting Responsibilities

Direct reporting is necessary as in any tumor. Mass effect and herniations increase the urgency of the report. Location is important and unusual presentations should prompt consideration of alternative diagnosis. Advanced imaging help in differentiating lymphoma from its mimics, and they should be suggested.

What the Treating Physician Needs to Know

• Location is important for treatment planning
• Is it safe to perform LP to exclude CSF seeding? Large masses and herniations may contraindicate LP

- Steroids should be withheld if PCNSL is a likely diagnosis by imaging criteria since steroid treatment can obfuscate histologic diagnosis

Answer

1. Intravascular lymphoma (IVL) is a rare presentation of PCNSL, and it is usually of B-cell lineage proliferating within lumens of capillaries, venules, and arterioles. The vascular occlusion results in ischemic features. The presence of associated nodular areas of enhancement should suggest an etiology besides typical ischemia. Dural and arachnoid enhancement is potentially present.

CLINICAL HISTORY *39-year-old female with strange sensations in her epigastric area radiating to her right shoulder. No frank weakness but some difficulty utilizing her right hand.*

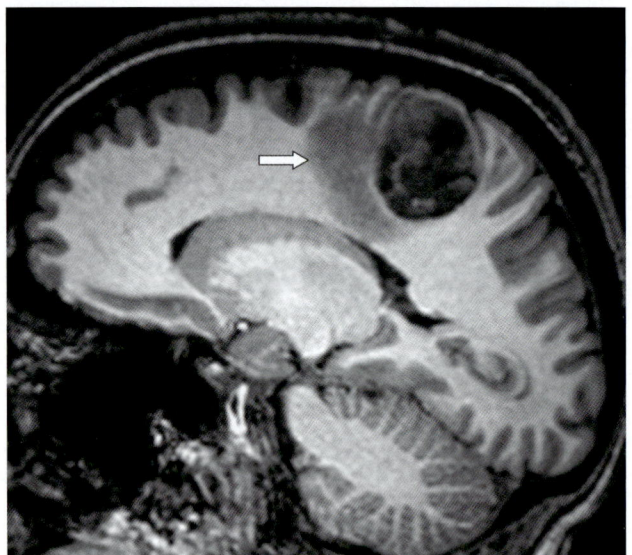

FIGURE 36-1

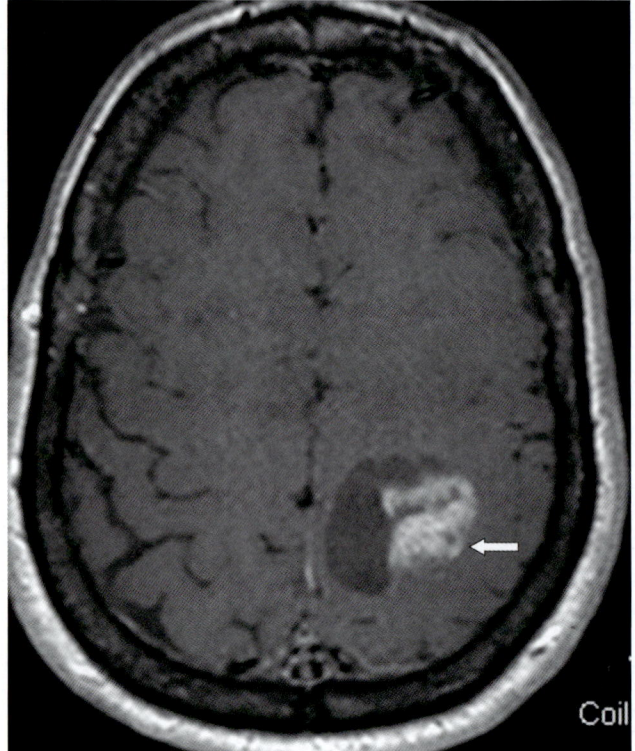

FIGURE 36-2

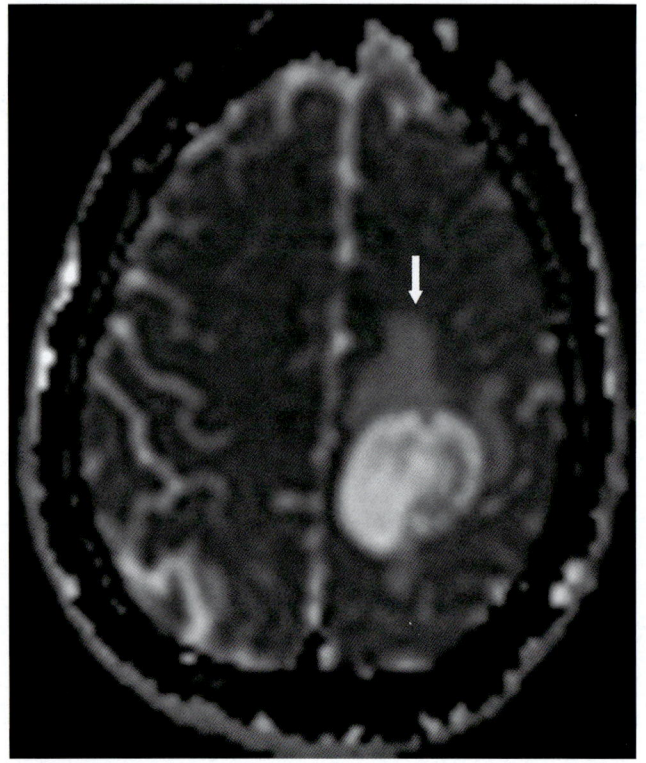

FIGURE 36-3

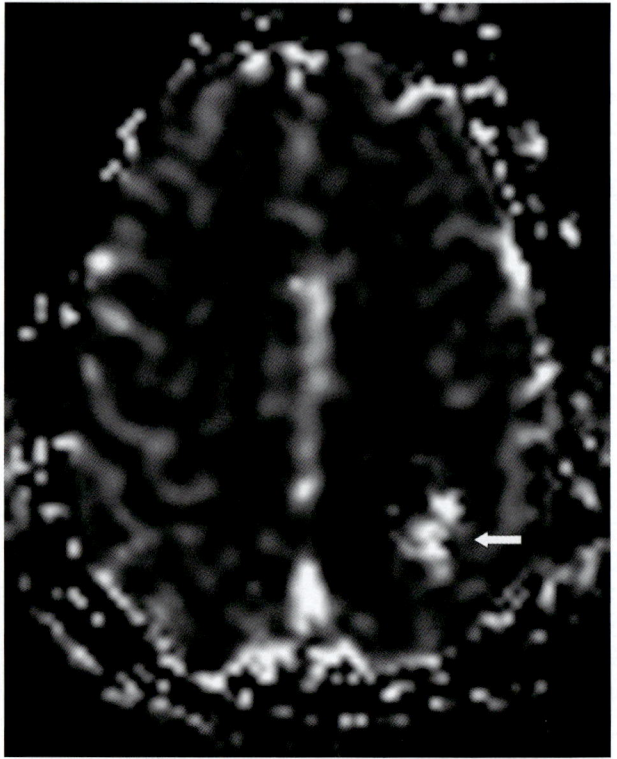

FIGURE 36-4

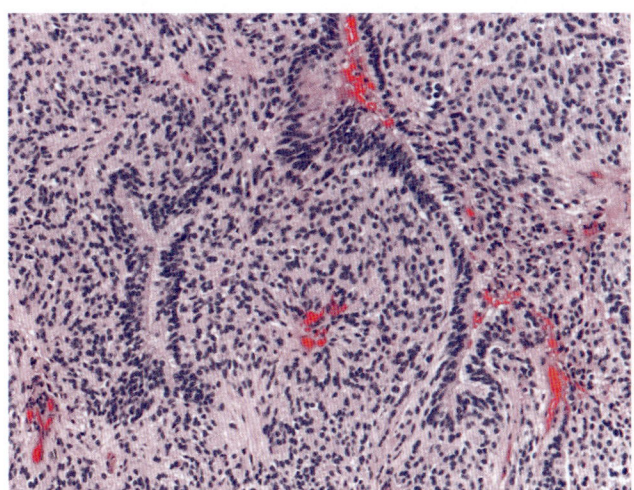

F‌IGURE 36-5

FINDINGS Figure 36-1. Left parasagittal non-contrast 3D T1WI. There is a well-defined posterior left frontal hypointense mass with mild vasogenic edema anteriorly (arrow). There is area of irregular isointensity within the lesion. Figure 36-2. Axial post-contrast T1WI through the mass. There is an avid contrast-enhancing portion laterally (arrow) with the rest showing a cystic appearance. Figure 36-3. Axial ADC map through lesion. There is an irregular, mild, low ADC within the solid component with the rest showing high ADC values. There is edema anteriorly to the mass (arrow). Figure 36-4. Axial relative Cerebral Blood Volume (rCBV) map through the mass. There is elevated rCBV in the lateral component of the mass (arrow). Figure 36-5. Photomicrograph shows tumor composed of monomorphic cells with mildly hyperchromatic nuclei. Central canal-like structures are present (H&E stain).

DIFFERENTIAL DIAGNOSIS
Metastasis, glioblastoma, astrocytoma, ganglioglioma (GG), pilocytic astrocytoma (PA), cortical ependymoma.

DIAGNOSIS
Cortical ependymoma.

DISCUSSION
Ependymoma is often cystic or multicystic with less common presentation as a solid tumor. Cortical ependymoma tends to enhance, and the enhancement has been described as having a popcorn appearance. Calcifications and hemorrhage occur within the tumor but have been reported to be variably present at imaging ranging from uncommon to common. On CT ependymoma is predominantly hypodense to isodense. T2WI demonstrates hyperintensity, and T1WI is more heterogeneously isointense to hypointense. When present the calcification is hyperdense on CT and is hypointense on MRI sequences. Extrapolating data from the pediatric population with a high percentage of infratentorial

ependymomas, we suggest that these tumors have elevated perfusion as seen in this case. MR spectroscopy demonstrates elevated choline and reduced NAA as is seen with many tumors. The ADC is elevated in ependymoma but not as high as in pilocytic astrocytoma. The mild surrounding edema and the pattern of enhancement are distinct from the thick irregular ring enhancement associated with a metastasis or glioblastoma. Edema is not a prominent component of cortical ependymoma. Other cortical tumors such as PA, dysembryoplastic neuroepithelial tumor (DNET), pleomorphic xanthoastrocytoma (PXA), GG, and oligodendroglioma could be considerations. Since cortical ependymoma is often present with a cyst and nodular appearance, this helps to differentiate it from ordinary WHO II astrocytoma and oligodendroglioma.

Cortical ependymoma is a rare tumor occurring more commonly in young adults often in the late second to early fourth decades. The tumor commonly presents with seizures because of its cortical location. Ependymoma is composed of monomorphic cells with round to oval nuclei with bland chromatin. It forms perivascular pseudorosettes and ependymal canals. Mitoses, necrosis, and vascular endothelial proliferation are present in the anaplastic lesion. Surgical resection is often curative for the WHO II ependymoma, and subtotal resection often results in worse outcome. WHO III ependymoma is known to recur locally despite radiation therapy.

Questions for Further Thought
1. Should postoperative radiation therapy be utilized?
2. Should there be continued posttreatment surveillance?

Reporting Responsibilities
Tumors deserve direct reporting so that treatment could begin in earnest. Location is important. Tumors located in eloquent areas may require functional imaging evaluation to determine resectability. Tumor growth should be reported in follow-up studies.

What the Treating Physician Needs to Know
- Location will determine resectability
- Presence of significant mass effect or herniations
- Rate of growth on surveillance or follow-up study
- Ependymoma recurrences are mostly local, and repeated surgery is often possible

Answers
1. There are limited data on utilizing radiotherapy in adult ependymoma. It is potentially not helpful in WHO II lesions, whereas in WHO III lesions it may be useful to add.
2. Surveillance imaging is justified to detect early evidence of recurrence that might allow reoperation or more effect salvage therapies.

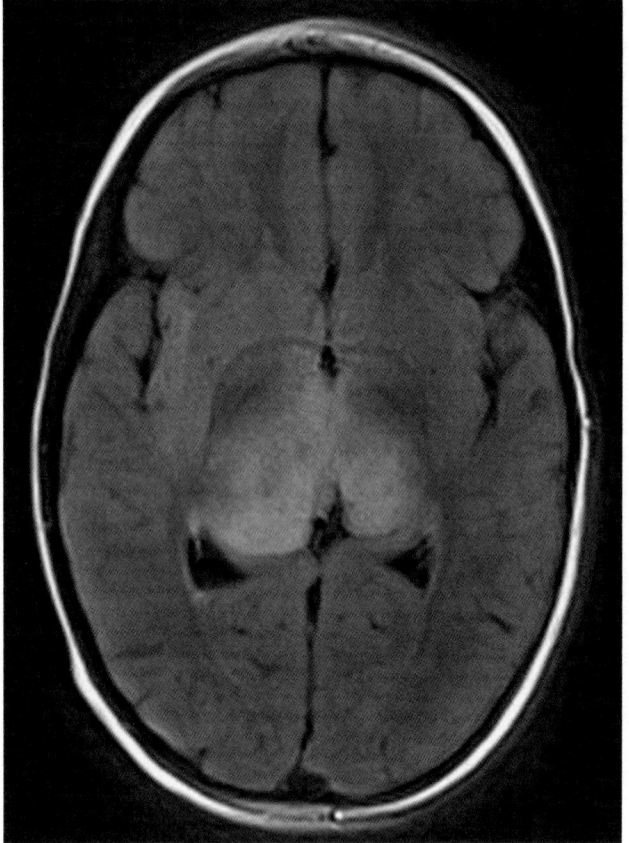

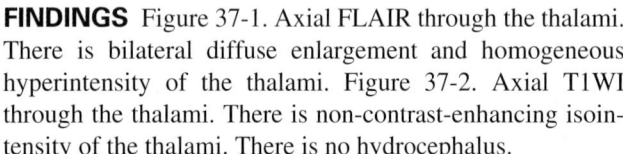

FIGURE 37-1

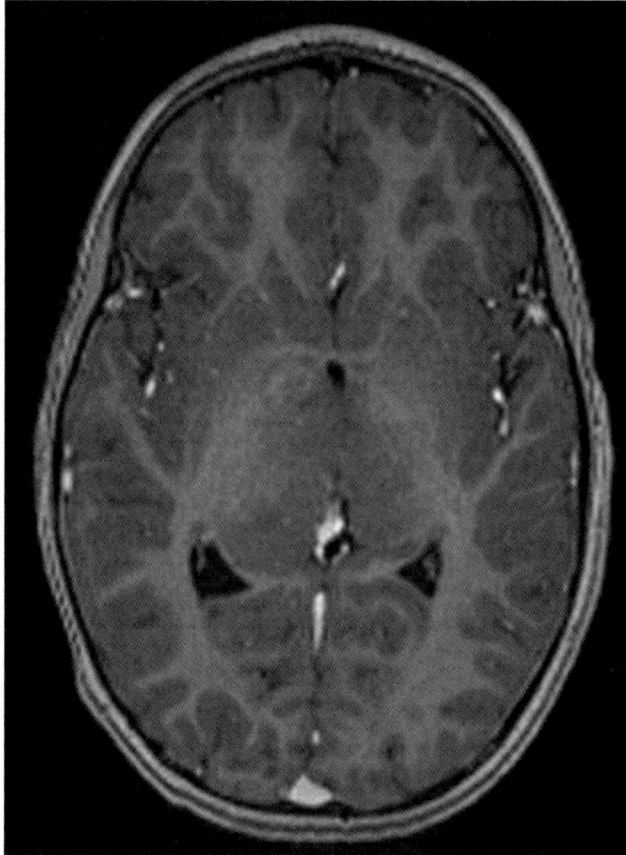

FIGURE 37-2

FINDINGS Figure 37-1. Axial FLAIR through the thalami. There is bilateral diffuse enlargement and homogeneous hyperintensity of the thalami. Figure 37-2. Axial T1WI through the thalami. There is non-contrast-enhancing isointensity of the thalami. There is no hydrocephalus.

DIFFERENTIAL DIAGNOSIS Encephalitis, mitochondrial encephalopathy, acute disseminated encephalopathy (rare without white matter involvement) or acute necrotizing encephalopathy of childhood, astrocytoma, germinoma (very rare).

DIAGNOSIS Primary bilateral thalamic astrocytoma.

DISCUSSION Bilateral thalamic astrocytoma results in symmetrical and diffuse enlargement of the thalami, showing homogeneous T2-weighted and FLAIR hyperintensity, T1WI isointensity, and generally no enhancement. These tumors tend to be of low grade when initially detected. MRS shows an elevated creatine-phosphocreatine peak, normal-to-low choline, high myoinositol on short echo time studies, and low *N*-acetyl aspartate. Characteristically, in sequential MRIs these tumors have stable features, without tumor progression,

preserving the integrity of the gray–white matter interface between the thalami and the adjacent posterior limbs of the internal capsule for long time. All the differentials have involvement of other parts of the brain outside the thalami.

Bithalamic gliomas are extremely rare tumors of the CNS, affecting children and young adults typically presenting with behavioral compromise ranging from personality changes to dementia (more common in adults). They are classified as low-grade tumors (WHO II). However, the outcome is very poor. Treatment is often radiation and chemotherapy given their deep location is not easily amenable to surgery. For a definitive diagnosis, biopsy is required. There is no logical explanation for bilateral involvement as no evidence exists for direct extension across the massa intermedia or other anatomic pathways. Infrequently, pineal region tumors, particularly germ cell neoplasms, may infiltrate bilateral thalami (a distinctive MRI finding might be restricted diffusion in these).

Questions for Further Thought

1. What is the relevance of biopsy?
2. Diagnosis can be delayed in the absence of symptoms. Which condition would cause an acute presentation?

Reporting Responsibilities

Direct reporting is essential as diagnosis could only be made by biopsy. Describe the extent of the abnormalities. Perform and interpret MRS results to improve diagnostic accuracy and offer a differential diagnosis.

What the Treating Physician Needs to Know

- Particular features of macroscopic appearance on MRI and possible differential diagnosis
- Extent of the lesion and complementary study for stereotaxic biopsy

Answers

1. Current imaging modalities are insufficient to accurately predict histologic diagnosis and prognosis. Tumors can have anaplastic areas that make them grade III or IV neoplasms.
2. Hydrocephalus can develop and needs prompt surgical treatment.

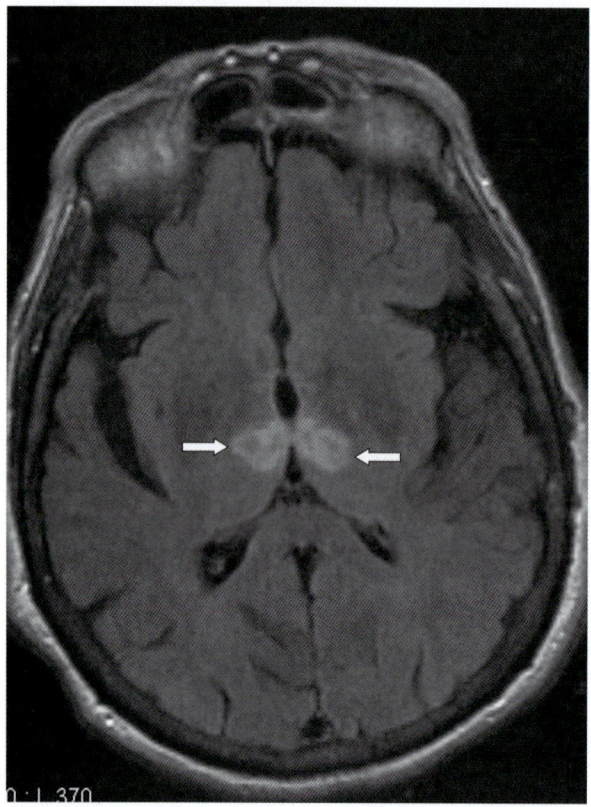

FIGURE 38-1

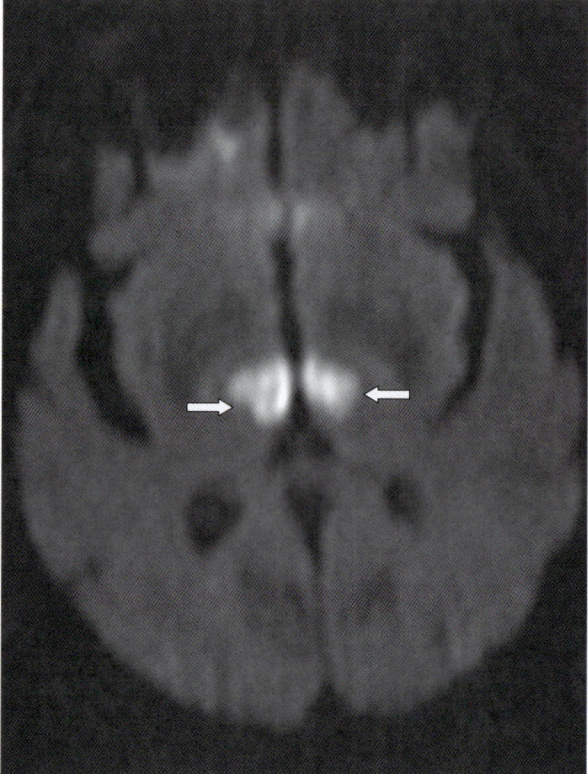

FIGURE 38-2

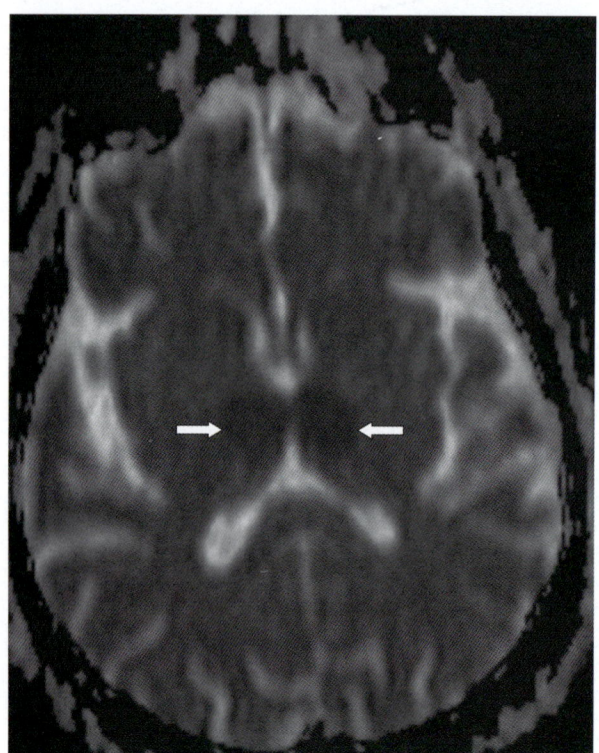

FIGURE 38-3

FINDINGS Figure 38-1. Axial FLAIR image through the thalami. There is bilateral almost symmetrical medial thalamic hyperintensity (arrows). Figures 38-2 and 38-3. Corresponding axial DWI and ADC map, respectively, through the thalami. The lesions restrict diffusion—hyperintense on DWI with low ADC—consistent with acute infarctions.

DIFFERENTIAL DIAGNOSIS Basilar artery thrombosis, deep cerebral venous sinus thrombosis, artery of Percheron infarctions.

DIAGNOSIS Bilateral paramedian thalamic infarcts from occlusion of the artery of Percheron.

DISCUSSION Acute arterial infarctions of both inferior and medial thalami most often result from occlusion of the rostral basilar artery, which also commonly affect the midbrain and portions of the temporal and occipital lobes (supplied by the posterior cerebral artery) or the cerebellum (supplied by branches of the vertebrobasilar arterial system).

One of the rare anatomical variants of the posterior circulation is the artery of Percheron (Table 38-1), an uncommon single dominant thalamoperforating artery arising from either of the P1 segments, which when occluded causes characteristic bilaterally symmetric paramedian thalamic

Table 38-1 The Vascularization of the Thalamus Is Rich, Being Fed by Multiple Perforating Arteries

Thalamic Territories	Fed By	Origin In
Anterior	Polar arteries	PcomA
Paramedian	Thalamoperforating arteries	P1 segment of the posterior cerebral artery (PCA)
Inferolateral	Thalamogeniculate arteries	P2 segment of the PCA
Posterior	Posterior choroidal arteries	P2 segment of the PCA

From Lazzaro NA, Wright B, Castillo M, et al. Artery of Percheron infarction: imaging patterns and clinical spectrum. *Am J Neuroradiol.* 2010;31:1283–1289.

Table 38-2 There Are Four Distinct Patterns of Artery of Percheron Infarctions, Which Reflect the Known Paramedian Artery Variations

Bilateral paramedian thalamic with rostral midbrain	43%
Bilateral paramedian thalamic without midbrain	38%
Bilateral paramedian and anterior thalamic with midbrain	14%
Bilateral paramedian and anterior thalamic without midbrain	5%

From Lazzaro NA, Wright B, Castillo M, et al. Artery of Percheron infarction: imaging patterns and clinical spectrum. *Am J Neuroradiol.* 2010;31:1283–1289.

infarcts, revealing hyperintense T2-FLAIR and restricted diffusion, with or without rostral midbrain involvement. The midbrain involvement occurs probably when the superior mesencephalic artery shares a common origin with the paramedian thalamic artery, determining a distinctive imaging finding that is a V-shaped hyperintensity on axial FLAIR and DWI along the pial surface of the midbrain in the interpeduncular fossa.

Questions for Further Thought

1. What are the clinical features at presentation and their anatomical correlation?
2. Is occlusion of the artery of Percheron perceived on MRI as a unique pattern?

Reporting Responsibilities

Direct reporting is necessary for these acute infarcts. Describe the extent of signal intensity abnormalities, referring to their specific locations within the thalami or midbrain, documenting a defined arterial territory of the paramedian or anterior thalamic arterial zones. It is necessary to exclude thrombosis of the basilar artery or the deep cerebral venous sinuses as these may require aggressive and different treatment than isolated occlusion of the artery of Percheron.

What the Treating Physician Needs to Know

- Exact localization of the infarct, excluding the anatomical appearance, other causes for the signal abnormalities,

like those referred in differential diagnosis section, which would imply a different clinical approach
- Occlusion of the artery of Percheron is generally treated systemically, but occlusion of the basilar artery, even its tip, may need interventional treatment

Answers

1. Bithalamic involvement generally causes agitation, obtundation or coma, and also memory dysfunctions and various types of ocular and behavioral changes. Occlusion of the artery of Percheron presents typically as a triad of altered mental status (variable severity), vertical gaze palsy (mesencephalic involvement), and amnesia (variable anterior polar territory involvement). Depending on which parts of the midbrain are affected (i.e., interpeduncular nucleus, decussation of the superior cerebellar peduncles, medial part of the red nucleus, nucleus of cranial nerve III, and anterior part of the periaqueductal gray matter), the neurologic signs may encompass other oculomotor disturbances, hemiplegia, cerebellar ataxia, and movement disorders.
2. The imaging pattern of artery of Percheron infarctions typically involves the bilateral median thalami with variable involvement of the midbrain (see Table 38-2).

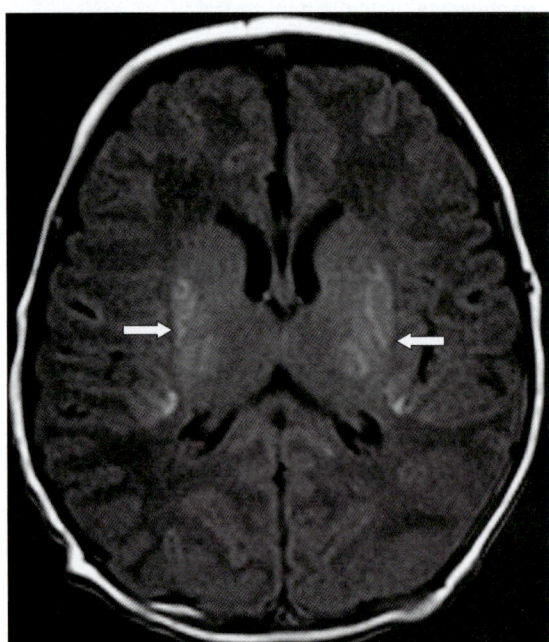

FIGURE 39-1

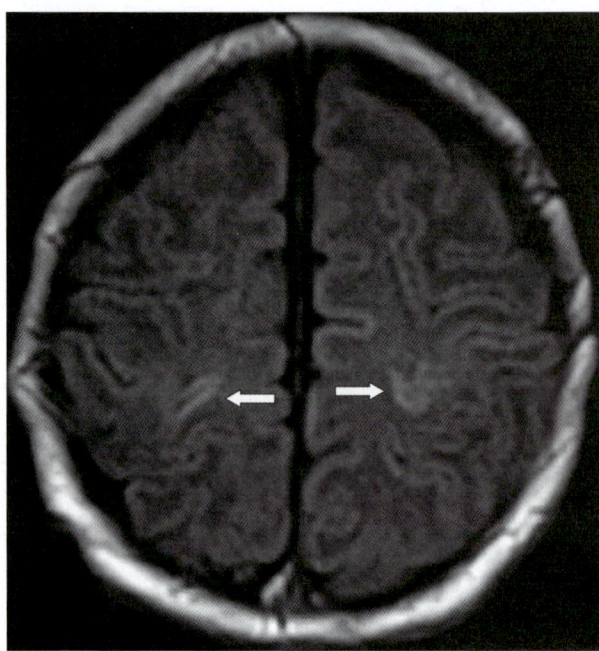

FIGURE 39-2

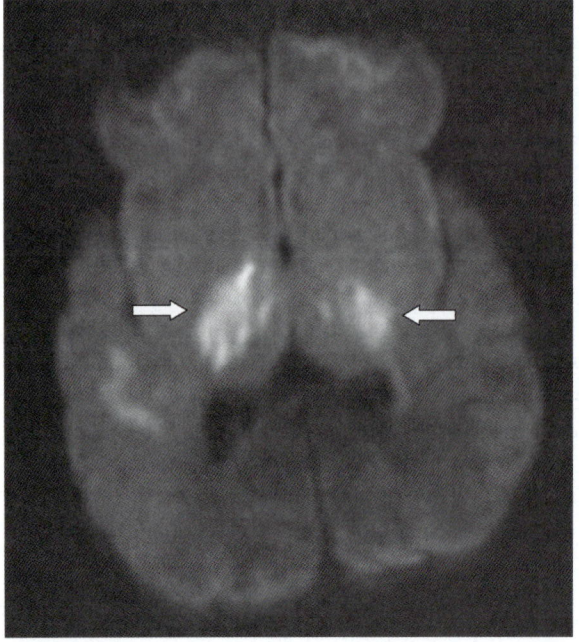

FIGURE 39-3

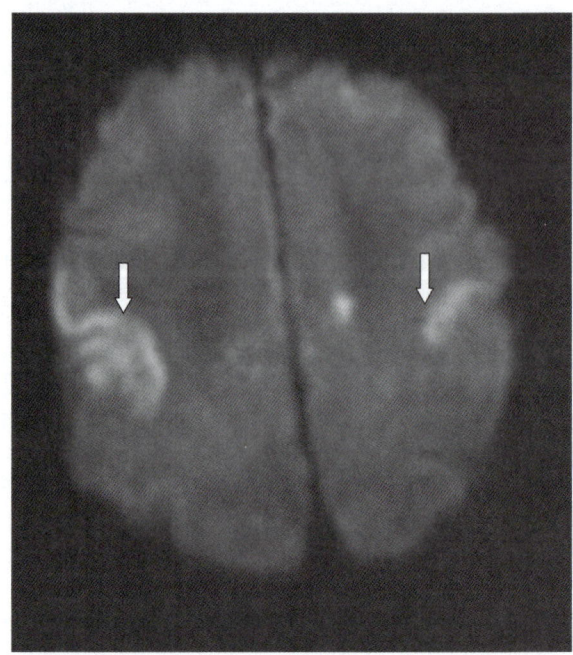

FIGURE 39-4

FINDINGS Figure 39-1. Axial non-contrast T1WI through the basal ganglia. There is bilateral symmetrical basal ganglia hyperintensity (arrows) with involvement of the internal capsules and lateral thalami. Figure 39-2. Axial non-contrast T1WI through the high convexities. There is bilateral perirolandic cortical gray matter (GM) hyperintensity (arrows). Figures 39-3 and 39-4. Axial DWI through the basal ganglia and the high convexities, respectively. There is diffusion restriction (arrows) in the bilateral basal ganglia and the perirolandic cortical GM as in Figures 39-1 and 39-2.

DIFFERENTIAL DIAGNOSIS Trauma with diffuse brain swelling, hypoglycemia, maple syrup urine disease, and nonketotic hyperglycinemia (NKHG), hypoxic-ischemic encephalopathy (HIE) in term baby.

DIAGNOSIS HIE in term infants.

DISCUSSION MRI remains the imaging technique of choice for the evaluation of infants with suspected HIE. On T1WI the abnormal GM may be hyperintense and the white matter (WM) hypointense, while on T2WI GM signal can be variable and WM may be hyperintense due to cytotoxic edema. DWI is sensitive for detecting acute HIE showing restricted diffusion. GRE and/or SWI detect hemorrhage. Proton MRS depicts the anaerobic metabolism revealing elevated lactate and diminished N-acetyl aspartate (NAA) (implying neuronal damage) concentrations. Transcranial ultrasound plays a limited role in the initial detection of HIE and may show increased echogenicity in the regions previously mentioned as will decreased blood flow on Doppler US. The changes in hypoglycemia and NKHG are very similar to HIE while trauma with diffuse brain swelling may show patchy nonsymmetrical changes.

Since the neonatal brain is extremely vulnerable to ischemia, the degree of brain maturity, and severity and duration of insult cause distinct patterns of brain lesions. The degree of brain maturation dictates the regional metabolism and configuration of the vascular system. In term infants the central nervous system's vascular supply is similar to that of adults and the hypermetabolic structures include the deep GM (lateral thalami, globus pallidus, posterior putamina, and hippocampi), the brainstem, the sensorimotor cortex, and the myelinated WM fibers. Ischemic lesions result from decreased arterial blood flow or difficulty in venous drainage. Severe arterial hypotension tends to involve these regions, while milder situations allow for redistribution of cerebral blood flow to these vulnerable structures and away from the watershed zones causing ischemic injuries at the watershed regions. Venous sinus thrombosis can cause ischemic injuries in the superficial venous system territory due to a mechanical injury during birth. The deep venous system territory may be involved due to systemic causes such as hypercoagulability, sepsis, or dehydration. A clinical history of peripartum asphyxia, traumatic delivery, neonatal resuscitation, seizures, abnormal neurologic status, and/or a low APGAR score can be associated with HIE. Clinical findings are related to the structures involved and vary from mild to severe neurologic impairment, seizures, and later, developmental delay.

The neonatal brain has a remarkable potential for recovery when therapeutic measures are promptly applied, including supportive care measures, hypothermia, and the use of neuroprotective agents such as calcium channel blockers, magnesium, and nitric oxide inhibitors.

Question for Further Thought

1. What is the distribution of ischemic lesions in the preterm brain?

Reporting Responsibilities

This is an acute situation and requires direct reporting. Identify the extent and pattern of the acute ischemic lesions and describe any associated complication such as hemorrhage.

What the Treating Physician Needs to Know

- Extent and pattern of changes
- Presence of complications such as parenchymal and intraventricular hemorrhage and brain swelling

Answer

1. In preterm infants with severe hypoperfusion the deep GM (especially the thalami) and the brainstem are usually affected as they are the most metabolically active structures. Mild or moderate ischemic episodes cause periventricular leukomalacia, because unlike the term infant, the vascular supply is ventriculopetal since penetrating arteries extend inward from the surface of the brain.

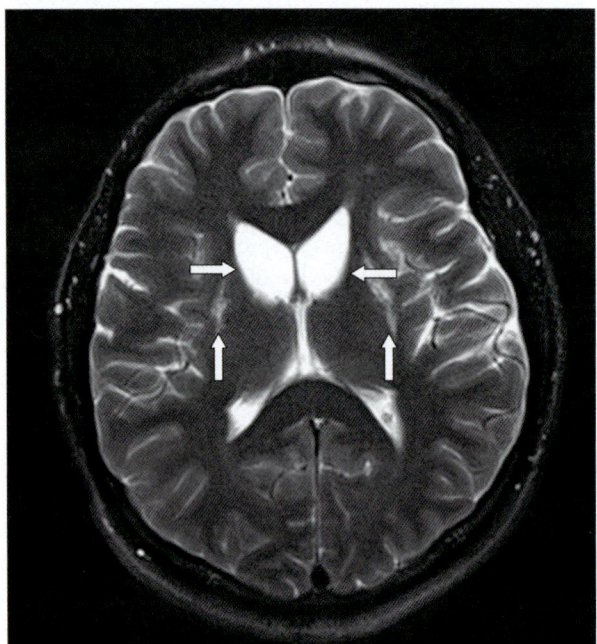

FIGURE 40-1

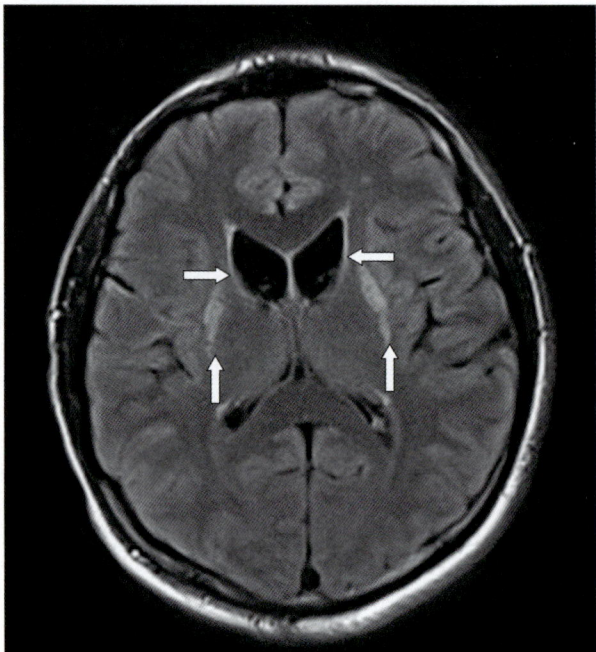

FIGURE 40-2

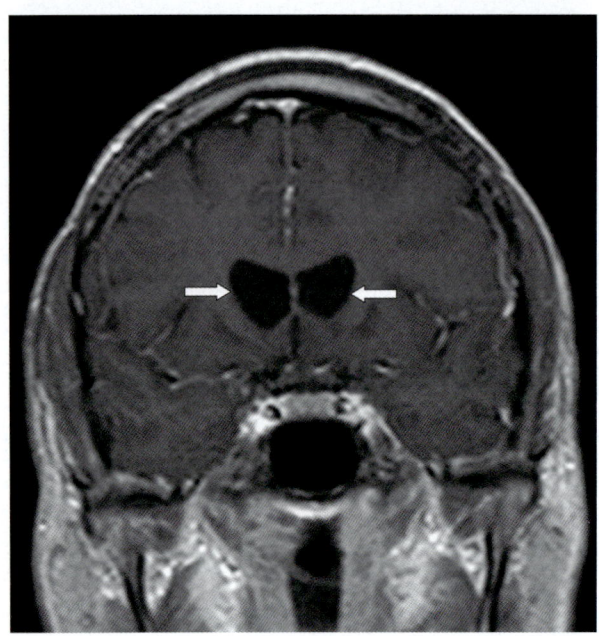

FIGURE 40-3

FINDINGS Figure 40-1. Axial T2WI through the caudate nucleus. There is outward bowing of the lateral walls of the frontal horns with nonvisualization of the heads of the caudate nuclei (arrows). There is hyperintensity of the putamina (vertical arrows). Figure 40-2. Corresponding FLAIR image shows similar findings (arrows). Figure 40-3. Coronal post-contrast T1WI shows the "box-like" configuration of

the frontal horns of the lateral ventricles (arrows). There is no contrast enhancement.

DIFFERENTIAL DIAGNOSIS Huntington disease, neuroacanthocytosis syndromes (McLeod, chorea-acanthocytosis), frontotemporal dementia, and Alzheimer disease.

DIAGNOSIS Huntington disease.

DISCUSSION MRI shows characteristic atrophy involving the head of the caudate nucleus and the putamen. Caudate atrophy results in the loss of the bulge of the inferior lateral borders of the frontal horns with enlargement of frontal horns of the lateral ventricles and flattening of their lateral contour giving them a "box-like" configuration. The brain is diffusely atrophic with white matter (WM) volume loss affecting both frontal lobes. DWI reveals increased ADC in the caudate nucleus, putamen, and WM which correlates with disease severity. Signal intensity abnormalities consisting of slight T2 hyperintensity in the atrophic neostriatum correlates with greater motor and cognitive impairments and usually seen in the juvenile form. Proton MRS shows low levels of *N*-acetyl aspartate (NAA) and creatine and presence of lactate peak in the basal ganglia as well as in the cortex of symptomatic patients. PET imaging shows abnormal neostriatal hypometabolism, especially in the caudate nuclei. Caudate atrophy is characteristic of neuroacanthocytosis syndromes (McLeod, chorea-acanthocytosis) as in Huntington disease. However, mild and generalized cortical and cerebellar atrophy and increased signal intensity lesions in the cerebral hemispheric WM on MRI are also common. Frontotemporal dementia and Alzheimer disease in later stages show predominance of brain atrophy, but atrophy in Huntington disease occurs in younger patients and affects predominantly the caudate nuclei.

Huntington disease is an autosomal dominant neurode-generative disorder caused by a CAG trinucleotide repeat expansion that lengthens a glutamine segment in the novel Huntington protein. The gene responsible for Huntington disease has been mapped to chromosome 4p16:3. The mutation leads to a selective neuronal loss, astrogliosis, and gross atrophy affecting the neostriatum, particularly the paraventricular portion of the caudate and putamen. Marked neuronal loss can also be seen in deep layers of the cerebral cortex, globus pallidus, thalamus, subthalamic nucleus, substantia nigra, and cerebellum, which may demonstrate varying degrees of atrophy depending on the pathologic grade.

Clinically, Huntington disease manifests with a triad of abnormal movement, emotional problems, and cognitive abnormalities which begin insidiously and progress over many years until the death of the individual. Movement abnormalities include disturbances of both involuntary and voluntary movements. Choreathetosis is an early sign present in over 90% of individuals. With advancing disease the chorea is superseded by bradykinesia, rigidity, and dystonia. There is global and progressive decline in cognitive capacity leading to dementia. Depression with suicide risk is the most common psychiatric symptoms. Individuals also develop significant personality changes, affective psychosis, or schizophrenic psychosis. Onset of symptoms is between 35 and 45 years of age resulting in death after 10 to 20 years. The juvenile form onset occurs in the first to second decades of life with survival of less than 15 years. This form accounts for 5% to 10% of Huntington cases, and its clinical presentation differs from the adult disease. There is severe mental deterioration, prominent motor and cerebellar symptoms, speech and language delay, and a rapid decline.

Questions for Further Thought

1. Which are the potential imaging biomarkers for detection of Huntington disease?
2. How can inheritance influence the severity and prognosis of the disease?

Reporting Responsibilities

This is a chronic disease, and routine reporting is in order. Identifying the typical pattern of the disease in an adequate clinical context helps to rule out other frequent causes of atrophy which can involve the striatum.

What the Treating Physician Needs to Know

- No single imaging technique is sufficient for diagnosis of Huntington disease, imaging findings are nonspecific and overlap with other conditions including aging; hence, the diagnosis must be confirmed by genetic tests
- Imaging plays a complementary role and is especially valuable for monitoring the disease progression

Answers

1. Potential neuroimaging biomarkers for detection of early neuronal dysfunction include MRS. Putaminal NAA and myoinositol are promising potential biomarkers of disease progression with low NAA and increased myoinositol levels seen in presymptomatic and early Huntington disease. Functional MRI has proven to be sensitive to changes in striatal function long before the emergence of motor symptoms showing decreased caudate activity and a compensatory increase in activity of the supplementary motor area and anterior cingulate during performance of a cognitive task.
2. Inheritance via the father can lead to earlier onset through succeeding generations, a phenomenon termed anticipation, and as a result most patients with juvenile Huntington disease inherit the disease from their fathers.

CLINICAL HISTORY *Liver transplant patient presenting with a rapidly progressive encephalopathy and seizures.*

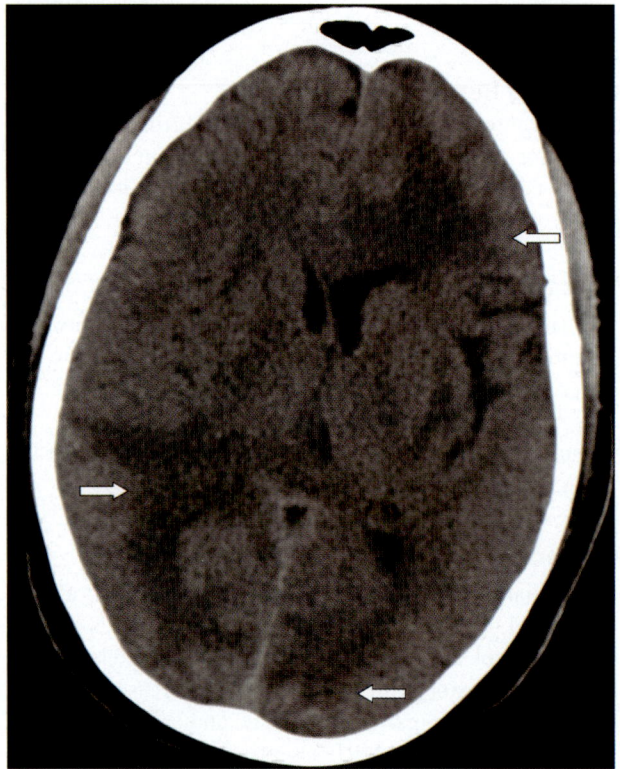

FIGURE 41-1

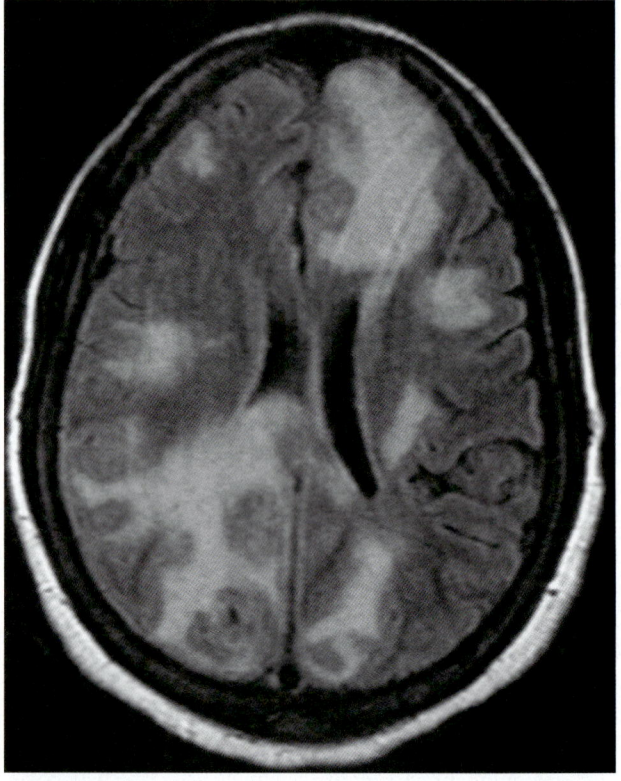

FIGURE 41-2

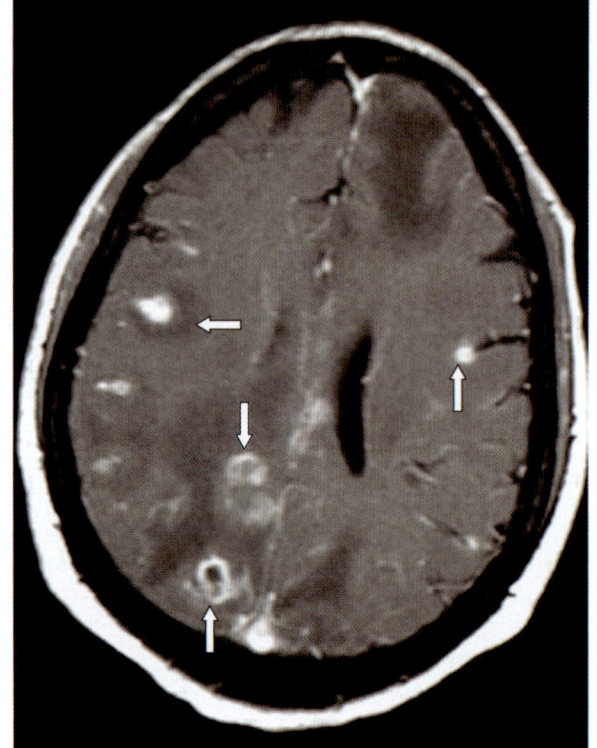

FIGURE 41-3

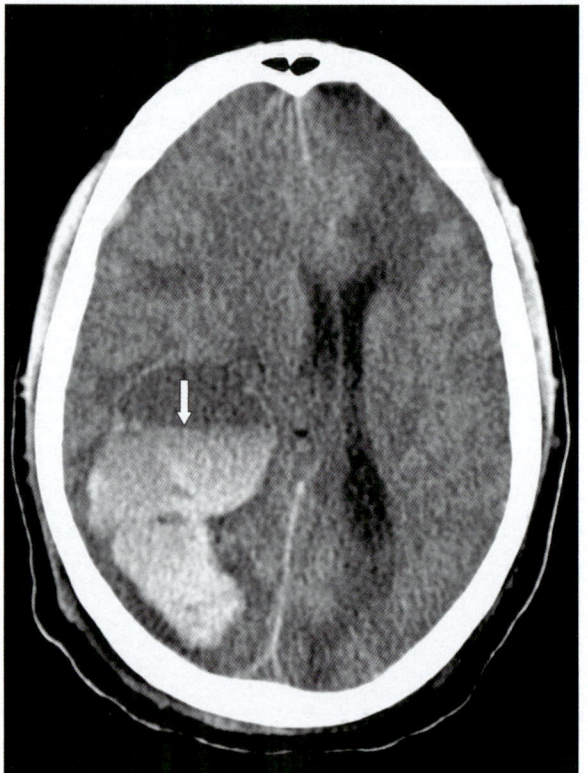

FIGURE 41-4

FINDINGS Figure 41-1. Axial NCCT through the basal ganglia. There are multiple patchy hypodense areas in the white matter (WM) (arrows). Figure 41-2. Axial FLAIR through the corona radiata. There are large hyperintense areas in bilateral cerebral WM with local mass effect. Figure 41-3. Corresponding axial post-contrast T1WI. There are multiple areas of enhancement mostly nodular and ring with surrounding edema (arrows). Figure 41-4. Axial NCCT in a different patient shows a large right parieto-occipital acute hemorrhage with an internal fluid level (arrow) as a complication of intracerebral posttransplant lymphoproliferative disorder (PTLD).

DIFFERENTIAL DIAGNOSIS Abscess, toxoplasmosis, and other neoplastic processes (other central nervous system [CNS] lymphomas), posttransplant lymphoproliferative disorder.

DIAGNOSIS Posttransplant lymphoproliferative disorder (PTLD).

DISCUSSION MRI offers the best imaging assessment of PTLD. The most common neuroimaging findings are multifocal disease with predominance for periventricular/basal ganglia regions, but also meningeal/ependymal and infratentorial involvement can occur. The pattern is very similar to AIDS-related lymphoma, usually iso- to hypointense on T1WI and heterogeneously hypo- to hyperintense on T2WI with heterogeneous patchy, nodular, or ring enhancement. Surrounding edema is common resulting in diffuse WM hyperintensity on FLAIR and T2WI. CT often shows patchy hypodensities with similar pattern of contrast enhancement as in MRI. It could be difficult to distinguish from opportunistic infections such as tuberculosis (TB) or toxoplasmosis. Biopsy is often required for definitive diagnosis.

PTLD is a complication of solid organ transplantation or hematopoietic stem cell transplantation, with higher incidence in children and a known association with Epstein-Barr virus (EBV). Typically, the lesions are B cell in origin, with common extranodal involvement. Isolated involvement of the CNS is rare. According to the WHO revised classification, there are four categories: early lesions, polymorphic PTLD, monomorphic PTLD, and classic Hodgkin lymphoma-type PTLD. Clinically patients present with headache, motor deficits, ataxia, aphasia, and seizures. Management often requires stopping immunosuppression. Prognosis is very poor indeed with mortality approaching 90% for those not responding to cessation of immunosuppression.

Questions for Further Thought

1. Are there risk factors for PTLD of the CNS?
2. Which is the best diagnostic approach?

Reporting Responsibilities

This is an emergency in view of the mimickers requiring direct reporting. Consider the possibility of PTLD in immunosuppressed and posttransplanted patients where you suspect infectious etiologies.

What the Treating Physician Needs to Know

- The extent and location of the lesions in order to program a biopsy

Answers

1. Yes, some factors increase the risk of PTLD such as transplantation type (lung and intestine are more commonly associated), type and intensity of immunosuppression (cyclosporine and tacrolimus), quantity of lymphoid tissue within the transplanted graft, and EBV infection and/or exposure.
2. As imaging and cerebrospinal fluid (CSF) abnormalities are nonspecific, and only a few patients have abnormal cytology and flow cytometry results, biopsy has been proven useful for a definite diagnosis. There is no optimal treatment for PTLD of the CNS. Without treatment the outcome is poor but with treatment survival times as long as 4 years have been reported.

CLINICAL HISTORY *3-month-old male with progressive encephalopathy, weakness, difficulty breathing, and cardiomyopathy.*

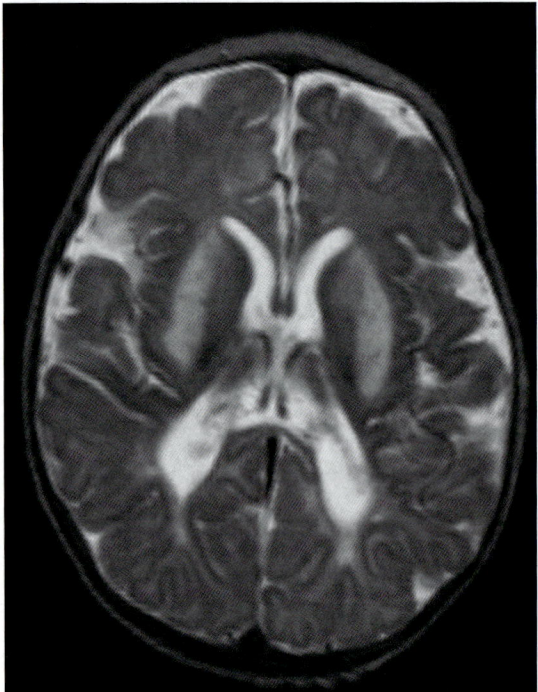

FIGURE 42-1

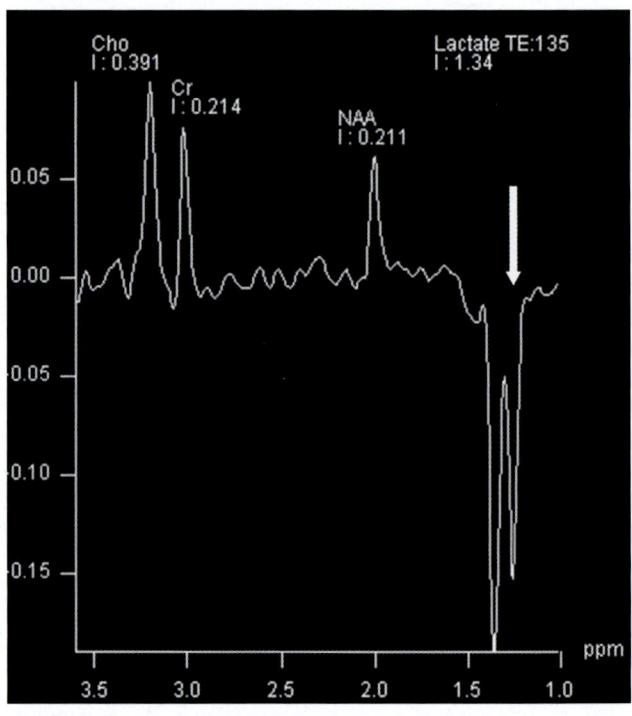

FIGURE 42-2

FINDINGS Figure 42-1. Axial T2WI. There are bilateral symmetrical hyperintense lentiform nuclei which appear swollen. There is high signal and atrophy of the occipital white matter (WM) and cortical sulci prominence. Figure 42-2. MRS at TE = 135 ms obtained at the level of the left basal ganglia. There are reduced overall concentrations of choline (Cho), creatine (Cr), and *N*-acetyl aspartate (NAA). The inverted peak of lactate is clearly seen (arrow).

DIFFERENTIAL DIAGNOSIS Diffuse anoxia (including inhalation of toxic gases), hypoglycemia, organic acidurias, acute necrotizing encephalitis (predominantly thalamic involvement), hemolytic uremic syndrome, and thrombotic thrombocytopenic purpura mitochondrial encephalopathy with lactic acidosis and strokes (MELAS).

DIAGNOSIS Mitochondrial encephalopathy with lactic acidosis and strokes (MELAS).

DISCUSSION MR T2WI and FLAIR image show high signal and swelling of the basal ganglia, thalami, and the midbrain. The WM may also show high signal intensity, and these areas may have restricted diffusion on ADC maps. As in this patient, cortical atrophy may be present.

MRS shows that all metabolites are low and presence of large inverted lactate doublet peak from a voxel obtained in the basal ganglia.

Mitochondrial disorders, also known as respirator chain disorders, are relatively common (1:10,000 live births). Most involve several organs including but not limited to the brain, heart, skeletal muscles, kidneys, and liver. Some mitochondriopathies present in newborns while others later in life when the energy demands overwhelm an already compromised energy pathway, thus presenting as exercise intolerance. One of the most common is MELAS which predominantly affects the deep gray matter structures but may also result in cortical and subcortical infarctions. In MELAS, MRS shows low metabolites and lactate even in the normal appearing brain. Another relatively common disorder is Kearns Sayre syndrome which presents with predominantly ophthalmoplegia, and thus, MRI shows pronounced abnormalities in the dorsal midbrain but also throughout the white matter. Leigh syndrome is caused by at least four different enzymatic defects, but on MRI their phenotypic manifestations are similar (basal ganglia, brainstem [especially the cranial nerve nuclei], and territorial infarctions) and do not permit their differentiation. Alper disease which is accompanied by liver cirrhosis and Menkes kinky hair syndrome are also considered as mitochondrial disorders. In the former, the brain abnormalities tend to be occipital, while in the latter there is diffuse white matter involvement, brain atrophy, and very tortuous intracranial arteries. Confirmation of all mitochondriopathies is a genetic one.

Questions for Further Thought

1. Why is the basal ganglia predominantly affected?
2. How can one be sure that one is looking at lactate on MR spectroscopy?

Reporting Responsibilities

Routine reporting is sufficient unless there is evidence of restricted diffusion. Suggest the diagnosis when the basal ganglia, thalamic or cerebral infarctions occur and suggest obtaining MRS to document the presence of lactate. You may suggest the type of mitochondrial disease according to the site of predominant involvement.

What the Treating Physician Needs to Know

- Extent of the disease and involvement of critical areas such as motor, visual, and auditory cortex
- Extent of brainstem involvement which may explain respiratory and swallowing difficulties

Answers

1. In any systemic disorder leading to energy failure, the basal ganglia and thalami are first affected because their metabolic rate is higher than that of the rest of the brain. Other regions with high metabolic rates such as the motor cortex, visual cortex, and brainstem cranial nerve nuclei are also acutely affected.
2. Lactate is located at 1.3 to 1.4 parts per million in the spectra and has the typical "doublet" peak configuration. It resonates below the baseline at TE of 135 to 145 ms and above the baseline at all other echo times.

CLINICAL HISTORY *35-year old male with a slowly progressive neurologic disorder characterized by tremor, abnormal gait, slow speech, and lately some trouble swallowing. His father had similar symptoms and died of an "unknown disease."*

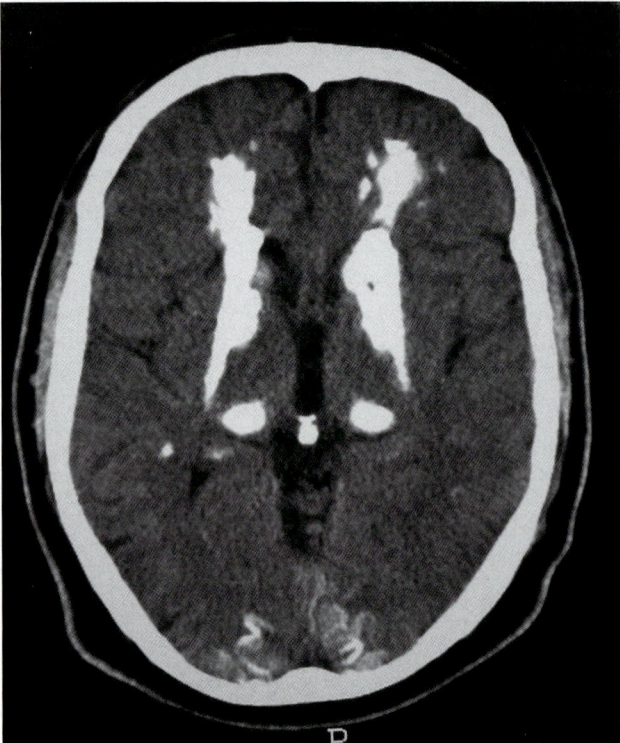

FIGURE 43-1

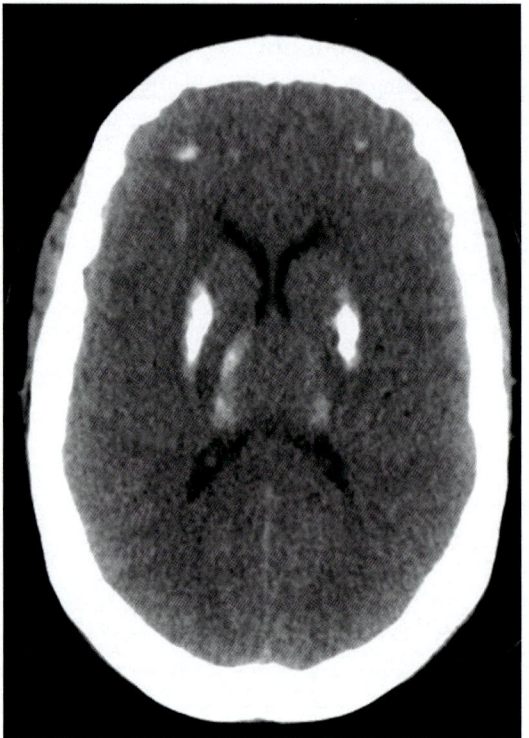

FIGURE 43-2

FINDINGS Figure 43-1. Axial NCCT through the basal ganglia. There are significant bilateral almost symmetrical calcifications in the basal ganglia, thalami, frontal white matter, and occipital cortex. There is no atrophy of the brain. Figure 43-2. Axial NCCT in a different patient. There is lesser degree of bilateral symmetrical calcifications in the basal ganglia, thalami, and subcortical frontal white matter.

DIFFERENTIAL DIAGNOSIS Hypoparathyroidism, pseudohypoparathryroidism, pseudopseudohypoparathyroidism, hypothyroidism, physiologic calcifications, Fahr disease (bilateral striopallidodentate calcinosis).

DIAGNOSIS Fahr disease (bilateral striopallidodentate calcinosis).

DISCUSSION CT of the head shows extensive and dense calcifications in the lentiform nuclei and heads of the caudate nuclei. Calcifications are also seen in the frontal white matter, posterior thalami, and occipital lobes. MRI shows GRE hypointensities in these areas of calcifications. All the differential diagnosis present with similar imaging findings except that physiologic calcifications tend to be relatively smaller and confined to the globus pallidus.

Patients with the very rare Fahr disease present with a progressive encephalopathy characterized by movement disorders, gait disturbances, tremors and other abnormal movements, headache, vertigo, syncope, and seizures and may also show psychiatric abnormalities particularly in the advanced stage of the disease. Rarely, the patients may be asymptomatic. They may have a family history of the disorder, and symptoms generally start between 30 and 50 years of age. Abnormalities in chromosomes 14, 8, and 2 have been suggested but remain unproven. The biologic abnormality is probably related to abnormal metabolism of phosphate transport leading to high calcium levels. Once calcification begins in the brain, it is progressive and may also affect the cerebellum. Anatomically, these calcifications occur intimately associated with arteries and not veins. Diffuse cerebral atrophy is common. The diagnosis is basically one of exclusion.

Questions for Further Thought

1. How common is it for extrapyramidal disorders to result in dementia?
2. What other findings can help you make the diagnosis of a systemic metabolic calcium disorder in the face of cerebral calcifications?

Reporting Responsibilities

This is a chronic disease, and routine reporting is sufficient. Identify features that may lead to the suspicion of a generalized disorder of calcium metabolism. Offer a differential diagnosis.

What the Treating Physician Needs to Know

- Are calcifications of the physiologic type and thus not important or are they pathologic and probably secondary to a disease?
- Are the hyperdensities truly calcifications or could they be related to other lesions such as hematomas?

Answers

1. Dementia is a very common long-term sequela of all extrapyramidal (movement) disorders, and most patients show progressive cognitive decline until they eventually reach a vegetative state.
2. Presence of extracranial calcifications such as sialoliths, ocular calcifications, extreme calcification of the pinnae, and skin calcifications all point to a systemic calcium disorder.

CLINICAL HISTORY *6-year-old female with a history of medulloblastoma.*

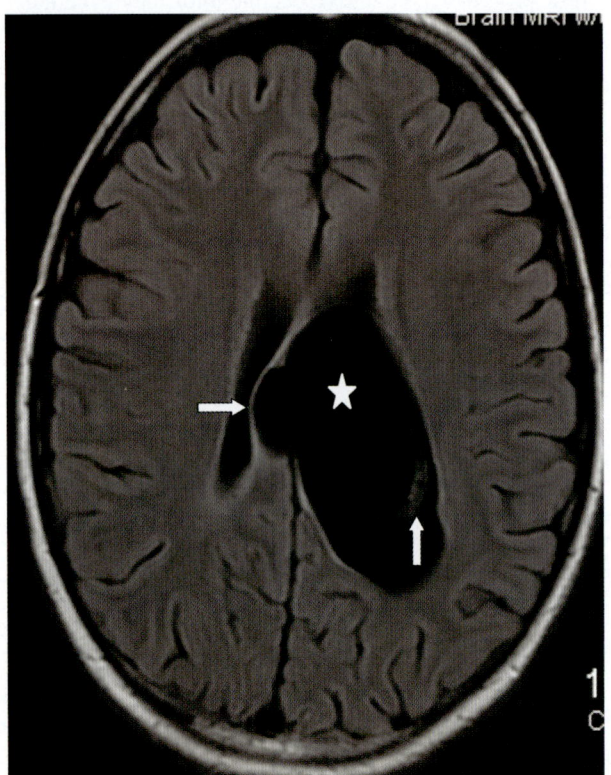

FIGURE 44-1

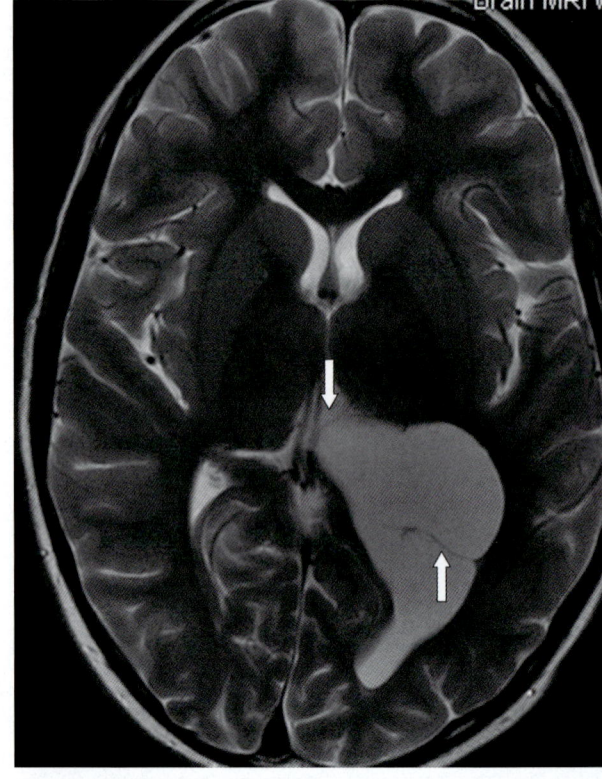

FIGURE 44-2

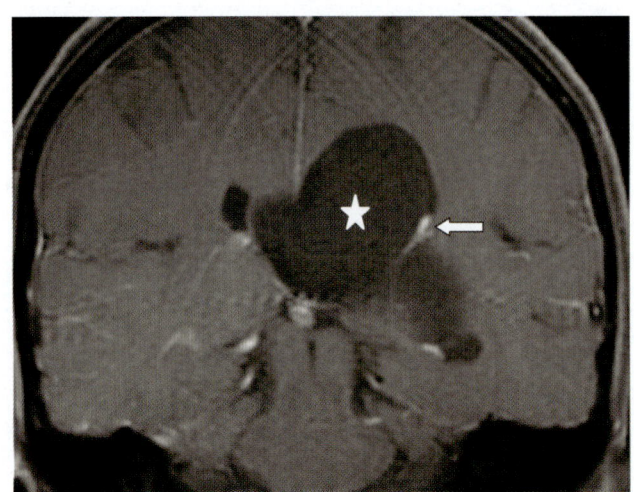

FIGURE 44-3

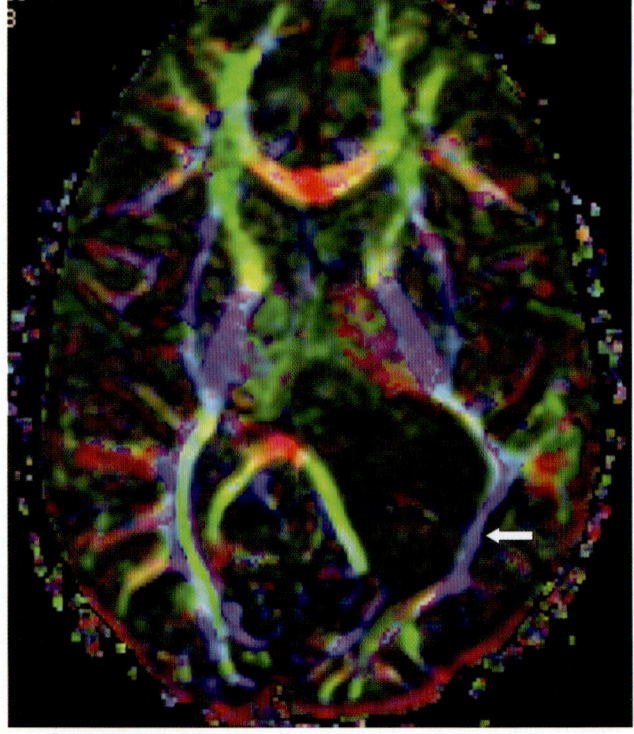

FIGURE 44-4

FINDINGS Figure 44-1. Axial FLAIR through the lateral ventricles. There is distension of the left lateral ventricle by a large CSF intensity cyst (star) which displaces the septum pellucidum medially (transverse arrow) and the left choroid plexus posterolaterally (vertical arrow). It is difficult to make out the cyst wall except where it compresses the ventricular walls laterally and medially. Figure 44-2. Axial T2WI through the trigones. The cyst is of CSF intensity with a very thin dark membranous wall (arrows). There is dilatation of the left occipital horn. Figure 44-3. Coronal post-contrast T1WI. The outline of the cyst (star) blends with the compressed lateral ventricular wall. The displaced enhancing left choroid plexus is compressed against the lateral ventricular wall (arrow). Figure 44-4. DTI color directional map through the lesion. There is compression and attenuation of the left inferior fronto-occipital fasciculus and the inferior longitudinal fasciculus (arrow).

DIFFERENTIAL DIAGNOSIS Intraventricular simple cyst, neuroepithelial cyst, intraventricular arachnoid cyst, choroid plexus cyst, intraventricular neurocysticercosis.

DIAGNOSIS Intraventricular simple cyst.

DISCUSSION Intraventricular simple cyst often called intraventricular arachnoid cyst could resemble all the entities listed in the differential diagnosis. There is no way of clearly distinguishing between them at imaging. Intraventricular neurocysticercosis, however, has been known to shift position on different images. This cyst follows CSF intensity on all MRI sequences and on CT. There is usually no restricted diffusion. Like other arachnoid cysts in the subarachnoid space (SAS), it could be complicated by hemorrhage, but this is unusual. They are mostly located in the trigone where they displace the choroid plexus and may rarely obstruct the temporal and occipital horns. Mass effect on surrounding structures as demonstrated on the DTI is frequent with large cysts. The CSF intensity on MRI with lack of restricted diffusion sets this cyst apart from epidermoid tumor and the lack of contrast enhancement excludes cystic neoplastic tumors.

Intraventricular cyst is generally asymptomatic and discovered incidentally as in this case which has been followed up for a number of years while the underlying medulloblastoma in this child is followed up. When a cyst becomes symptomatic, the patient may present with headache, signs and symptoms of obstructive hydrocephalus, focal neurologic deficit, or seizures. Intraventricular cyst represents a number of different simple cystic structures differing only in the histology of the wall. If treatment is ever desired on account of being symptomatic, simple endoscopic fenestration or removal has been recommended.

Question for Further Thought

1. What is the origin of intraventricular simple cyst?

Reporting Responsibilities

These are usually benign nonneoplastic lesions. Routine reporting is sufficient. Location, size, and presence of obstruction to CSF pathway or complication should be reported. Change in size and geography on follow-up should also be noted.

What the Treating Physician Needs to Know

- Location and size
- Presence of obstruction or complication
- Usually requires no treatment if asymptomatic

Answer

1. The origin of the cyst is controversial. It may derive from arachnoid tissue within the ventricular system or as an extension of an arachnoid cyst in the contiguous choroidal fissure lined by flattened arachnoid epithelial tissue. It has also been suggested that it could originate from vascular mesenchyme or from the ependyma as ependymal cyst which are lined by tall columnar epithelium or by cuboidal choroidal cells.

CLINICAL HISTORY *14-month-old female with hypotonic cerebral palsy.*

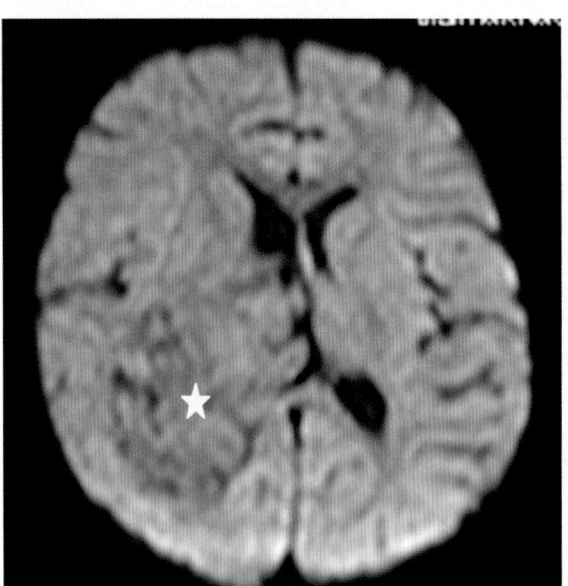

FIGURE 45-1

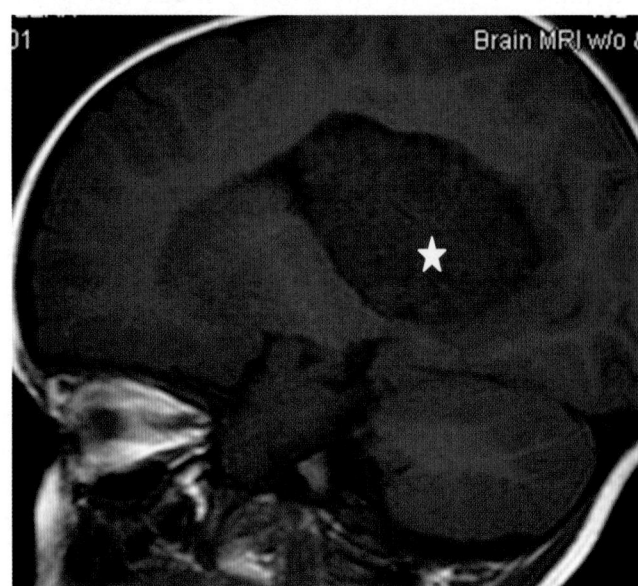

FIGURE 45-2

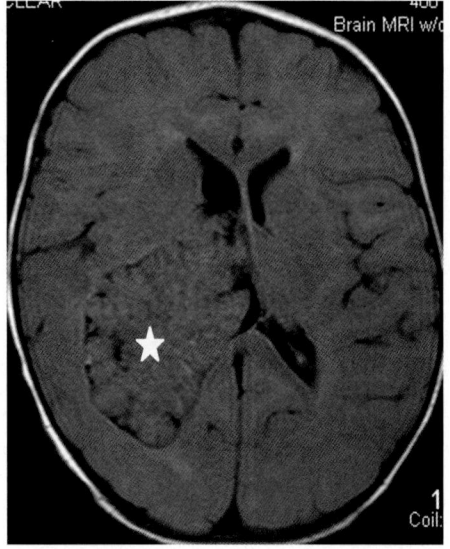

FIGURE 45-3

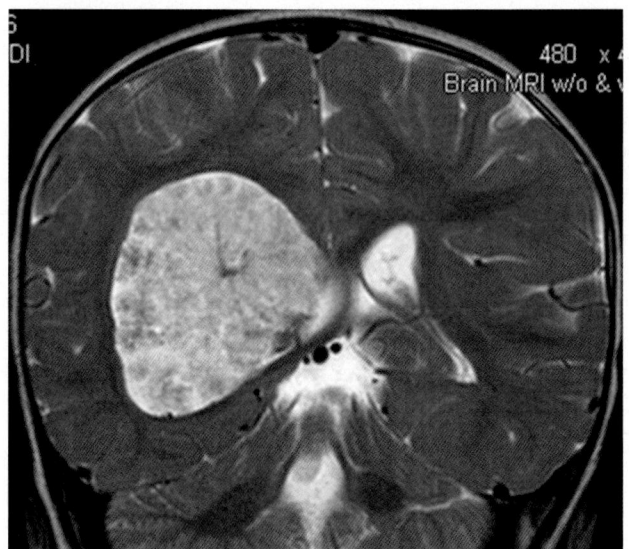

FIGURE 45-4

FINDINGS Figure 45-1. Axial DWI. There is a large isointense mass occupying the trigone and body of the right lateral ventricle (star). Figure 45-2. Right parasagittal T1WI. The large intraventricular mass is hypointense (star) to surrounding white matter (WM). Figure 45-3. Axial FLAIR. The right intraventricular mass is isointense (star). There is mild asymmetry of the lateral ventricles with mild displacement of the septum pellucidum to the left. There is no hydrocephalus. Figure 45-4. Coronal T2WI through the trigones. The mass

is hyperintense with myriads punctate and linear hypointense areas. Figure 45-5. Post-contrast axial T1WI. There is avid contrast enhancement with lobulation of the outline of the mass. Some punctate and short linear hypointensities are within the mass.

DIFFERENTIAL DIAGNOSIS Choroid plexus carcinoma (CPC), choroid plexus meningioma, choroid plexus papilloma (CPP).

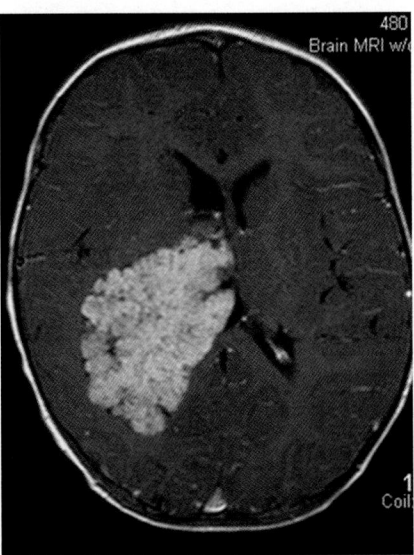

FIGURE 45-5

DIAGNOSIS Choroid plexus papilloma (CPP) WHO I.

DISCUSSION CPP is usually a well-marginated intraventricular mass sometimes with irregular mildly lobulated outline. CPP generally does not restrict diffusion, is isointense to hypointense on T1WI, isointense to hyperintense on FLAIR and T2WI, and avidly contrast enhancing. The punctate and linear hypointense areas on T2WI reflect vascular signal voids of the rich vasculature, hemorrhage, and/or calcifications. Hydrocephalus is common usually due to overproduction of CSF or CSF pathway obstruction. CPP could also occur in the cerebellopontine angles with extraventricular and cystic CPP being very rare. CSF dissemination is a well-known complication resulting in nodular leptomeningeal enhancement and CSF pathway obstruction. The CT usually shows avidly contrast enhancing iso- to hyperdense intraventricular mass with lobulated margin. Calcification and hemorrhage impart some degree of heterogeneous hyperdensity to the mass. Hydrocephalus may also be present on CT. About 50% of CPP occur in the lateral ventricles, 5% in the third, and 40% in the fourth ventricle, with 5% multi-ventricular. It usually does not infiltrate the ventricular walls or produce periventricular edema like meningioma and CPC.

CPP is a WHO I tumor of children and along with other choroid plexus tumors constitutes about 10% to 20% of all brain tumors in the first year of life but less than 1% of all brain tumors.

CPP usually presents with symptoms and signs of raised intracranial pressure such as headache, nausea, and vomiting. Enlargement of the head is common in infants. CPP arises from the epithelium of the choroid plexus. The pathology mirrors normal choroid plexus architecture, usually a cauliflower, well-defined mass which may adhere to the ventricular wall but no infiltration. Increased vascularity, cysts, xanthomatous degeneration, hemorrhage, and calcifications may be present. Surgical removal is usually curative with a very low recurrence rate. Rare transformation to CPC has been reported, and dissemination into the CSF spaces is not unknown.

Questions for Further Thought
1. What is the etiology of CPP?
2. What is atypical CPP?

Reporting Responsibilities
Direct reporting is necessary because this is a tumor and may present with hydrocephalus, and early treatment may be curative. Location, presence of hydrocephalus, and leptomeningeal enhancement should be reported.

What the Treating Physician Needs to Know
- Location, number if more than one, presence of hydrocephalus, leptomeningeal enhancement

Answers
1. It has been postulated that the simian virus 40 (SV40) plays a role in the etiology of CPP. SV40 DNA sequences were found in populations exposed to SV40-contaminated polio vaccine but not in those who received noncontaminated polio vaccine. It is also determined that the incidence of CPP in both populations is the same, suggesting that SV40 may therefore not play a causal role in the development of CPP but a bystander infection due to an enabling microenvironment that allows replication of the virus in the tumor. CPP has also been reported in the rhabdoid predisposition syndrome and as part of the Aicardi syndrome; a triad of infantile spasm, CC agenesis, and chorioretinal lacunae that occur almost exclusively in female as an X-linked dominant syndrome. Multi-ventricular CPP occurs in about 1% of Aicardi syndrome.
2. Atypical CPP represents about 15% of all choroid plexus neoplasm. It is a CPP with increased mitotic activity with a malignancy status higher than CPP WHO I but lower than CPC WHO III. It is a histologic grading with no differentiating imaging findings from CPP.

CLINICAL HISTORY *11-year-old female diagnosed with neurofibromatosis type 2 (NF2) has a growing intraventricular mass.*

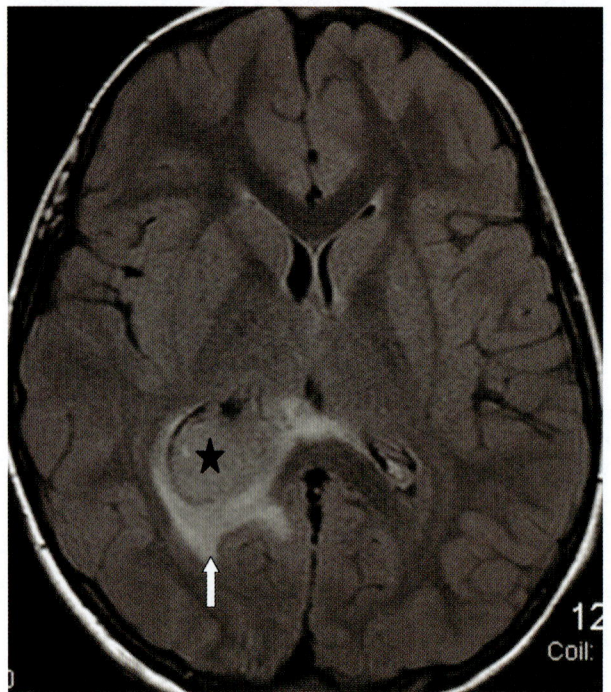

FIGURE 46-1

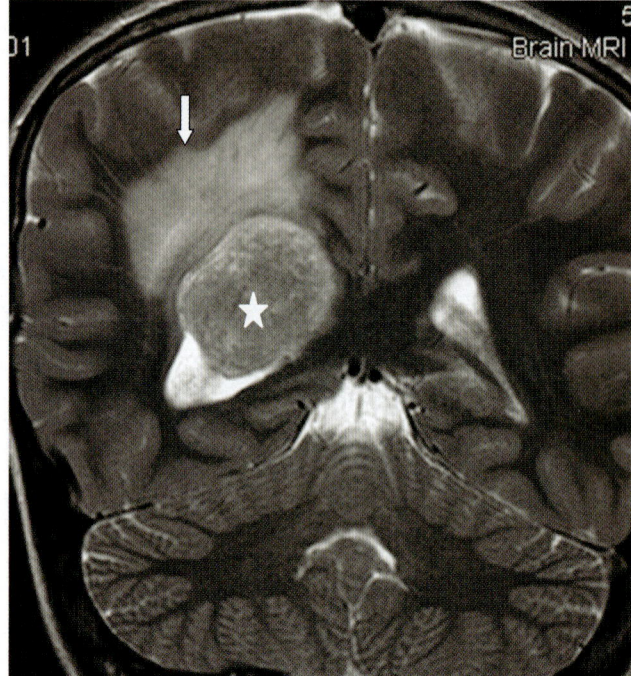

FIGURE 46-2

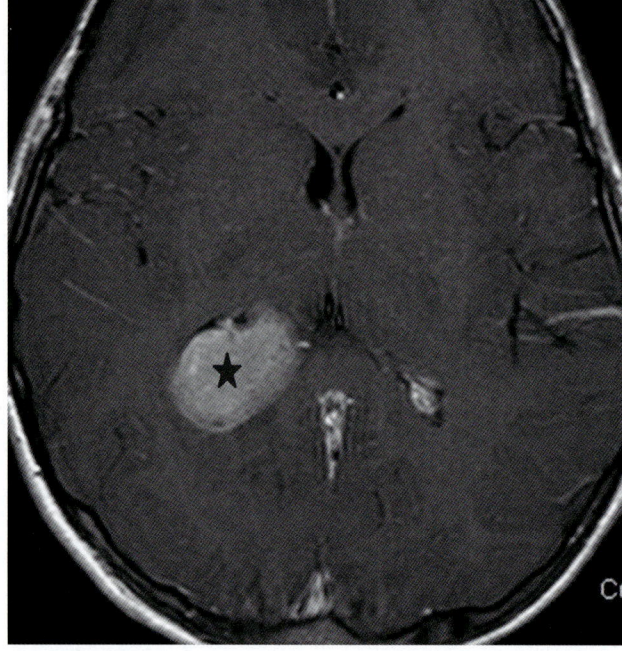

FIGURE 46-3

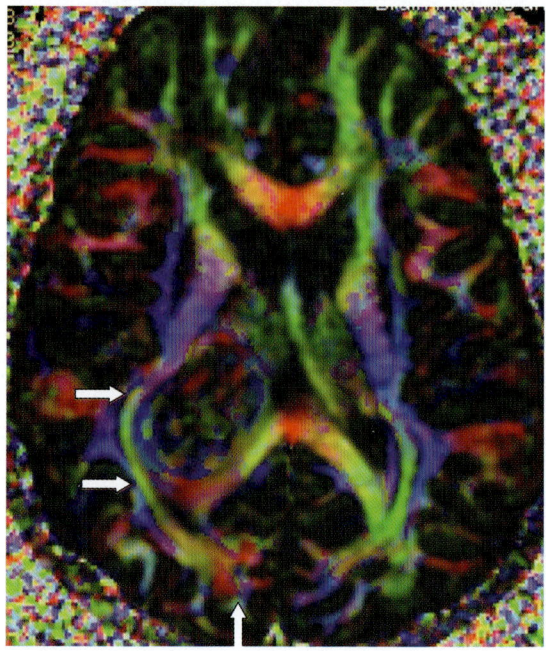

FIGURE 46-4

FINDINGS Figure 46-1. Axial FLAIR through the trigones. There is a homogeneous isointense (to gray matter [GM]) mass within the right trigone measuring 3.8 cm × 2.6 cm at the widest point (star). There is periventricular hyperintensity extending into the white matter (WM) consistent with parenchymal vasogenic edema (arrow). Figure 46-2. Coronal T2WI through the mass. Mass (star) is mildly heterogeneous but isointense to GM. Peripherally superiorly and medially the mass is as hyperintense as the adjacent periventricular hyperintense vasogenic edema (arrow). Figure 46-3. Post-contrast T1WI. There is homogeneous contrast enhancement of the smooth marginated mass (star). Figure 46-4. DTI color directional map. There is mass effect on the right inferior fronto-occipital fasciculus and inferior longitudinal fasciculus (transverse arrows) which have been compressed laterally. There is also posterior displacement of the fibers in the right splenium with disorganization of the right forceps major (vertical arrow).

DIFFERENTIAL DIAGNOSIS Choroid plexus carcinoma (CPC), choroid plexus papilloma (CPP), intraventricular meningioma, ependymoma.

DIAGNOSIS Intraventricular meningioma.

DISCUSSION Like most meningiomas, intraventricular meningioma has unique imaging features on MRI. It is mostly isointense to GM on T1WI and isointense to hyperintense on T2WI, usually smooth marginated and avidly contrast enhancing. Calcifications impart some heterogeneity to the signal pattern with multifocal hypointensities on T2WI. Meningiomas generally exhibit local mass effect dilating the ventricle and compressing adjacent structures but rarely producing perilesional edema as in this case. DTI may show attenuation of surrounding fiber tracts and reduced Fractional Anisotropy (FA). The trigone is the most common location of intraventricular meningioma. About 77.8% of intraventricular meningiomas occur in the lateral ventricles closely followed by the third ventricle in 15.6% and the fourth ventricle in 6.6%. On NCCT meningiomas are isodense to slightly hyperdense with avid contrast enhancement following contrast administration. Angiogram usually shows increased vascularity and tumor blush with most of the supply coming from the posterior choroidal artery and some from the anterior choroidal artery. CPP is usually lobulated, more heterogeneous on T2WI with flow voids, and more frequently associated with hydrocephalus even when it is not obstructing the CSF pathways. CPC in more poorly marginated with a tendency to infiltrate ventricular walls and cause perilesional edema. Ependymomas are generally more heterogeneous in signal characteristics and avidly contrast enhancing.

Intraventricular meningioma is rare accounting for between 0.5% and 3% of all intracranial meningiomas.

Menigiomas are designated WHO I tumors with very few histologic subtypes atypical WHO II or anaplastic WHO III. NF2-associated meningiomas have a higher mitotic index and a more aggressive clinical behavior than sporadic meningiomas. All histologic subtypes of meningiomas have been reported within the ventricles. They are more common in adults than in children except in NF2. There is no gender preference unlike hemispheric menigiomas that are more common in females. Clinical presentation is usually not specific and may include headache, mental status changes, focal neurologic deficit, vertigo, and gait disturbance. Intraventricular menigiomas tend to grow very large before presenting because of the vague symptoms unless it is situated where it could obstruct the CSF pathways. Total excision by piecemeal reduction in tumor volume with ultrasonic aspiration has been advocated as providing a safe surgical treatment and providing cure.

Question for Further Thought

1. Apart from meningioma, what other intracranial tumors occur in NF2?

Reporting Responsibilities

Direct reporting is desirable. CSF pathway obstruction makes direct reporting more urgent. Early treatment of intraventricular meningioma is very important to achieve favorable outcome. Location, size, and number if more than one should be reported. Presence of periventricular edema which might suggest an aggressive tumor or confuse location of tumor should be mentioned.

What the Treating Physician Needs to Know

- Location and size of tumor
- Effect on surrounding structures
- Presence of hydrocephalus
- Differential diagnosis

Answer

1. Bilateral vestibular schwannomas are the hallmark of NF2. Other tumors include schwannomas of the trigeminal nerves, and gliomas which include ependymomas and astrocytomas (mostly pilocytic). Other nontumoral intracranial lesions may include menigioangiomatosis and cerebral calcifications.

CLINICAL HISTORY *68-year-old male undergoing restaging for non-small cell carcinoma of the lung.*

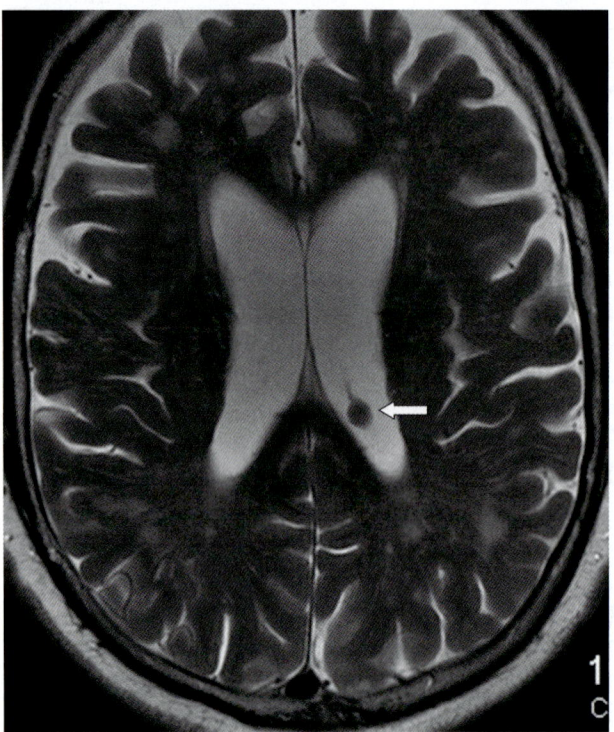

FIGURE 47-1

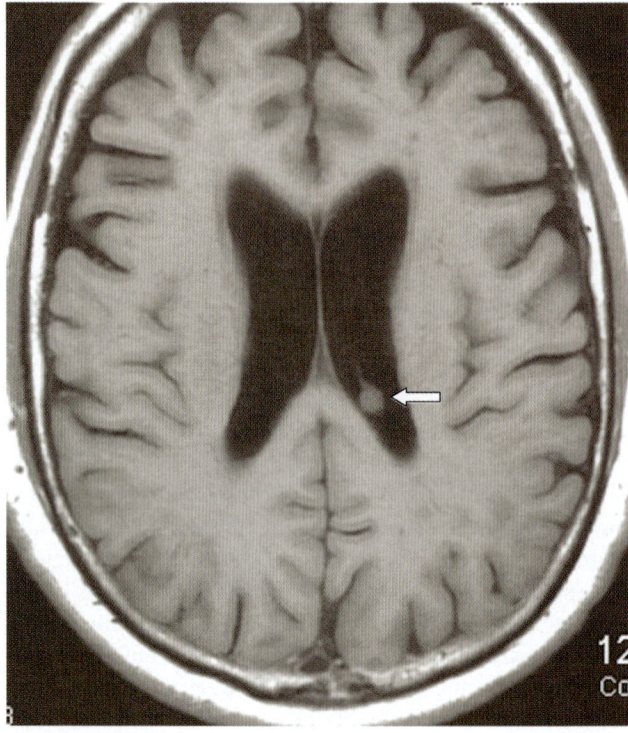

FIGURE 47-2

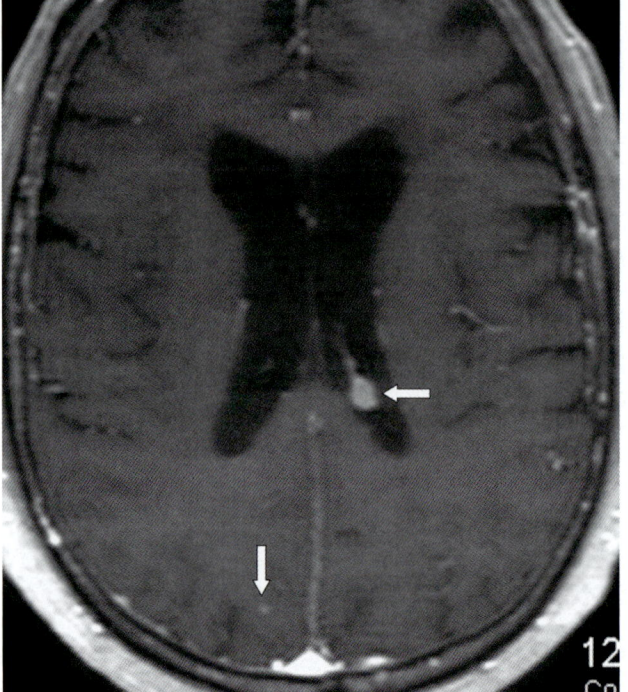

FIGURE 47-3

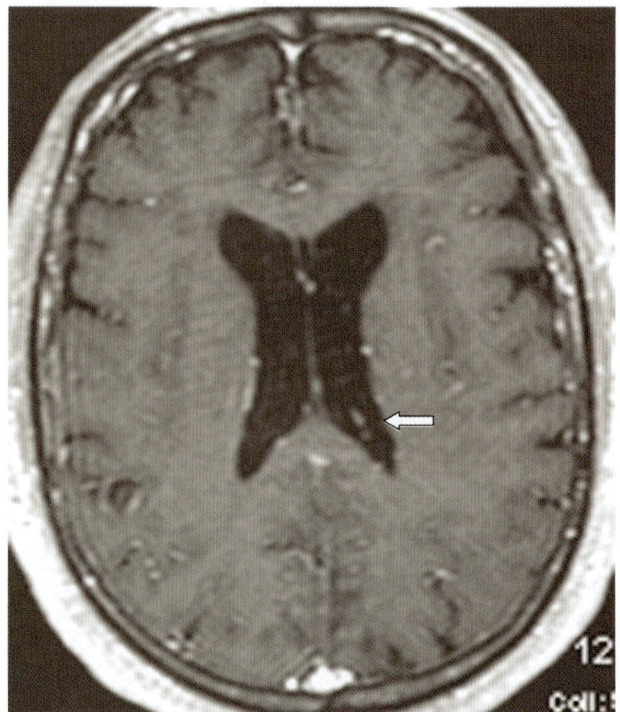

FIGURE 47-4

FINDINGS Figures 47-1 to 47-3. Axial T2WI, non-contrast T1WI, and post-contrast T1WI through the lateral ventricles, respectively. There is a small left lateral ventricle round T1 and T2 isointense (to white matter [WM]) avidly contrast-enhancing choroid plexus mass (arrows). There is also a punctate metastasis in the right parasagittal parietal lobe (vertical arrow in Figure 47-3). Numerous new punctate contrast-enhancing metastases are present in other areas of the brain (not shown). Figure 47-4. Axial post-contrast T1WI through same level 7 months before. There is no significant mass in the choroid plexus.

DIFFERENTIAL DIAGNOSIS Intraventricular meningioma, colloid cyst, xanthogranuloma, choroid plexus metastasis.

DIAGNOSIS Metastasis non-small cell lung carcinoma.

DISCUSSION Metastasis to the choroid plexus is rare. It could be isolated but most often associated with multifocal metastases to the brain. It is more common in the lateral ventricular trigones than elsewhere. It usually presents as an avid contrast-enhancing mass of varying sizes on CT or MRI. Signal pattern is variable on T1WI and T2WI. NCCT often shows a hypodense to isodense mass. It may be complicated by hemorrhage and hydrocephalus. Presence of hemorrhage may alter the density pattern on CT and intensity pattern on MRI. Third ventricular choroid plexus metastases have been reported to mimic a colloid cyst except that the metastases showed vivid contrast enhancement. Ependymal contrast enhancement has been reported with choroid plexus metastases indicating ependymal spread. Ventricular wall invasion with peritumoral edema has also been reported mimicking intraventricular meningioma, carcinoma, or xanthogranuloma. Choroid plexus metastasis could be difficult to diagnose when they are small, mimicking normal contrast-enhancing choroid plexus. Comparison with prior study and index of suspicion helps in catching this very difficult lesion.

The most common metastasis to the choroid plexus is from renal cell carcinoma. Tumors of origin have included lung carcinoma, melanoma, and colon carcinoma. Metastases are seen most commonly in adults, although they have also been found in children with extracranial childhood tumors. When they form part of multifocal brain metastases, the presentation could be mute. Headache or symptoms and signs of hydrocephalus are present in obstructive lesions. Visual symptoms may arise as a result of periventricular invasion and edema. Treatment includes surgical removal, radiation treatment, or chemotherapy. Isolated choroid plexus metastases have been known to be indolent for a long period.

Question for Further Thought

1. What are the common metastatic tumors to the brain?

Reporting Responsibilities

Direct reporting is essential. Location, number, other parenchymal metastases, hydrocephalus or hemorrhagic, and/or periventricular complications are all worth reporting.

What the Treating Physician Needs to Know

- Location, number, and complications
- Is it safe to perform lumbar puncture for CSF sampling?

Answer

1. The most common sources of metastases to the choroid plexus are kidney, lung, and colon. There are a few reports of thyroid, melanoma, stomach, breast, bladder, and lymphoma. The sources in children are leukemia, lymphoma, and sarcoma. 11% of brain metastases have no known origins at the time of diagnosis. Despite the very high blood flow to the choroid plexus, it is very rare to find choroid plexus metastases accounting for less than 5% of intracranial metastases in autopsy series and less than 1% of clinically evident cerebral metastases.

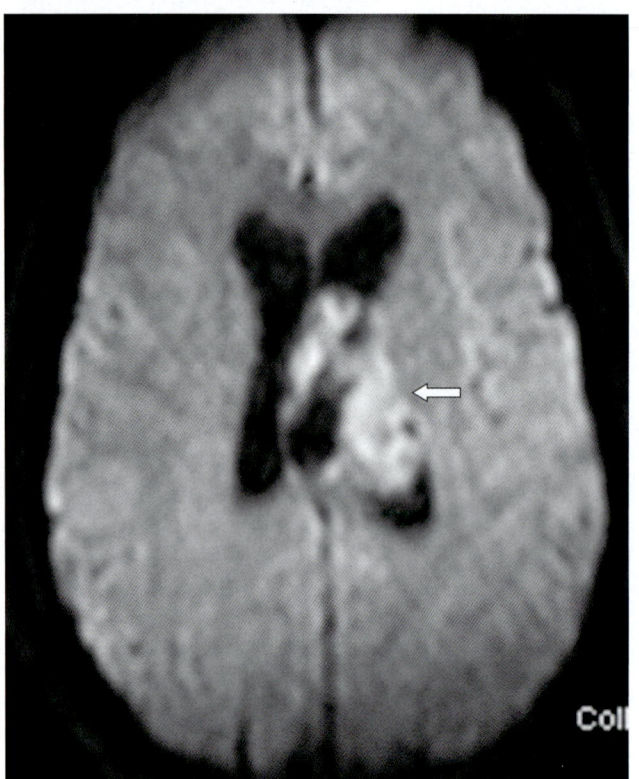

FIGURE 48-1

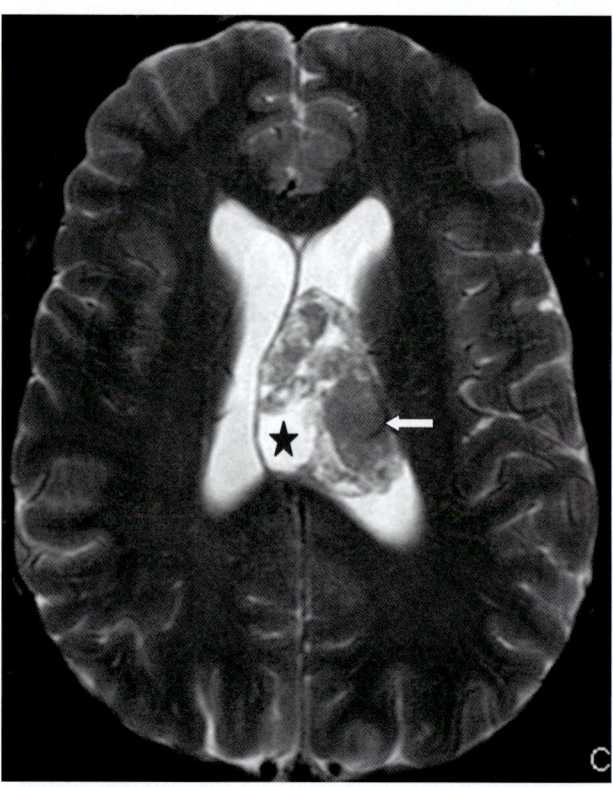

FIGURE 48-2

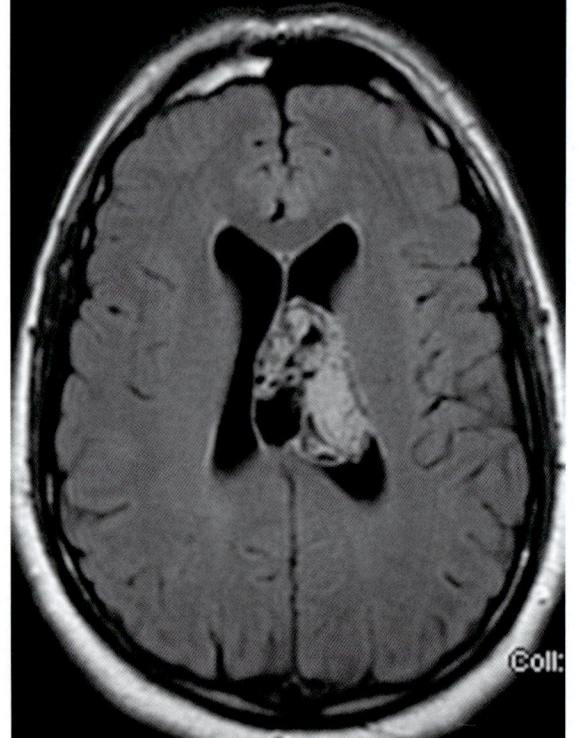

FIGURE 48-3

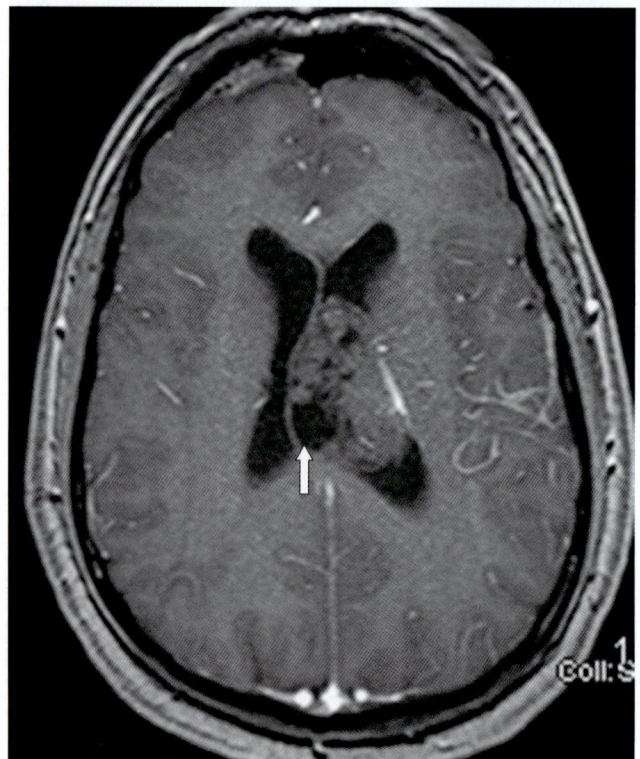

FIGURE 48-4

FINDINGS Figure 48-1. Axial DWI through the lateral ventricles. There is a 4.7 cm × 3.3 cm ovoid cystic solid mass in the left lateral ventricle with local mass effect on the lateral ventricular walls. The solid component is hyperintense (arrow). The corresponding ADC map (not shown) shows hypointense solid component consistent with restricted or reduced diffusion. There is mild ventricular dilatation. Figure 48-2. T2WI through the lateral ventricles. The solid components (arrow) are isointense with cortical gray matter (GM) somewhat slightly higher than white matter (WM) intensity. The cystic portion has cerebrospinal fluid (CSF) intensity (star). Figure 48-3. Axial FLAIR. The solid areas are mildly hyperintense. Figure 48-4. Axial post-contrast T1WI. There is no contrast enhancement. Mass has isointense solid areas with hypointense (or CSF intensity) cystic components (arrow).

DIFFERENTIAL DIAGNOSIS Oligodendroglioma, pilocytic astrocytoma, giant cell astrocytoma, ependymoma, central neurocytoma.

DIAGNOSIS Central liponeurocytoma.

DISCUSSION Central neurocytoma is a rare intraventricular predominantly lateral ventricular mass, but extraventricular neurocytoma (EVN) is not unknown. Third and fourth ventricular neurocytomas are rare. It is a cystic/solid mass in 85% of the cases, inhomogeneously isointense on T1WI with hypointense areas representing vessels (62%) or calcifications (69%) or hemorrhagic product. It is iso- or hyperintense on T2WI with mild-to-moderate contrast enhancement. Cystic degeneration is common and is hypointense or CSF intensity on all sequences. Neurocytoma may show significantly increased choline, decreased N-acetyl aspartate (NAA), and creatine at MRS with lower Normalized apparent diffusion coefficient (NADC) values; findings that may resemble high-grade glioma. Hydrocephalus may be a feature depending on its location and usually due to foramen of Monro obstruction. Periventricular CSF permeation may be present in such a situation. The presentation here is therefore somewhat different from the majority of neurocytomas. Our tumor shows mild restricted diffusion but no contrast enhancement. NCCT shows iso- to slightly hyperdense mass with mild-to-moderate heterogeneous contrast enhancement in most neurocytomas. About 51% show hyperdensity consistent with calcifications. DSA may show tumor blush or very vascular tumor. Most of the differential diagnosis could mimic neurocytoma. They are also cystic and solid with calcifications or hemorrhagic components.

Neurocytoma is designated a WHO II neuroepithelial tumor mostly occurring in adolescent and young adults with a mean age of 29 years with about 70% presenting between 20 and 40 years. It has no gender preference. Headache and visual disturbance are the prevalent presenting symptoms with papilledema and ataxia as the most frequent presenting signs. Neurocytomas account for between 0.25% and 0.5% of all intracranial tumors. Tumor is usually composed of uniform round cells within a fibrillary matrix with focal glial fibrillary acidic protein (GFAP) reactivity in less than half the cases. Treatment is by surgical removal with chemotherapy and radiation treatment reserved for incomplete resection and recurrence.

Question for Further Thought

1. Are EVNs different from intraventricular neurocytomas?

Reporting Responsibilities

Direct reporting is necessary because this is a tumor. Size, location, and number if more than one and the presence of hydrocephalus should be reported.

What the Treating Physician Needs to Know

- Location, size, and number if more than one
- Presence of hydrocephalus
- Leptomeningeal enhancement that may suggest metastases
- Is there a need for craniospinal axis imaging? This is always necessary in all high-grade intraventricular tumors

Answer

1. EVNs are similar but show some variation in the biologic and histologic features compared to the intraventricular lesions. There could be some imaging differences arising from disruption of the blood–brain barrier resulting in perilesional edema in hemispheric lesions, but not all hemispheric lesions show surrounding edema. Hemispheric lesions are also usually well defined with cystic degeneration, calcifications, hemorrhage, and varying degrees of contrast enhancement and could mimic a high-grade tumor such as high-grade astrocytoma, Primitive neuroectodermal tumor (PNET), or oligodendroglioma. EVNs are also more frequently associated with poorer outcome compared to their intraventricular counterparts.

CLINICAL HISTORY *47-year-old right-handed female presenting with seizures. These are follow-up images after subtotal resection of original lesion.*

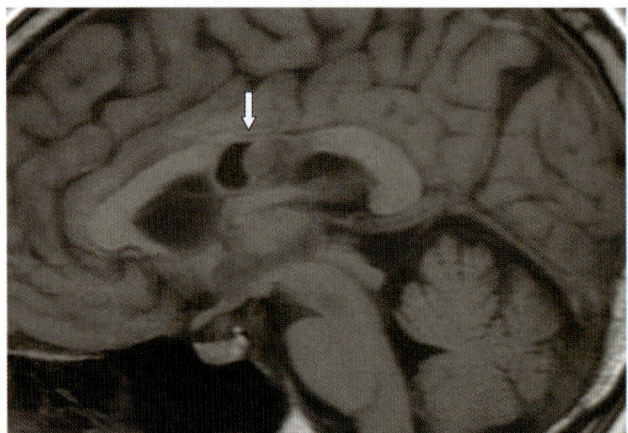

FIGURE 49-1

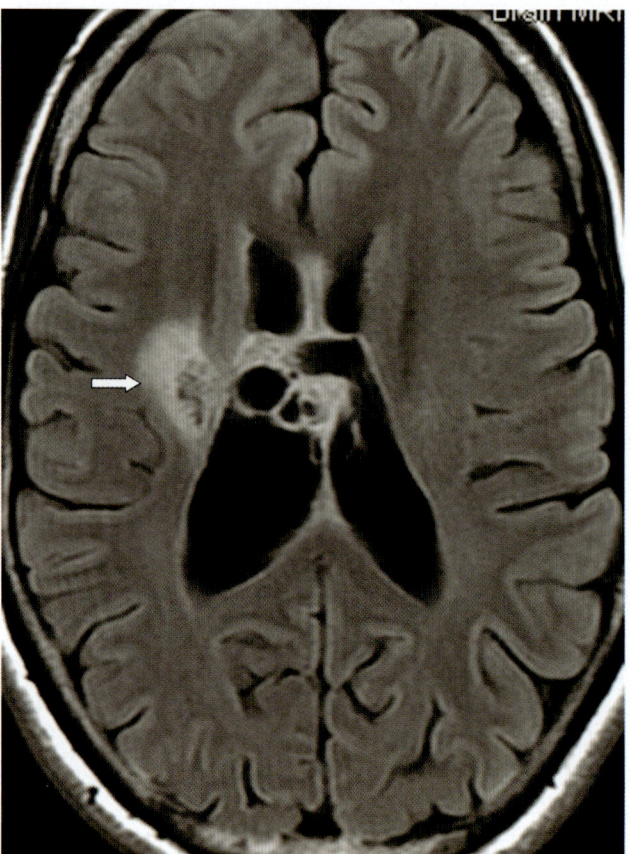

FIGURE 49-2

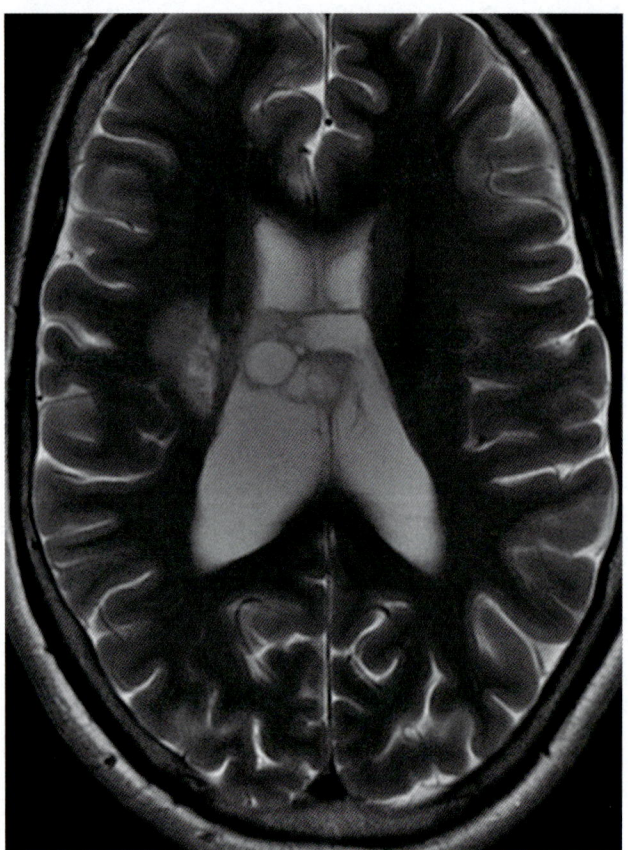

FIGURE 49-3

FINDINGS Figure 49-1. Sagittal T1WI through the corpus callosum (CC). There is a mixed cystic anteriorly (cerebrospinal fluid [CSF] intensity) and solid hypointense (posteriorly) mass in the midbody of the CC (arrow) projecting to the septum pellucidum inferiorly. Post-contrast T1WI (not shown) demonstrated very minimal contrast enhancement. Figure 49-2. Axial FLAIR through the corona radiata. The

solid components are hyperintense and project into the right corona radiata (arrow), while the cystic components show CSF hypointensity. Figure 49-3. Axial T2WI through the corona radiata. The solid components are somewhat hyperintense but brighter than surrounding white matter (WM). Figure 49-4. Axial DTI color directional map through the CC. There is disruption of the red CC fibers (vertical arrows) and the adjacent right superior fronto-occipital fasciculus and the superior internal capsule (transverse arrows).

DIFFERENTIAL DIAGNOSIS Glioblastoma (GB), lymphoma, tumefactive or toxic demyelination, oligodendroglioma.

DIAGNOSIS CC oligodendroglioma II (ODG II) recurrent.

DISCUSSION CT and MRI are complementary techniques for imaging ODG. Tumor calcification is better defined on CT scans than on MRI, but MRI is till the examination of choice. Conventional MRI of the brain is crucial in the diagnosis, staging, treatment, and follow-up of brain tumors. ODGs are relatively hypointense on T1WI and hyperintense on T2WI. Peritumoral edema, uncommon with ODG, is depicted as hyperintensity on T2WI and FLAIR. Mixed

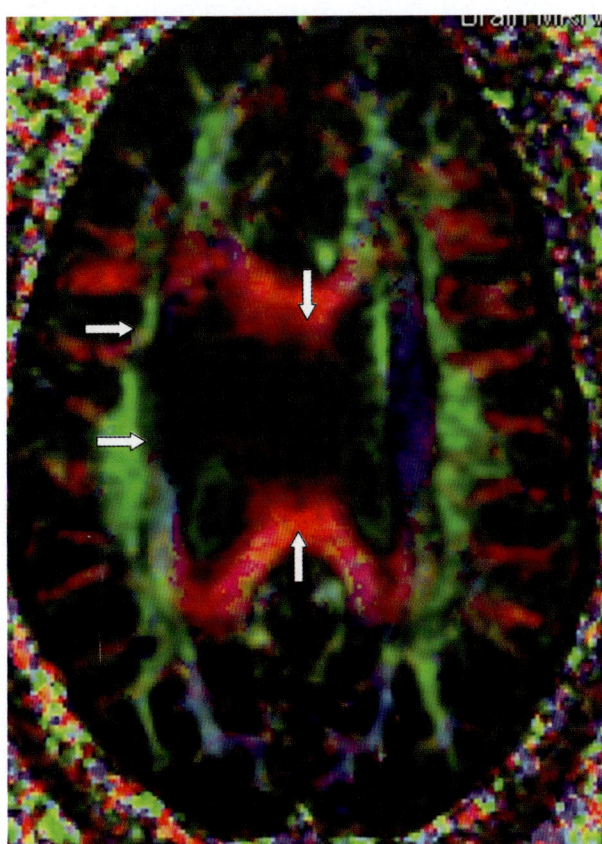

Figure 49-4

cystic and solid regions could be present. Hemorrhage and calcifications may be present in the mass depicted as areas of blooming on GRE. Post-contrast MRI is always performed as it has a prognostication value; completely resecting enhancing tissue (more common in ODG III) independently improves outcome irrespective of histologic grade or genetic status. Physiologic MRI techniques such as perfusion, diffusion, and functional MRI add information to the microscopic architecture of the tumor but might not necessarily differentiate between the different types of tumors or the differential diagnosis.

Primary ODG of the CC is rare. Initial imaging of the brain showed a right frontoparietal tumor (images not shown). She had a subtotal resection, and histology was that of ODG II. Follow-up MRI showed an increase in the size of the residual lesion, with the latest MRI showing infiltration of the CC and the contralateral hemisphere. The patient had a repeat stereotactic biopsy confirming ODG II. Fluorescence In Situ Hybridization analysis (FISH) analysis on the tissue demonstrated co-deletion of 1p/19q. As the lesion was not amenable to resection, she was offered chemotherapy with temozolomide and radiation.

Questions for Further Thought

1. What is the treatment of ODG?
2. What is the survival rate of patients with ODG?

Reporting Responsibilities

Direct reporting is essential in a recurrent tumor. Changes in the original location of tumor should be mentioned, while changes of aggressive behavior, crossing CC and infiltrating the corona radiata, should be reported.

What the Treating Physician Needs to Know

- Extent and progression of tumor along with possible complications of herniation or hydrocephalus
- Although this was an ODG II, the imaging behavior of invasion and crossing the CC and involvement of the contralateral hemisphere suggest anaplastic ODG; hence, the treatment recommendation is that for aggressive ODG
- Tumors with 1p/19q co-deletion benefit particularly from the addition of procarbazine/lomustine and CCNU are the same/vincristine (PCV) chemotherapy to radiation therapy. Side effects of PCV is, however, very significant and probably translate into reduced quality of life for long-term survivors. Therefore, temozolomide which has less severe side effects is replacing PCV in the treatment of these tumors. The long-term benefit of temozolomide is unknown

Answers

1. The treatment of an ODG should be individualized depending on the presence or absence of symptoms, location, and biologic aggressiveness of the tumor, extent of possible surgical resection, histopathology, and degree of anaplasia. Treatment options vary from conservative treatment with serial imaging studies and no intervention to aggressive multimodal treatment including surgical resection, radiotherapy, and chemotherapy.
2. Overall, as many as 75% of patients with nonanaplastic tumors have a median reported survival duration of 6 to 10 years. For those with anaplastic ODGs, median survival is about 3 to 4 years.

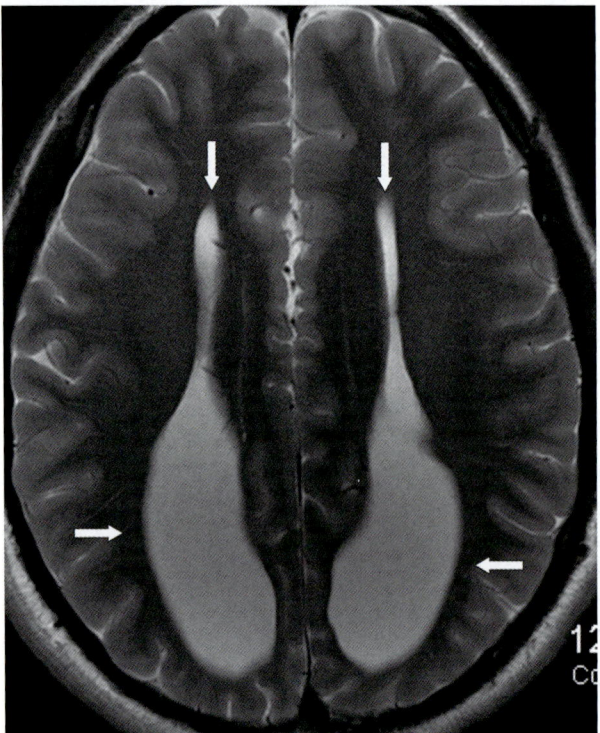

FIGURE 50-1

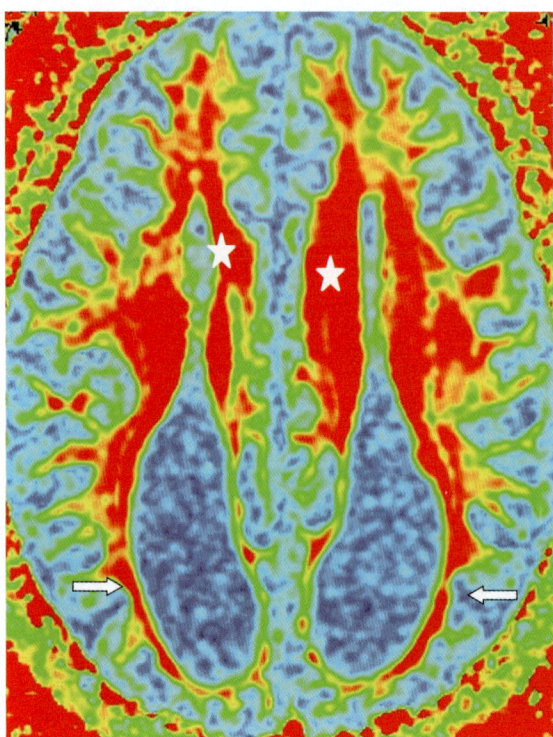

FIGURE 50-2

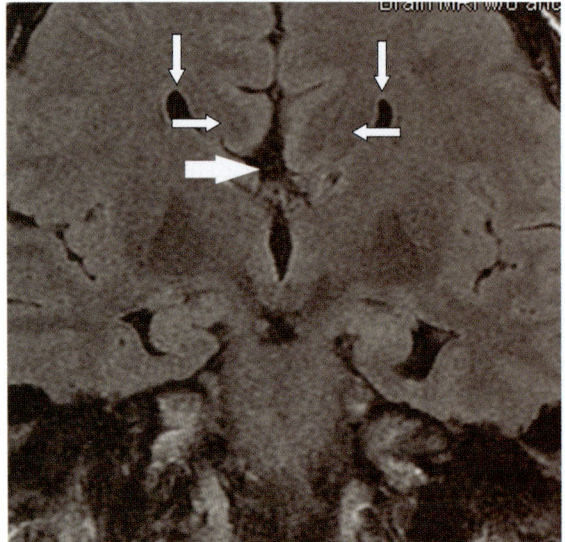

FIGURE 50-3

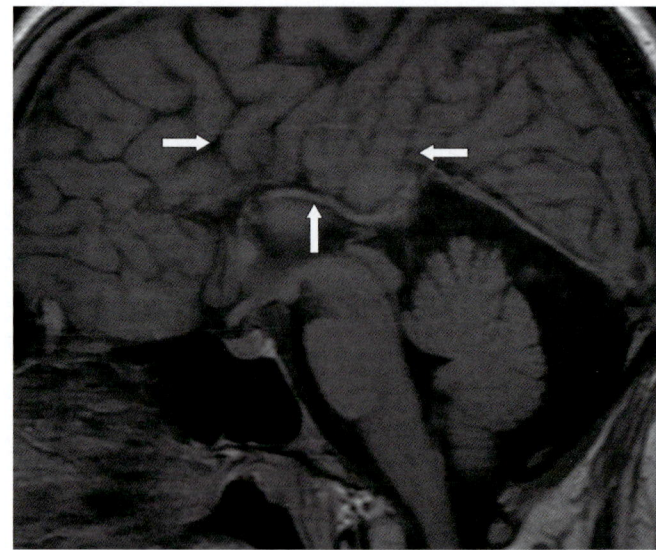

FIGURE 50-4

FINDINGS Figure 50-1. Axial T2WI through the lateral ventricles. The lateral ventricles are widely separated and parallel with bilateral tapering of the frontal horns (vertical arrows) and dilated occipital horns (colpocephaly) (transverse arrows). The interhemispheric fissure separates the two lateral ventricles with well-formed subcortical white matter (WM) tract (Probst bundle) and cortical gray matter (GM) separating the lateral ventricles from the interhemispheric fissure. The septum pellucidum and corpus callosum (CC) are absent. Figure 50-2. Axial DTI Fractional Anisotropy (FA) map through the lateral ventricles. The WM tract around the colpocephaly is thin suggesting hypoplasia (arrows). WM tracts do not cross the midline. Probst bundles are medial to the ventricles (star). Figure 50-3. Coronal T2 FLAIR through the frontal horns. There is wide separation of the tapered frontal horns (vertical arrows). WM Probst bundle project medially to the frontal horns (transverse arrows). The interhemispheric fissure extends down to the third ventricular roof (hatched arrow). Figure 50-4. Sagittal T1WI. There is radiating cortical bundles, so-called spoke wheel gyri, in the midline (transverse arrows). The CC and the cingulate gyrus are missing. The internal cerebral vein lies in the inferior aspect of the interhemispheric fissure, the expected location on the velum of the third ventricle (vertical arrow).

DIFFERENTIAL DIAGNOSIS N/A.

DIAGNOSIS Agenesis of corpus callosum (ACC).

DISCUSSION MRI is superior to CT in demonstrating the features of ACC because of its multiplanar and tissue characterization capabilities. Axial MRI demonstrates parallel lateral ventricles separated by brain tissue bundle on either side of the interhemispheric fissure. There is no midline crossing of the WM. Coronal and axial MRI and DTI demonstrate the longitudinal callosal bundles of Probst. They represent nondecussated callosal fibers that deviate at the interhemispheric fissure to run along the medial borders of the lateral ventricles instead of crossing the midline. Coronal images demonstrate widely separated anterior horns of the lateral ventricles with the interhemispheric fissure extending unto the roof of the third ventricle (trident sign) or in some cases unto a midline cyst resembling a "Viking helmet" or "mouse head." ACC is typically accompanied by a characteristic dilatation of occipital horns or colpocephaly. The sagittal image shows radiating brain folds on either side of the midline. The cingulate gyrus is not visualized. DTI confirms lack of midline connectivity.

The CC develops between 8 and 20 weeks of gestation and is made of four parts with the rostrum anteriorly followed by the genu, body, and splenium in that order. The development of the CC is thought to progress craniocaudally, with the exception of the most anterior part, the rostrum, that develops later. Some studies suggest that the development of the CC starts with the formation of the anterior body and progresses bidirectionally. The four components of the CC are best viewed on sagittal MRI although its relationship to the cerebral hemispheres is best shown on coronal images. DTI/tractography demonstrates the midline connectivity of the hemispheres through the CC. The CC is a densely packed WM structure and therefore has the expected hypointensity on T1WI and T2WI after the age of 24 months. Up until that age, MRI shows that myelination is more advanced in the posterior part of the CC when compared to the anterior region. CC dysgenesis can be partial or complete (or agenesis).

Questions for Further Thought

1. What is the etiology of CC dysgenesis or agenesis?
2. What are the clinical findings associated with CC dysgenesis/agenesis?

Reporting Responsibilities

Routine reporting is sufficient. Degree of dysgenesis and other associated anomalies should be described.

What the Treating Physician Needs to Know

- Pattern of CC dysgenesis
- ACC can be isolated or associated with other brain abnormalities
- As many brain structures form concurrently, other brain malformations and syndromes such as interhemispheric cysts, pericallosal lipomas, lissencephaly, polymicrogyria and pachygyria, neuronal heterotopias, Dandy-Walker malformation, midline facial malformation, and syntelencephaly (fusion of the dorsal part of the brain) might be present
- Dysgenesis of the CC can be screened for in utero using ultrasound or MRI

Answers

1. CC dysgenesis can be sporadic or result from genetic (chromosomal abnormalities such as trisomies 8 and 18 and genetic syndromes such as Andermann and Aicardi), infectious (prenatal rubella, toxoplasmosis, CMV, influenza), vascular, or toxic (fetal alcohol syndrome) causes.
2. The clinical presentation of CC dysgenesis is very broad and ranges from none in two-thirds to three-quarters of the cases to borderline/moderate and severe disability with learning disability, mental retardation, seizures, and psychiatric disorders. Most importantly, the prognosis does not seem to be different in isolated and complex cases.

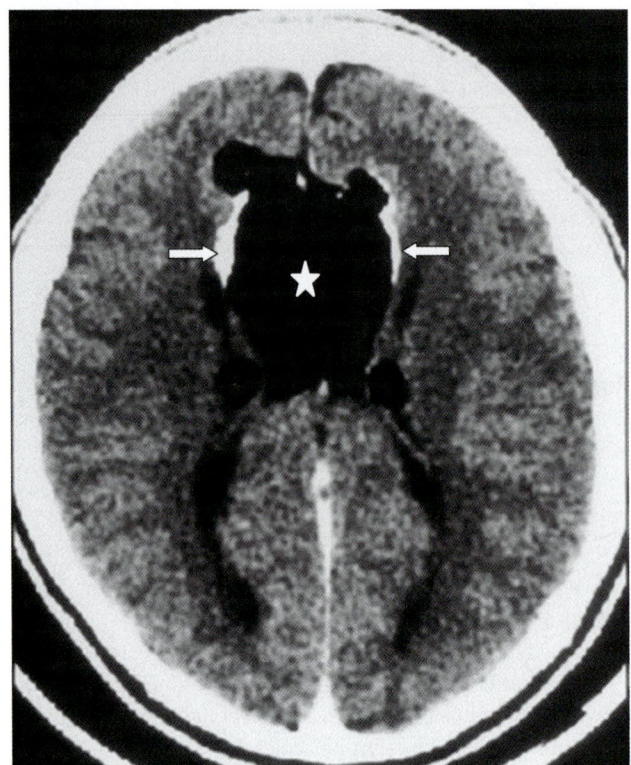

FIGURE **51-1**

FINDINGS Figure 51-1. Axial NCCT through the lateral ventricles. There is a large hypodensity (HU in the region of fat) (star) surrounded by thick irregular linear peripheral hyperdensity—calcification—(arrows) replacing the genu and body of the corpus callosum (CC). There is wide separation of the frontal horns.

DIFFERENTIAL DIAGNOSIS Midline cyst in agenesis of CC, lipoma in agenesis of CC, abscess.

DIAGNOSIS Lipoma in agenesis of CC.

DISCUSSION NCCT of intracranial (IC) lipomas present a well-defined hypodensity that does not enhance with contrast. Calcifications might be present peripherally as hyperdensity surrounding the hypodense lipoma mostly in the interhemispheric fissure or replacing the CC. Depending on the history, it may be pertinent to distinguish this hypodensity from pneumocephalus or midline cyst. Hounsfield measurement usually shows a lipoma in the range of -100 to -200 HU, air in pneumocephalus is usually in the range of -900 to -1000 HU, and midline cyst always correlate with cerebrospinal fluid (CSF) measurement at or near 0.

MRI shows a homogeneous, hyperintense mass on T1WI and T2WI, hypointense with fat suppression and usually without contrast enhancement. The surrounding calcification is hypointense on GRE. TOF MRI might show some vascular abnormalities.

IC lipoma is a rare and benign congenital malformation of the brain rather than a neoplasm. They develop due to abnormal persistence and maldifferentiation of the embryonic meninx primitiva during development of the subarachnoid cisterns and are composed of adipose tissue that is not normally present in the central nervous system (CNS). They are generally asymptomatic and generally do not require any treatment. The symptomatic ones might cause compressive symptoms or seizures depending on the location. Most lipomas occur at or near the midline typically in the pericallosal cistern as in this patient accounting for 45% of all cases. Large CC lipomas may sometimes extend into the lateral ventricles and choroid plexus. There are two types of IC lipomas, tubulonodular and curvilinear. Tubulonodular is anteriorly situated, round or cylinder-shaped generally greater than 2 cm in diameter and have a high incidence of CC dysgenesis, frontal lobe anomalies, and frontal cephaloceles. Curvilinear lipoma is thin, posteriorly situated, and "curving" around the splenium and is generally associated with a normal CC with a low incidence of associated anomalies. The remainder of the IC lipomas tends to be found in the quadrigeminal/superior cerebellar cistern (25%) suprasellar/interpeduncular cistern (14%), cerebellopontine angle cistern (9%), and sylvian cistern (5%). Rarely, they can be found on the surface of the cerebral hemispheres.

Question for Further Thought

1. What is the differential diagnosis of the hyperdensity surrounding the lipoma?

Reporting Responsibilities

Routine reporting is sufficient. It is however important to distinguish this from pneumocephalus and to identify the associated CC dysgenesis.

What the Treating Physician Needs to Know

- Location and associated anomalies
- Associated congenital CNS abnormalities may include agenesis or dysgenesis of the CC (most frequent abnormality), absence of the septum pellucidum, cranium bifidum, spinal bifida, encephalocele, myelomeningocele, hypoplasia of the vermis, and malformation of the cortex as the lipoma may interfere with the growth of cortical tissue. Abnormal or prominent drainage has been described

together with cortical dysplasia. Associated arterial abnormalities such as azygos ACA, aneurysms, arteriovenous malformations, and veins with abnormal drainage have been reported

- Treatment is generally not necessary. Symptoms are generally not due to the lipomas but the underlying associated anomaly

Answer

1. The differential diagnosis of surrounding hyperdensity includes calcification and hemorrhage. It is important in the context of trauma to exclude pneumocephalus with surrounding hemorrhage simply by taking the Hounsfield measurement.

CLINICAL HISTORY *28-year-old female who presented with 6-month history of vertigo followed by headache, left arm and leg numbness, and left lower homonymous quadrantanopia.*

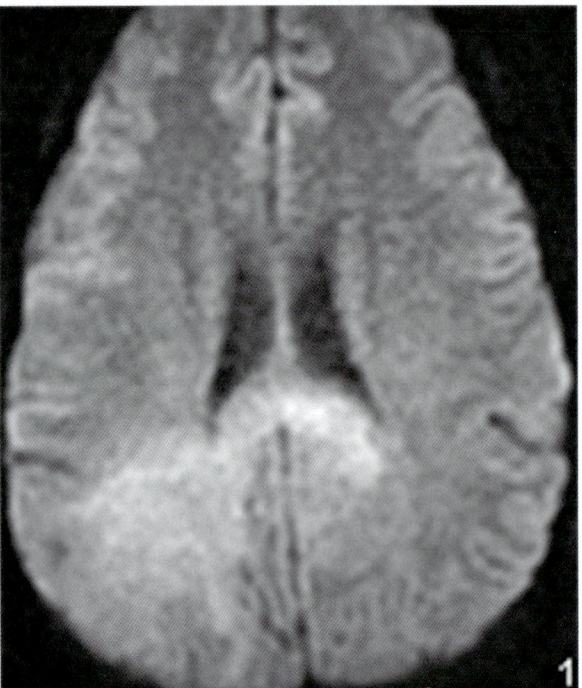

FIGURE 52-1

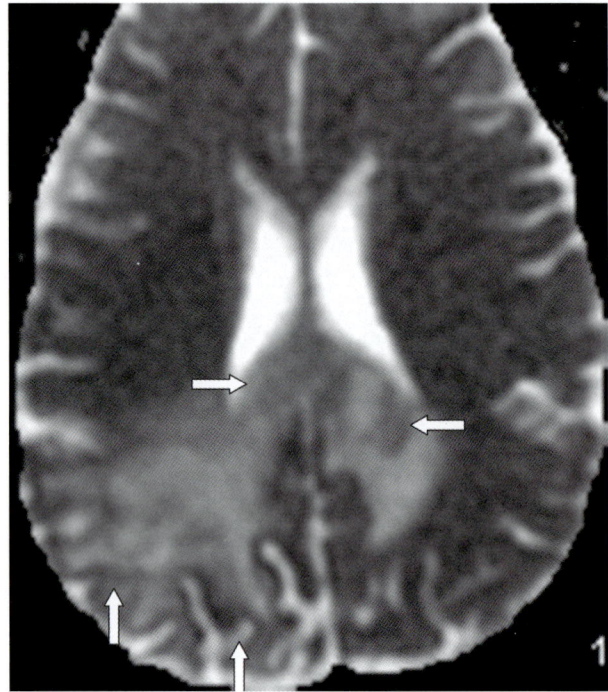

FIGURE 52-2

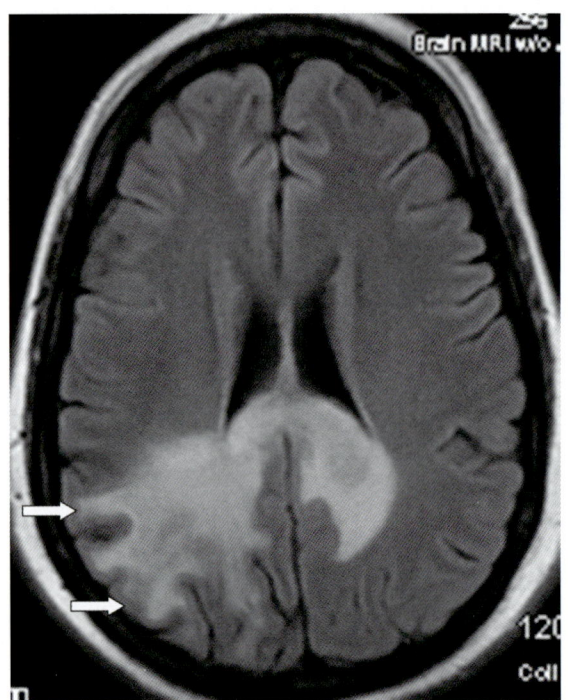

FIGURE 52-3

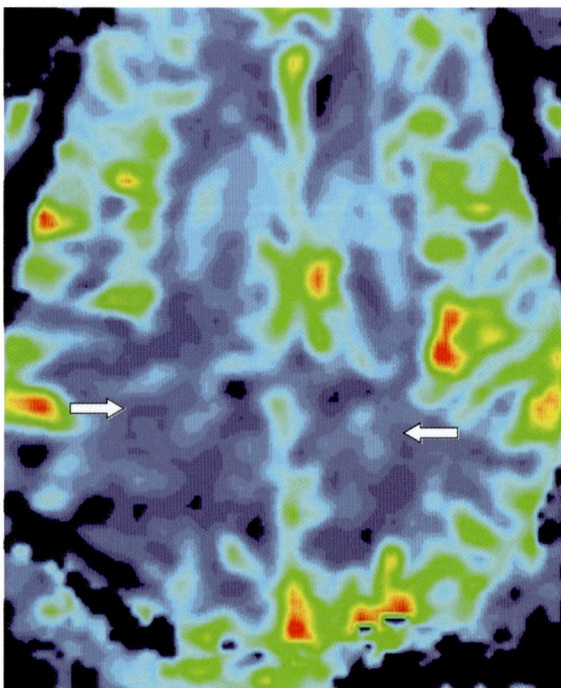

FIGURE 52-4

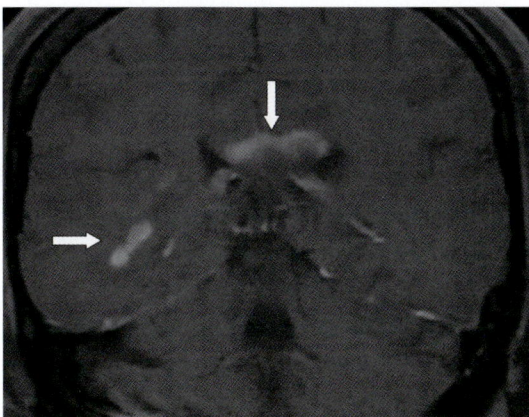

FIGURE 52-5

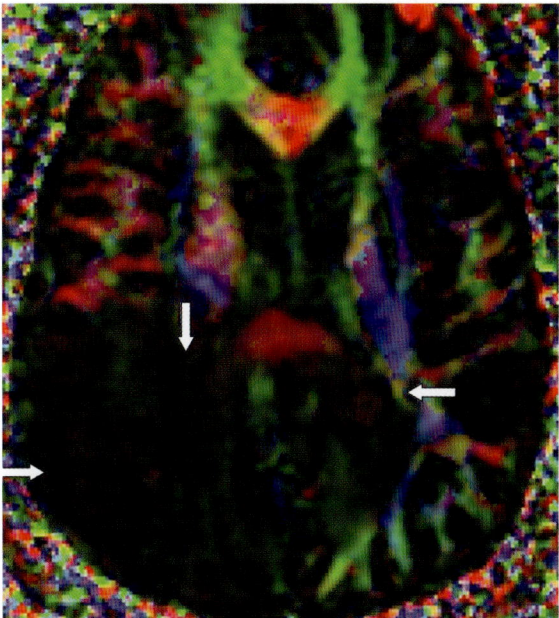

FIGURE 52-6

FINDINGS Figures 52-1 and 52-2. Axial DWI with ADC map through the corpus callosum (CC) and bilateral forceps major showing confluent asymmetric bilateral hyperintensity larger on the right than left crossing the splenium of the CC. There is involvement of the subcortical U fibers on the right (vertical arrows in Figure 52-2). Some areas of subtle restricted diffusion are seen within the splenium of CC (transverse arrows) in Figure 52-2. Figure 52-3. Axial FLAIR through the same level showing splenium and bilateral forceps major confluent hyperintensity surrounding isointense core extending into the subcortical region on the right (arrows). There is no significant mass effect. Figures 52-1 to 52-3 show enlargement of the splenium. Figure 52-4. Axial MRI perfusion relative Cerebral Blood volume (rCBV) map through the lesion showing low blood volume in the splenium and bilateral forceps major (arrows). Figure 52-5. Post-contrast coronal T1WI through the splenium showing patchy nodular contrast enhancement through the splenium and lateral to the right trigone (arrows). Figure 52-6. Axial DTI color orientation map through the splenium showing disruption of fiber tracts with reduced FA in the splenium, bilateral forceps major, and the right posterior corona radiata (arrows).

DIFFERENTIAL DIAGNOSIS Demyelinating process, lymphoma, butterfly glioma.

DIAGNOSIS Tumefactive demyelinating lesion (TDL).

DISCUSSION MR findings of demyelination include white matter (WM) T2 hyperintensity anywhere in the brain including the CC, minimal surrounding edema and mass effect, nodular, patchy, incomplete ring, and arc patterns of contrast enhancement on post-contrast T1WI. However, contrary to popular belief, TDL can be associated with mass effect and edema. Diffusion restriction could be subtle but not common and usually indicates acute lesions. Low relative blood volume and flow on perfusion studies have been

reported in demyelination. The definition of "tumefactive demyelination" is not consistent in the literature and may refer to various combinations of the following: WM location, large size (>2 cm), little mass effect or edema, and/or typical enhancement patterns (nodular, patchy, thin open or incomplete ring, heterogeneous). The butterfly pattern fits any of the listed differential diagnoses. Butterfly glioma tends to be necrotic and has a thick irregular ring contrast enhancement with surrounding large vasogenic edema and increased blood flow and volume on perfusion studies. Lymphoma on the other hand is highly cellular and may show restricted diffusion and avid contrast enhancement. Necrosis is not a component of lymphoma except in the setting of HIV. It has been suggested that NCCT may be able to differentiate TDL from GB and lymphoma on the basis of attenuation pattern on CT; lymphoma is usually hyperdense.

Cerebrospinal fluid (CSF) analysis prior to biopsy showed minimal increase in protein and an increase in IgG synthesis rate. There were no pleocytosis or oligoclonal bands. Bacterial, viral, and fungal studies were negative. MRI of the cervical and thoracic spine was normal. The diagnosis was made by stereotactic brain biopsy through the right parietal lesion. TDL of the central nervous system (CNS) can be solitary or multiple. In the presence of preexisting demyelinating lesions such as multiple sclerosis (MS) the diagnosis may be easy. Dissemination in time and space is necessary to convert to diagnosis of MS. Scrutinization of the history and prior imaging if available becomes important in this regard. TDL has been described rarely in association with astrocytoma. Solitary TDL has preceded the appearance of lymphoma, and therefore, longitudinal monitoring of single TDL is warranted.

Question for Further Thought

1. What other lesion could be confused with the histology of TDL?

Reporting Responsibilities

Direct reporting is required of a mass lesion. In the presence of a single solitary intracranial lesion suspicious for demyelination, imaging of the spinal cord should be recommended to exclude other lesions that could confirm presence of a demyelinating process elsewhere.

What the Treating Physician Needs to Know

- Is this a single lesion or are there other lesions that may suggest MS?

- Other imaging studies that may narrow the list of differential diagnosis include MR spectroscopy, MRI of the spinal cord, and MR of the orbits in the presence of visual disturbance to exclude other forms of demyelination

Answer

1. TDL may be misinterpreted as a neoplasm given its hypercellular nature and the frequent presence of atypical reactive astrocytes and mitotic figures.

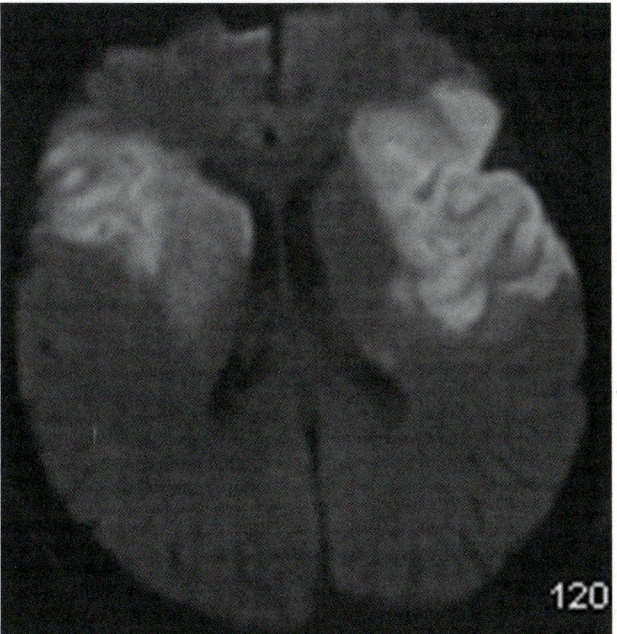

FIGURE 53-1

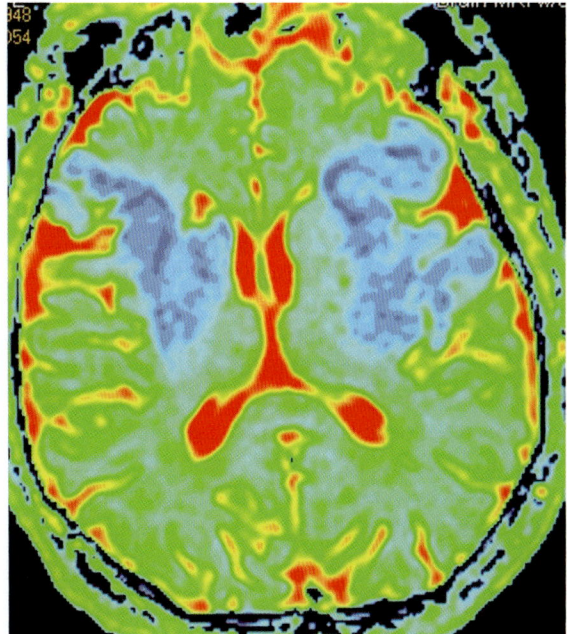

FIGURE 53-2

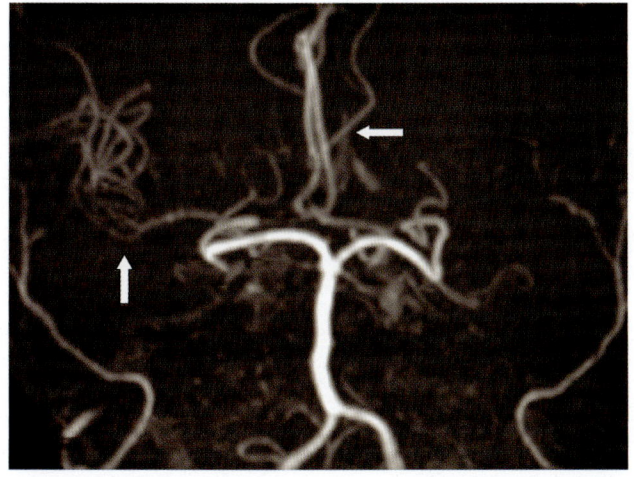

FIGURE 53-3

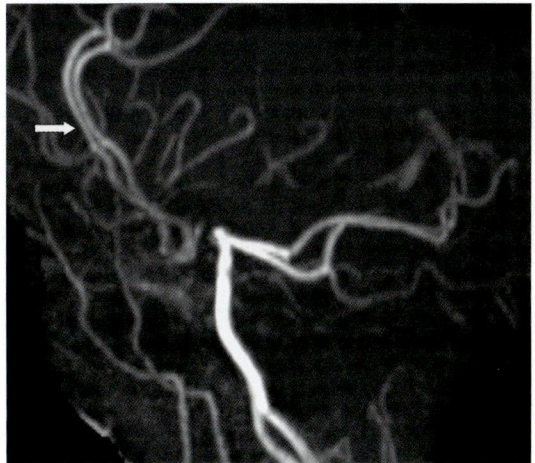

FIGURE 53-4

FINDINGS These images were obtained on the second day of admission. Day 1 images (not shown) showed a left perisylvian area of restricted diffusion. Figures 53-1 and 53-2. Axial DWI and corresponding ADC map through the lateral ventricles. There is bilateral perisylvian restricted diffusion. The right basal ganglia is involved, while the left posterior lentiform nucleus and the adjacent left corona radiata are involved as well. Inferior extension into the anterior temporal lobes (not shown) was present bilaterally. Figures 53-3 and 53-4. 3D time of flight MRA of the head obtained on day 1 showing nonvisualization of bilateral internal carotid arteries and the left middle cerebral artery (MCA). The right MCA (vertical arrow) is attenuated. Its occlusion is probably responsible for the new infarct on the right side. Bilateral anterior cerebral arteries (ACAs) (transverse arrows) show robust intensity.

DIFFERENTIAL DIAGNOSIS N/A.

DIAGNOSIS Bilateral MCA territory acute infarction.

DISCUSSION The classical MRI finding of acute/ subacute ischemic infarct is the restricted diffusion— hyperintense on DWI with low ADC. This becomes evident within the first 30 minutes before the FLAIR and T2WI changes are clearly visible. It may take up to 2 hours for FLAIR and T2WI changes to be seen. The initial mass effect is local. Simultaneous acute bilateral MCA territorial infarcts are unusual. CT may show hypodensity in the same locations. The MCA is the largest vascular territory in the brain and the most common location for infarcts. Embolic phenomenon tends to be common in the MCA territory since it receives a disproportionate share of the blood. Atherothrombotic changes and in this situation Internal carotid artery (ICA) occlusion are not uncommon.

There is a necessity to evaluate the neck vasculature either by CTA or by contrast MRA in this patient in order to prescribe appropriate management. Large MCA infarction has been found to be associated with cardiogenic embolism, ICA occlusion, and ICA dissection. Subsequent CTA of the neck revealed an occluded left ICA at origin with a (presumably recanalized) 95% stenosis of the right ICA origin. There appear to be significant collaterals to the MCA territory since only the perisylvian territories are affected despite occlusion of M1 on the left and significant disease on the right.

MCA infarcts present with aphasia, hemiparesis, mental status changes, and coma. The prognosis of a complete MCA territory stroke is very poor. Life-threatening MCA infarction, that is the so-called malignant infarction, occurs in up to 10% of all stroke patients with the main cause of death being severe edema leading to raised intracranial pressure, clinical deterioration, coma, and death. Brain swelling with mass effect develops rapidly and appears to peak within 5 days of the ictus. Uncal, subfalcine, and transtentorial herniations and hemorrhagic transformations are not uncommon complications. Large MCA infarction is a major predictor of death and severe disability.

Question for Further Thought

1. How does blood get to the ACAs despite complete occlusion of bilateral ICA?

Reporting Responsibilities

Direct reporting is always necessary in acute infarcts. Locations of infarcts, presence of mass effect, and hemorrhage should be mentioned. The vascular changes if MRA is obtained should be enumerated. MRA or CTA of the head and neck should be recommended if not already done.

What the Treating Physician Needs to Know

- Size and location of infarcts
- Complications such as mass effect, herniations, hydrocephalus, hemorrhage
- Complete MRA or CTA of the head and neck is necessary for evaluation of vascular structures

Answer

1. A patent circle of Willis (COW) ensures adequate compensation for occlusions. The posterior communicating arteries are present, thus routing blood from the posterior circulation to the ACA via the supraclinoid ICA. Anastomosis of the ECA and ICA via the ophthalmic artery is another route of blood from the extracranial circulation to the intracranial circulation. Other collateral circulations include the posterior/anterior pericallosal arteries around the splenium of CC and leptomeningeal collaterals not necessarily visualized in this case. Contrast-enhanced MRA or CTA may be useful in demonstrating these collaterals.

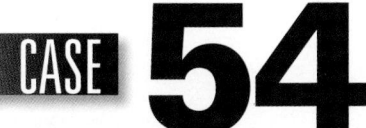
CLINICAL HISTORY *71-year-old male suddenly became bradycardic, hypoxic, and unresponsive following esophagoscopy to dislodge impacted meat.*

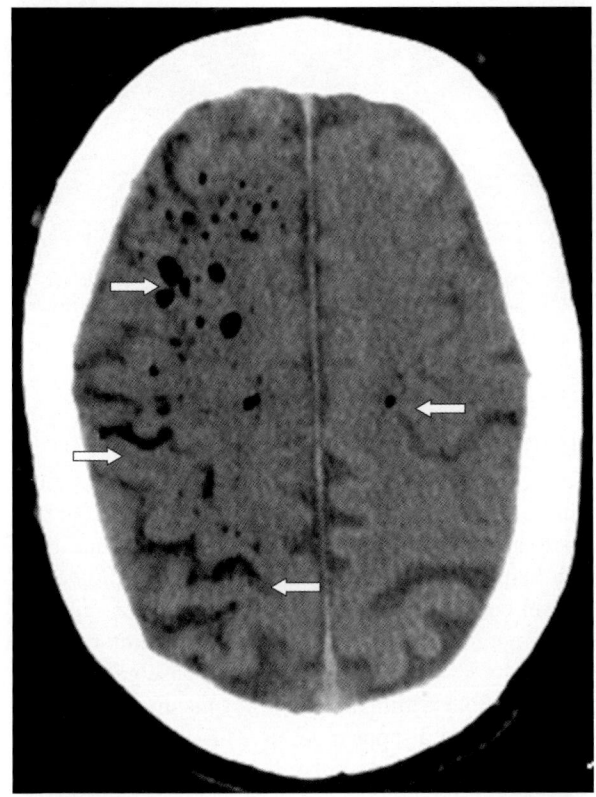

FIGURE 54-1

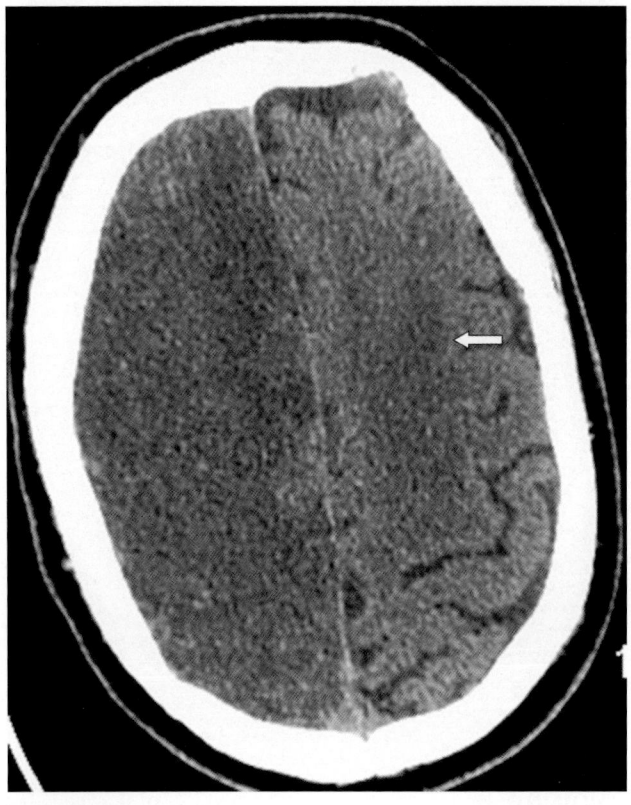

FIGURE 54-2

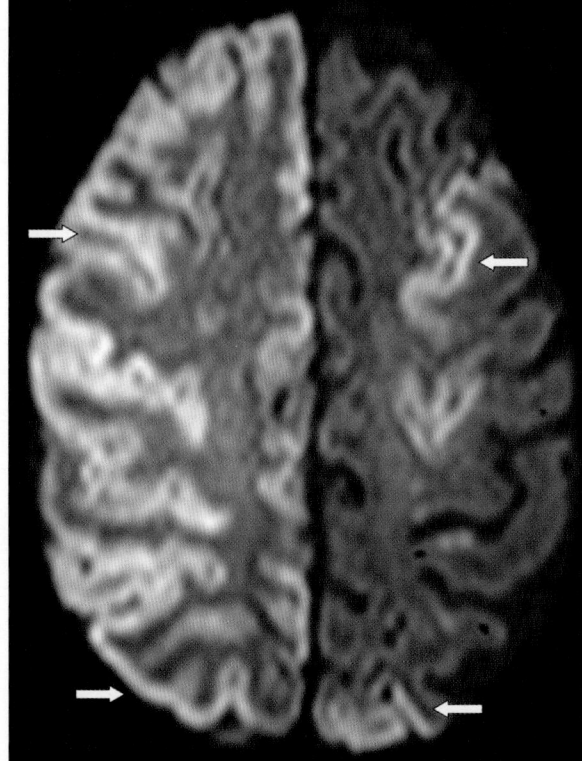

FIGURE 54-3

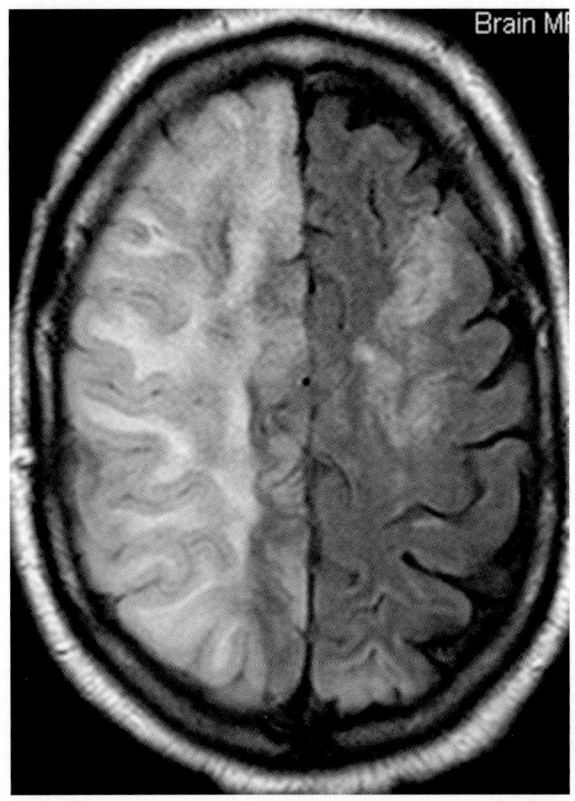

FIGURE 54-4

111

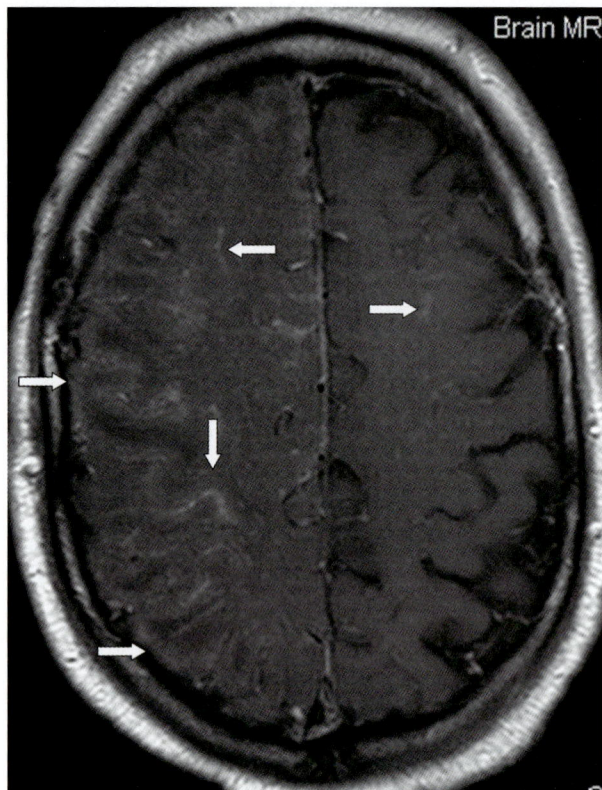

FIGURE 54-5

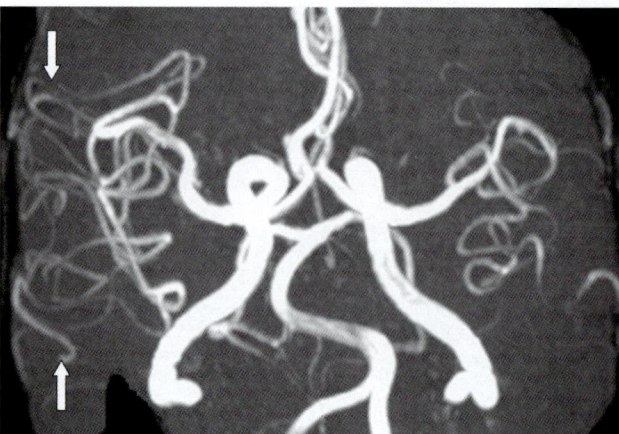

FIGURE 54-6

FINDINGS Figure 54-1. Axial NCCT through the centrum semiovale. There are multiple gas bubbles measuring up to −450 HU in the right cerebral parenchyma and within the right convexity sulci (arrows). Fewer similar gas bubbles are present in the left frontal lobe. Figure 54-2. Axial follow-up NCCT within 24 hours. There is resolution of the gas bubbles. There is diffuse right cerebral hemisphere hypodensity with no gray matter (GM)–white matter (WM) differentiation. There is effacement of the right convexity sulci. Similar but less prominent hypodensity is present in the left cerebral hemisphere (arrow). Figure 54-3. Axial DWI a few hours following Figure 54-2. There is extensive right hemispheric cortical ribbon hyperintensity consistent with cortical laminar necrosis (arrows). There is underlying WM smudgy hyperintensity. Similar but patchy changes are present in the left hemisphere. Figure 54-4. Axial FLAIR. There is smudgy right hemispheric hyperintensity with patchy changes on the left. Figure 54-5. Axial post-contrast T1WI. There is extensive right hemispheric linear sulcal and patchy parenchymal contrast enhancement with similar but less prominent changes on the left (arrows). Figure 54-6. 3D TOF MRA. There are more prominent right MCA territory branches (arrows) compared to the left suggesting increased right hemispheric perfusion.

DIFFERENTIAL DIAGNOSIS Gas embolus, fat embolus.

DIAGNOSIS Cerebral arterial gas embolism (CAGE).

DISCUSSION The hallmark of CAGE on NCCT is hypodense gas bubbles within the brain parenchymal measured in this instance −450 HU. The HU measurement differentiates gas from fat. There are also gas bubbles outlining the right hemispheric sulci presumably within leptomeningeal vessels or subarachnoid space (SAS). There appears to be a preponderant involvement of the right cerebral hemisphere by CAGE in the literature. These gas bubbles are usually visible within a very short time after the occurrence. They tend to disappear within 24 hours at which time the affected cerebral hemisphere becomes hypodense with mass effect consistent with cerebral swelling and infarctions. DWI demonstrates gyriform cortical ribbon hyperintensity consistent with cortical laminar necrosis with underlying WM edema visualized on FLAIR and T2WI. Diffuse mass effect is present. Contrast enhancement both within the sulci and brain parenchyma is in keeping with blood–brain barrier breakdown.

CAGE is a rare complication of endoscopy and has been reported following upper gastrointestinal (GI) endoscopy of various types. CAGE has variable clinical presentations which include altered mental status, confusion, headache, dizziness, seizures, visual field defect, and coma during or shortly after the procedure. Autopsy report has demonstrated edematous brain with changes of diffuse hypoxic ischemic damage at microscopy. Brain herniations have also been reported. There is no evidence-based treatment since very few cases have been reported. The recommended treatment is administration of hyperbaric oxygen (HBO2). This patient had six HBO2 therapy treatments but did not regain consciousness.

Question for Further Thought

1. How does air get into the cerebral arterial circulation during endoscopy?

Reporting Responsibilities

This is an acute event that requires direct reporting. Immediate HBO2 administration has been suggested as life-saving.

What the Treating Physician Needs to Know

- Location of the air bubbles
- Presence or otherwise of brain swelling or herniations

Answer

1. Gas entry into the circulation requires an open vessel and a pressure gradient. The presence of severed veins at the site of the procedure coupled with high pressure gas insufflation allows gas to enter the venous circulation into the right atrium. Presence of intraatria shunt allows gas into the arterial circulation and onward propagation to the brain and other organs. It is also suggested that in the absence of intraatrial shunt, overwhelming amount of pulmonary venous gas in excess of 30 mL could result in systemic arterial gas embolism. Echocardiogram did not reveal intraatrial shunt in this patient. A patent foramen ovale is present in 33% of the normal population until the third decade and in 27% in all age groups.

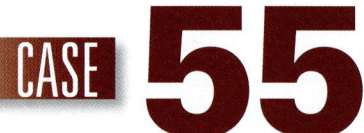
CLINICAL HISTORY *28-year-old female with postpartum headache. She was readmitted 4 days later following seizure at home.*

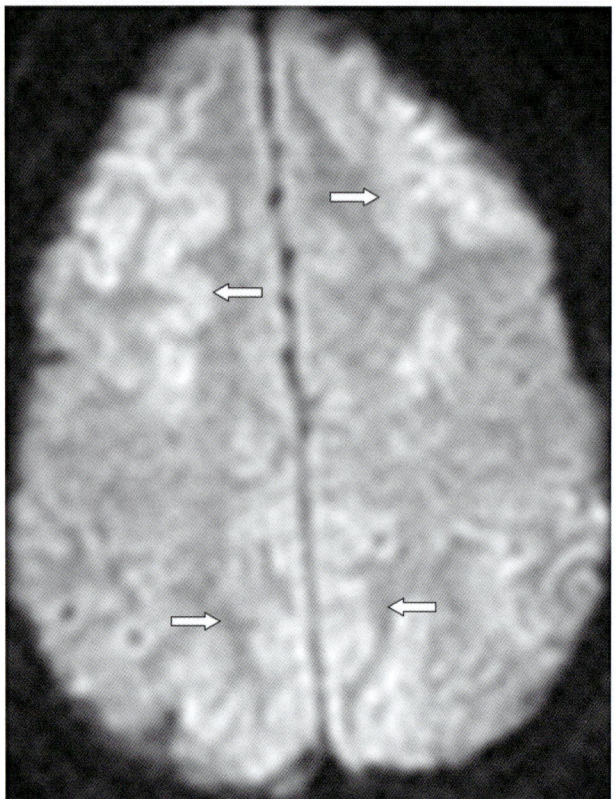

FIGURE 55-1

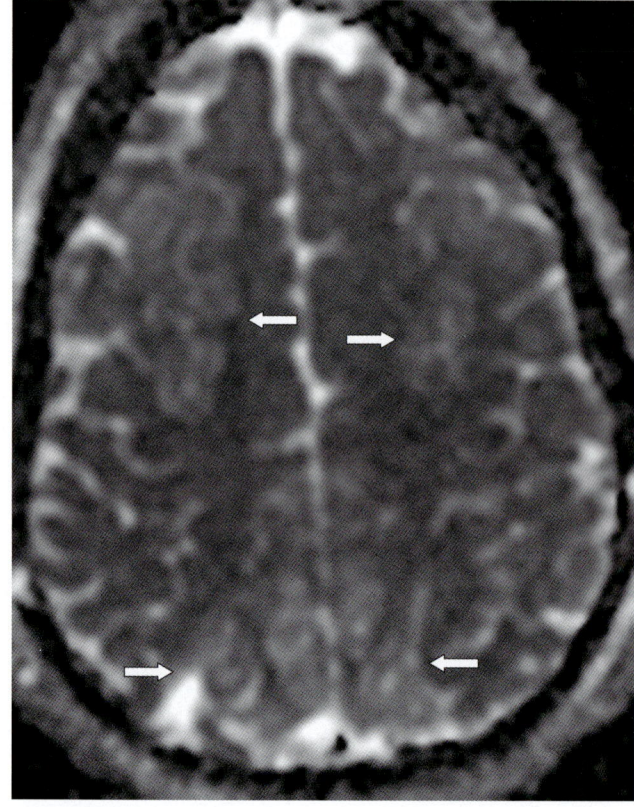

FIGURE 55-2

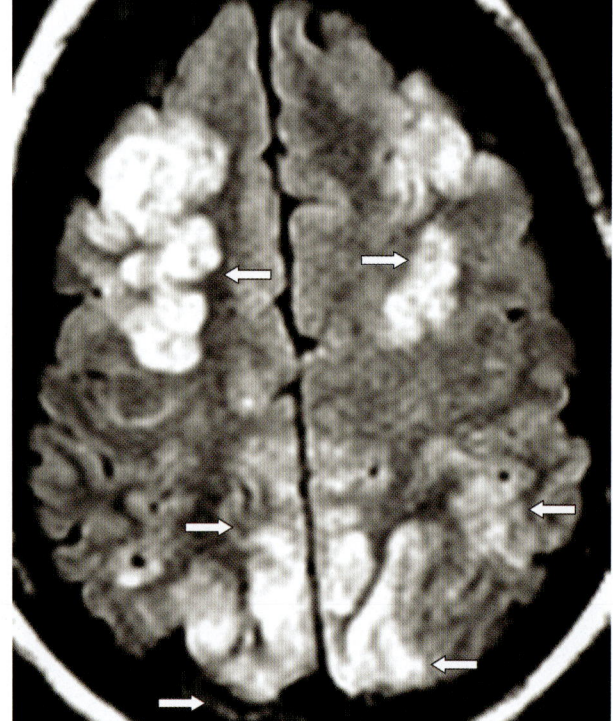

FIGURE 55-3

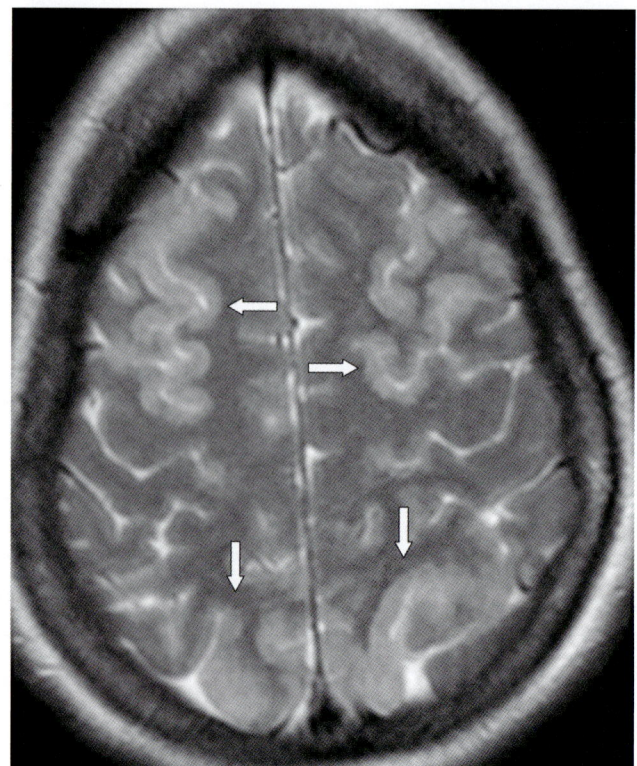

FIGURE 55-4

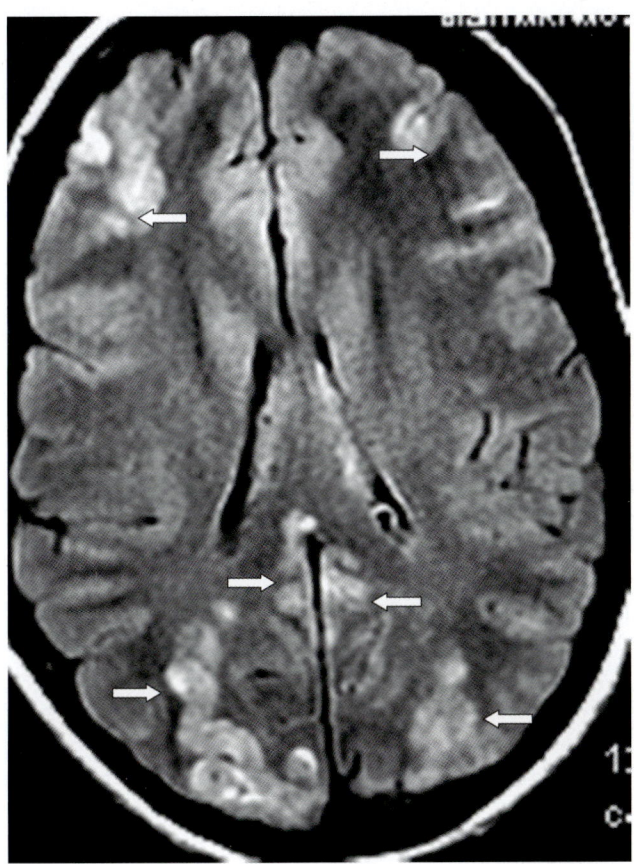

FIGURE 55-5

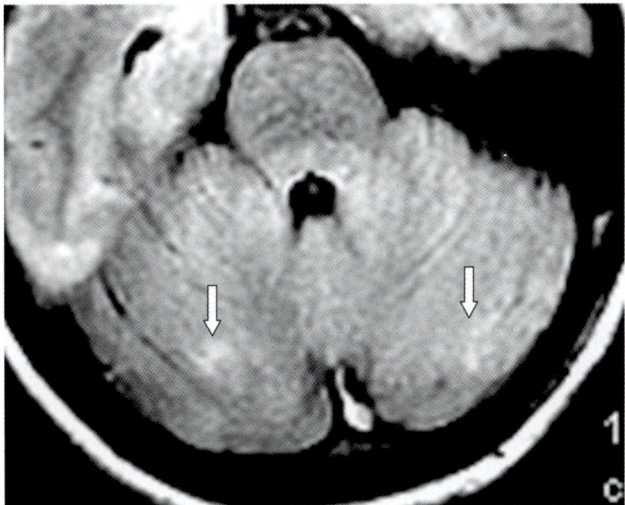

FIGURE 55-6

FINDINGS Figures 55-1. Axial DWI through the upper centrum semiovale showing patchy bilateral almost symmetrical frontoparietal cortical hyperintensity with corresponding ADC hyperintensity in Figure 55-2 (arrows). Figures 55-3 and 55-4. Axial FLAIR and T2WI, respectively, through same level confirm cortical patchy hyperintensity with mild effacement of sulci in the involved areas consistent with cortical swelling (arrows). Subcortical U fibers are intact. Figure 55-5. Axial FLAIR through the lateral ventricles. There is almost symmetrical cortical ribbon multifocal hyperintensity in bilateral frontal and parieto-occipital lobes (arrows). Temporal lobes (not shown) are also involved. Figure 55-6. Axial FLAIR through the cerebellum. There is patchy bilateral almost symmetrical cerebellar hyperintensity (arrows). Subtle changes are also present in the bilateral brachium pontes and tegmentum. Follow-up MRI 4 months after these images demonstrated complete resolution of the lesions.

DIFFERENTIAL DIAGNOSIS Posterior reversible encephalopathy syndrome (PRES), multifocal watershed subacute infarcts, multifocal cortical edema, acute demyelinating encephalomyelitis (ADEM), cerebral venous sinus thrombosis.

DIAGNOSIS Posterior reversible encephalopathy syndrome (PRES).

DISCUSSION The most important diagnostic workup for PRES is imaging. NCCT shows diffuse hypodense areas in subcortical and cortical bilateral temporal occipital and parietal lobes. MRI lesions of PRES appear as bilateral cortical and/or subcortical iso- or hypointensities on T1WI and hyperintensities on T2WI and FLAIR predominantly posteriorly in the temporal, occipital, and parietal lobes. Bilateral frontal lobes particularly superiorly are also affected as in this patient. The parietal or occipital lobes are involved in 98% of cases, frontal lobes (68%), the temporal lobes (40%), and the cerebellar hemispheres (30%). A bilateral and symmetrical appearance is highly typical. DWI generally show increase diffusion consistent with vasogenic edema. Occasional areas of restricted diffusion indicate ischemic changes. The lack of restricted diffusion in the classical areas tends to exclude multifocal watershed infarcts. Hemorrhages, ischemic lesions, and contrast enhancement are unusual but do occur in a small percentage of patients. Perfusion imaging may show a reduction in relative Cerebral Blood Volume (rCBV) and Cerebral Blood Flow (CBF) consistent with hypoperfusion. MR spectroscopy may show increase choline and creatine peaks with decreased N-acetyl aspartate (NAA). MRA and MRV are normal, thus excluding vasculopathy and venous sinus thrombosis. However, there has been some angiographic demonstration of vascular irregularities and string-of-bead appearance that may suggest some form of vasculopathy.

The clinical presentation of PRES includes headache, confusion, visual impairment, nausea, vomiting, and seizures. Other findings include status epilepticus, focal neurologic deficits, cerebellar syndrome, and coma. PRES triggers include arterial hypertension in the classic setting of hypertensive encephalopathy, eclampsia or pre-eclampsia, chemotherapy agents such as cisplatin and methotrexate, immunosuppressant such as cyclosporine and tacrolimus in organ transplant patients, septicemia and severe infections, chronic renal failure and dialysis, autoimmune diseases such as systemic lupus erythematosus (SLE), scleroderma, and

Wegener's granulomatosis. Moderately to severely elevated blood pressure is reported in 75% of patients.

The pathophysiology of PRES is poorly understood. These include (1) a breakdown of cerebral autoregulation due to a rapid rise in blood pressure leading to disruption of the blood–brain barrier, (2) endothelial dysfunction due to circulating toxins which is more pertinent for triggers such as cytotoxic and immunosuppressive drugs, sepsis, and autoimmune disease and pre-eclampsia, and (3) focal vasospasm leading to decreased blood flow and ischemia with resultant edema. Usually all blood tests are normal. Cerebrospinal fluid (CSF) may be normal or have a slightly raised protein level. Abnormal blood tests when they occur are nonspecific for PRES and may reflect underlying pathology. Laboratory evidence of endothelial injury with thrombocytopenia, red cell fragmentation with schistocyte formation and increased lactate dehydrogenase may be present especially in pre-eclampsia/eclampsia.

Management usually consists of removal and/or treatment of triggers, airways support, and seizure control. Complete recovery is the rule unless there are complications. Complications may include infarcts, hydrocephalus, and unabated seizures. Epilepsy has been reported as a long-term complication in a few cases. Recurrent forms of PRES have been reported in about 10% of cases.

Questions for Further Thought

1. What is the reason of the parieto-occipital predilection of PRES on imaging?

2. What is the relationship between PRES and NMO antibodies?

Reporting Responsibilities

PRES is an emergency and requires direct reporting of findings to the referring physician to allow prompt withdrawal or treatment of any known triggers.

What the Treating Physician Needs to Know

- MRI is the definitive imaging investigation of PRES
- Atypical imaging features include involvement of the basal ganglia, deep white matter and splenium of the corpus callosum, isolated brainstem lesions, and unilateral involvement. Hydrocephalus can complicate swelling in the posterior fossa

Answers

1. The predominance of posterior involvement is explained on the basis of poor sympathetic innervation of these lobes and the posterior fossa structures.
2. The increased occurrence of PRES in patients with Neuromyelitis optica (NMO) and positive aquaporine-4 (AQP4) water channel autoantibodies have led to hypothesis that an alteration in water flux due to AQP4 autoimmunity may predispose to PRES. There is no proof of this yet.

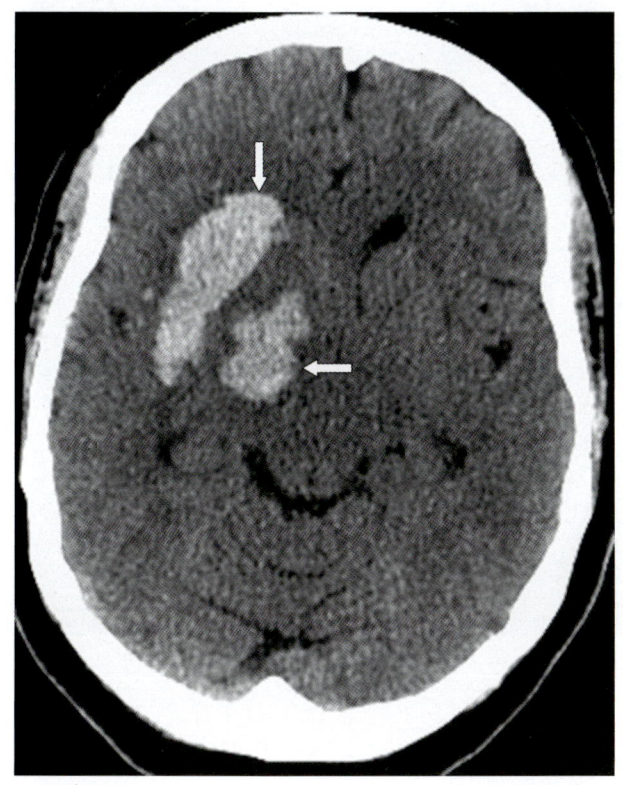

FIGURE 56-1

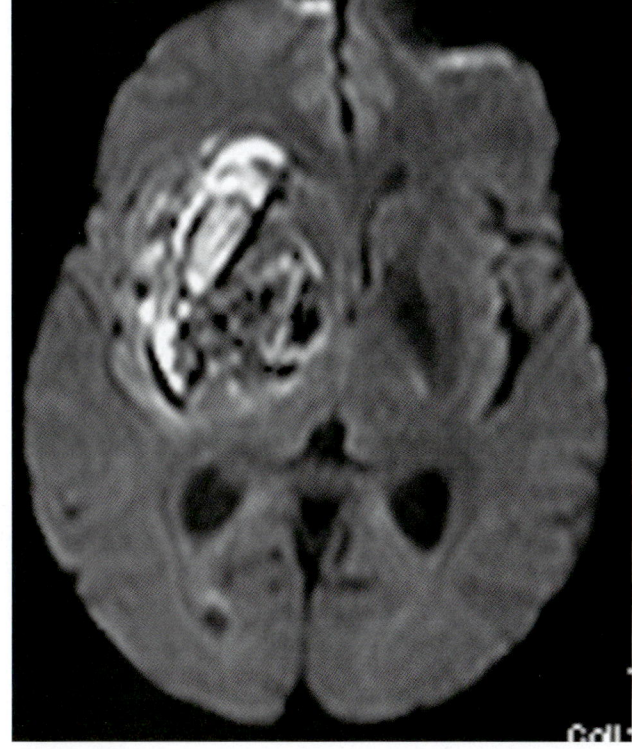

FIGURE 56-2

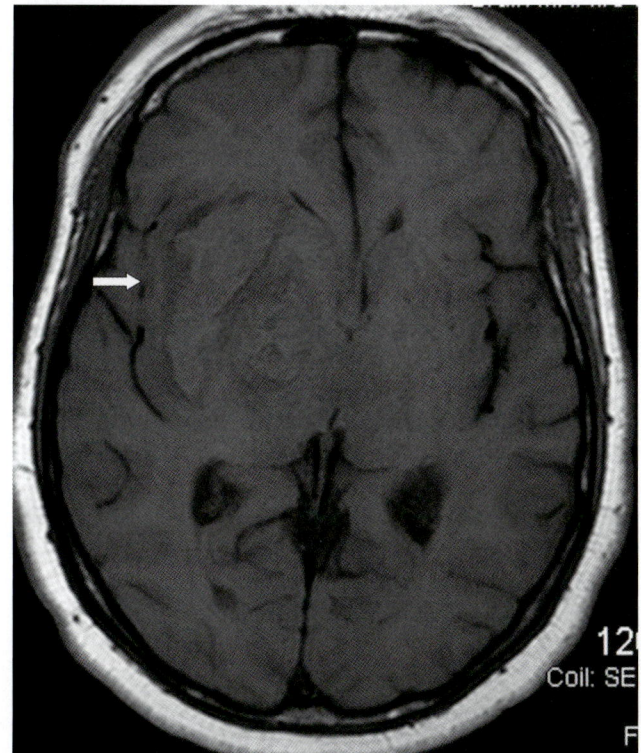

FIGURE 56-3

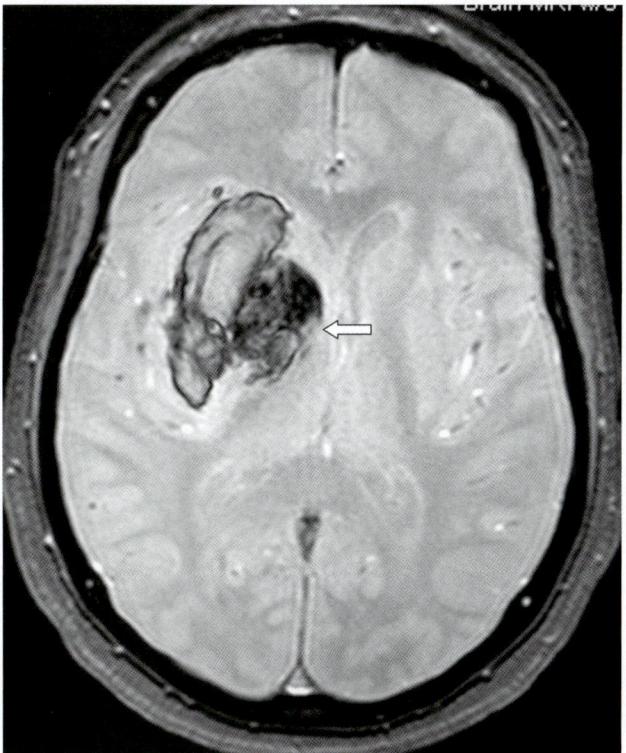

FIGURE 56-4

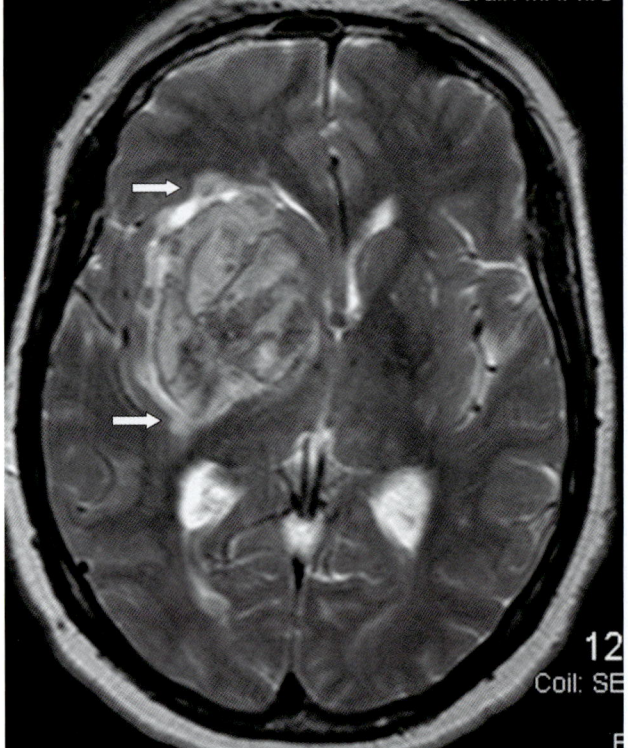

FIGURE 56-5

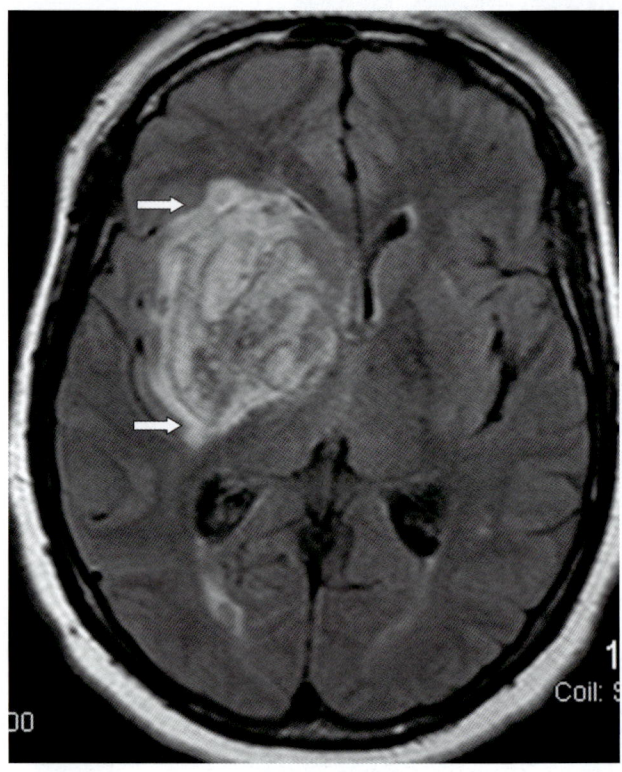

FIGURE 56-6

FINDINGS Figure 56-1. Axial NCCT through the basal ganglia. There are two hyperdense masses in the right basal ganglia, one in the right globus pallidus (transverse arrow) and the larger lateral one straddles the putamen and external capsule (vertical arrow). Both communicate superiorly (not shown). There is effacement of the right frontal horn due to mass effect. Figure 56-2. Axial DWI through the basal ganglia. There is heterogeneous area of restricted diffusion in the right basal ganglia. Figure 56-3. Axial T1WI through the basal ganglia. The right basal ganglia mass is mainly isointense with thin surrounding hypointense halo. There is effacement of the right sylvian fissure (arrow). Figure 56-4. Axial GRE through the basal ganglia. There is heterogeneous blooming of the mass (arrow). Figures 56-5 and 56-6. Axial T2WI and FLAIR through the mass. The mass has similar heterogeneous pattern of mixed hyperintensity and isointensity with local mass effect and midline shift. There is mild surrounding hyperintensity consistent with vasogenic edema (arrows).

DIFFERENTIAL DIAGNOSIS N/A.

DIAGNOSIS Acute hypertensive right basal ganglia hematoma.

DISCUSSION CT remains the fastest and the most efficient way to image acute bleed. The NCCT obtained within hours of the ictus shows a homogeneous hyperdense mass typical of acute hemorrhage. Fluid levels can occur in the hyperacute stage or if a bleed occurs into an existing mass. Acute bleed could be hypodense in the anemic patient since the density is due to the hemoglobin protein. Presence of mass effect depends on the size of the hematoma. The basal ganglia are one of the classical locations of hypertensive hematoma. Other locations include the brainstem, thalamus, and the cerebellum. However, up to 20% of hypertensive hematoma occurs elsewhere in the brain outside these primary areas. MRI is useful for further characterization of the hemorrhage and to visualize presence of associated lesions such as microhemorrhages, lacunar infarcts, and white matter (WM) changes that may not have been well characterized by CT. The MRI pattern of hematoma depends on the age of the hematoma primarily due to the state of the hemoglobin. In this case, MRI was obtained within 24 hours of the ictus, and the pattern is somewhere between the hyperacute and acute stages. The typical hyperacute hematoma contains intracellular oxyhemoglobin which has diamagnetic property and is hyperintense on T2WI and hypointense on T1WI. The acute hematoma contains intracellular deoxyhemoglobin with paramagnetic property. It is hypointense on T2WI and GRE and isointense on T1WI. Usually in the hyperacute/acute stages, surrounding edema and mass effect begin to develop. If the hematoma is large enough, it may result in herniations and dissect into the ventricles. Hydrocephalus is a complication of intraventricular hemorrhage (IVH).

Chronic hypertension is the most common cause of primary nontraumatic intracerebral hematoma (PICH) with the location mostly central in the brain. Other causes of PICH include amyloid angiopathy, mostly subcortical in location. Use of street drugs such as cocaine, amphetamines, and other stimulants can cause intracerebral hematoma (ICH). The classic clinical presentation of acute hemorrhage is that of acute neurologic deficits, mental status changes, and coma. This patient has a history of hypertension, hyperlipidemia, coronary artery disease, and diabetes mellitus type 2. The basis for hypertensive bleed remains debated. It is generally believed that chronic hypertension results in intimal hyperplasia and hyalinization of the end or penetrating arteries in the brainstem, cerebellum, thalamus, and basal ganglia. These hyalinized vessels become narrow predisposing to necrosis and formation of small pseudoaneurysms known as Charcot-Bouchard aneurysms. These aneurysms rupture giving rise to hemorrhage. The hemorrhage is interstitial in location splitting tissue; hence, the appearance is more often ovoid and linear than round. The prognosis depends on size and location with brainstem lesions generally fairing the worst.

Question for Further Thought

1. What are the MRI changes in subacute and chronic hematoma?

Reporting Responsibilities

Direct reporting is essential. Complications such as mass effect, herniations, IVH, or subarachnoid hemorrhage (SAH) should be reported.

What the Treating Physician Needs to Know

- Location and size of hematoma
- Complications
- Associated lesions such as WM changes, microhemorrhages and their location, and other suspicious signs of secondary intracerebral hematoma (SICH)
- Further evaluation by MRA or CTA in the appropriate situation

Answer

1. Early subacute ICH contains methemoglobin within the red cells resulting in hypointensity on T2WI and GRE and hyperintensity on T1WI. The mass effect is persistent. The late subacute stage has extracellular methemoglobin resulting in hyperintensity on all sequences. It may begin to show peripheral contrast enhancement. Chronic hematoma contains mostly ferritin, and hemosiderin which are isointense to hypointense on all sequences. The edema and mass effect have resolved with a central cleft mainly containing cerebrospinal fluid (CSF) or residual methemoglobin.

CLINICAL HISTORY *40-year-old female with right-sided weakness.*

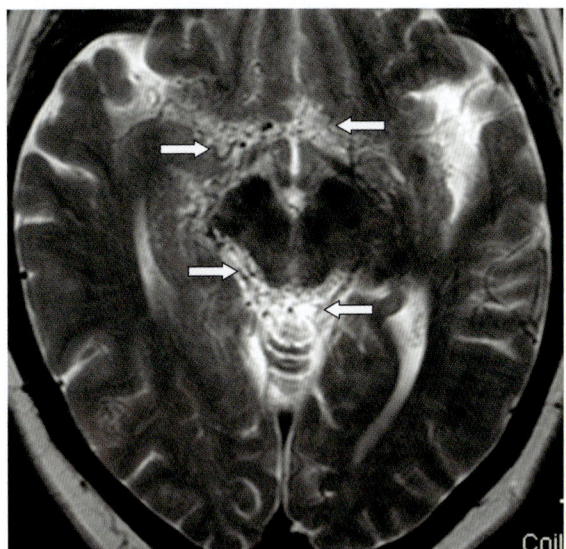

FIGURE 57-1

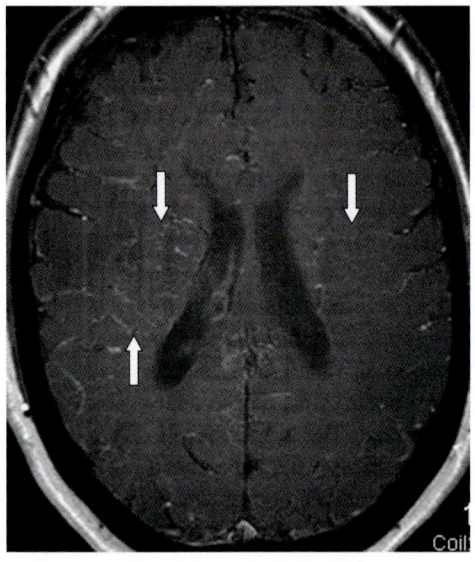

FIGURE 57-2

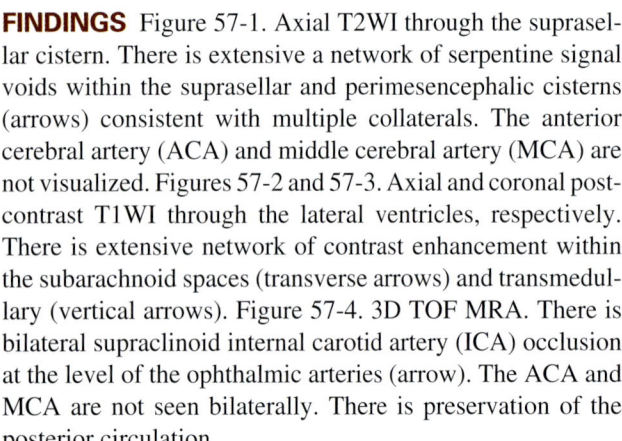

FIGURE 57-3

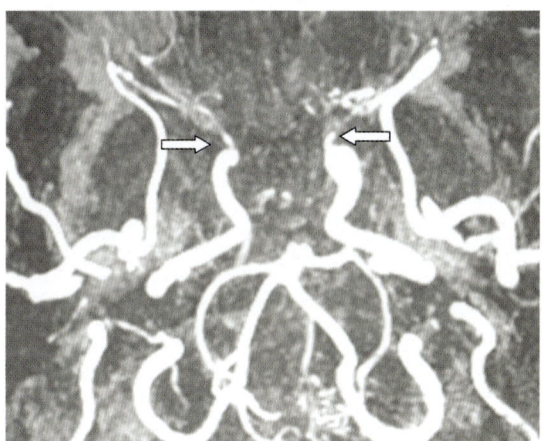

FIGURE 57-4

FINDINGS Figure 57-1. Axial T2WI through the suprasellar cistern. There is extensive a network of serpentine signal voids within the suprasellar and perimesencephalic cisterns (arrows) consistent with multiple collaterals. The anterior cerebral artery (ACA) and middle cerebral artery (MCA) are not visualized. Figures 57-2 and 57-3. Axial and coronal postcontrast T1WI through the lateral ventricles, respectively. There is extensive network of contrast enhancement within the subarachnoid spaces (transverse arrows) and transmedullary (vertical arrows). Figure 57-4. 3D TOF MRA. There is bilateral supraclinoid internal carotid artery (ICA) occlusion at the level of the ophthalmic arteries (arrow). The ACA and MCA are not seen bilaterally. There is preservation of the posterior circulation.

DIFFERENTIAL DIAGNOSIS N/A.

DIAGNOSIS Moyamoya disease (MMD).

DISCUSSION The classical finding in MMD is the bilateral supraclinoid ICA occlusion with preservation of the posterior circulation. To compensate for the occlusions, there is development of a rich network of collaterals at the base of the brain, within the basal ganglia and thalami, in the subarachnoid spaces and transmedullary within the cerebral WM seen as multiple serpentine network of vessels, leptomeningeal enhancement, and transmedullary streaky contrast enhancement on CT and MRI as demonstrated in this case. Prominent sulcal linear hyperintensity on FLAIR which represents leptomeningeal collaterals is known as "ivy sign." The classical DSA findings in MMD are those of intracranial ICA occlusions with prominent collaterals at the base of brain likened to "something hazy, like a puff of cigarette smoke," which, in Japanese, translates into moyamoya. Transdural collaterals from extracranial circulation are usually present. The posterior circulation is usually intact. MRA and CTA demonstrate the occlusion of the ICA but may not demonstrate the "puff of smoke" as reliably as DSA. The occlusion or in some cases severe stenosis could be unilateral with eventual bilaterality of lesions in most cases. Complications include subarachnoid and parenchymal cerebral hemorrhage (hyperdense on CT) due to rupture of the fragile collaterals. Ischemic infarcts, hypodense parenchymal lesions on CT, and hyperintense DWI and FLAIR/T2WI lesions on MRI are also common due to the arterial occlusions. Aneurysms are also common.

There are two peaks for the occurrence of MMD at age of 5 years and in the mid-40s. It is more common in women than men. MMD is more common in Asian population but has been described in people of all races. Down syndrome, sickle cell disease, and cranial radiation particularly for pituitary and parapituitary lesions present special risk factors. Headache, transient ischemic attack (TIA), seizures, movement disorders, mental status changes, and focal neurologic deficits are some of its presenting features. An ophthalmologic finding occasionally seen in association with moyamoya is the "morning glory disk," an enlargement of the optic disk with concomitant retinovascular anomalies. Six grades of MMD have been recognized. There is no known cure, but revascularization surgery has been promising.

Question for Further Thought

1. What is moyamoya syndrome?

Reporting Responsibilities

Direct reporting is necessary in view of the vascular occlusions. Complications when present should be categorized.

What the Treating Physician Needs to Know

- The pattern of intracranial arterial occlusions
- Presence or otherwise of subarachnoid and parenchymal hemorrhages

Answer

1. Patients with supraclinoid ICA occlusion and associated risk factors (Down syndrome, sickle cell disease, and cranial radiation) are said to have moyamoya syndrome while those without associated risk factors are regarded as having moyamoya disease. Those with unilateral findings have the moyamoya syndrome, even if they do not have other associated risk factors.

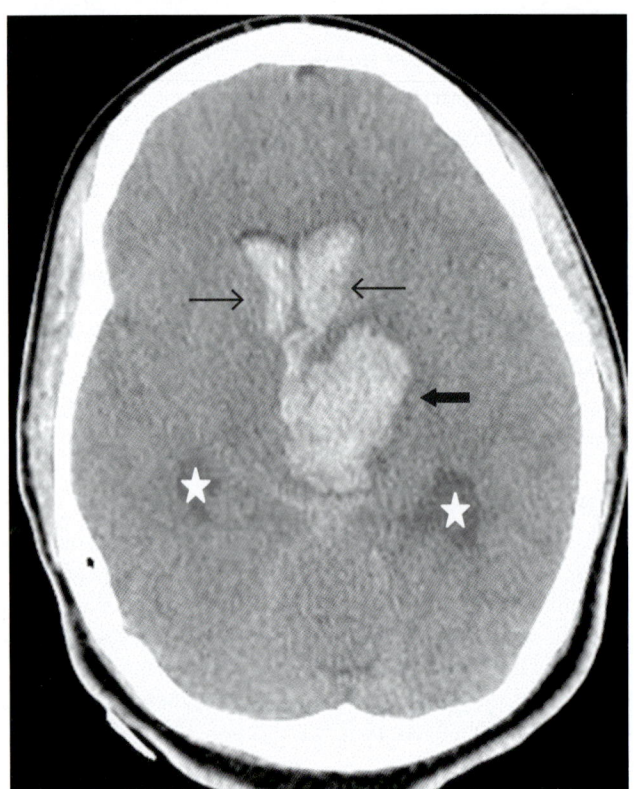

FIGURE 58-1

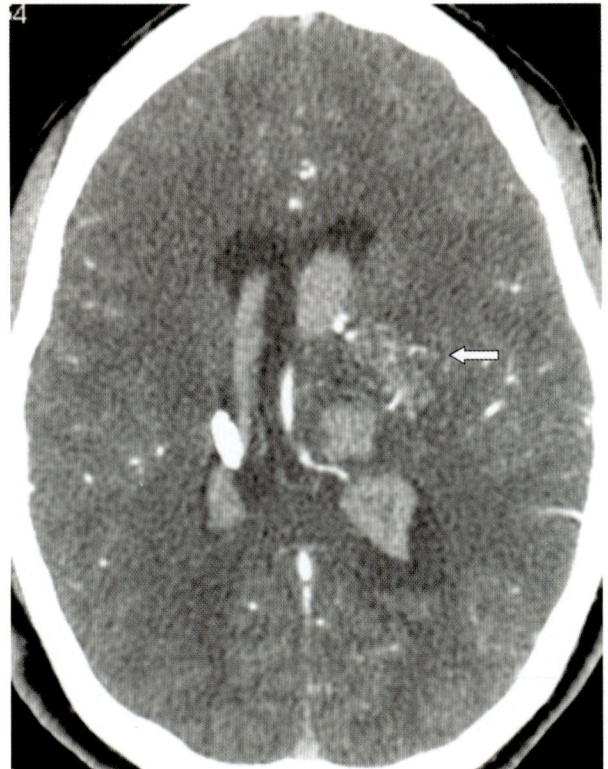

FIGURE 58-2

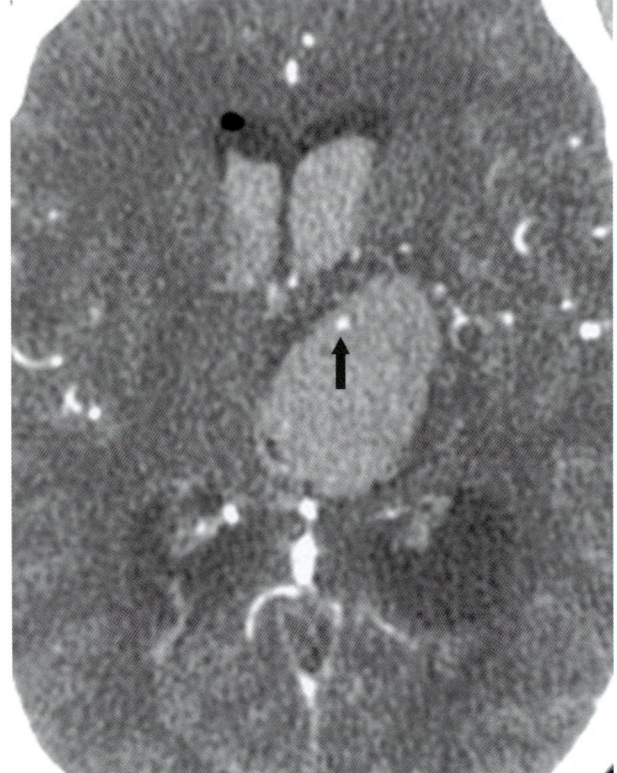

FIGURE 58-3

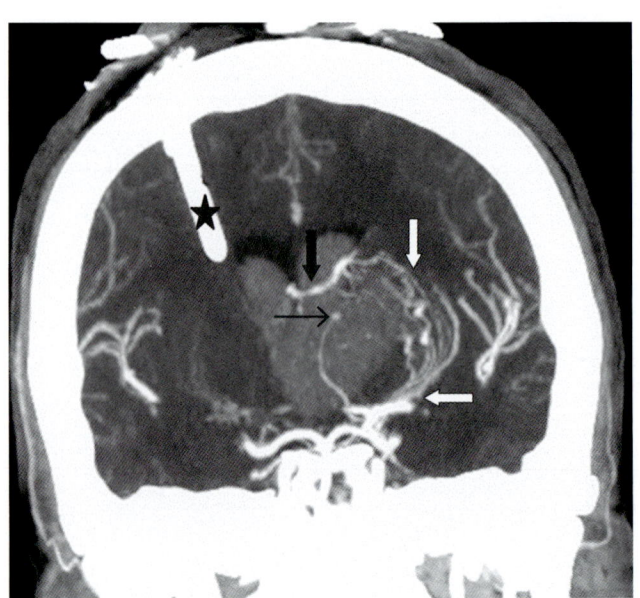

FIGURE 58-4

FINDINGS Figure 58-1. Axial NCCT through the thalami. There is a large left thalamic well-defined homogeneous hyperdensity consistent with acute hematoma with surrounding hypodense halo (black arrow)—edema. There is similar hyperdensity within the dilated bilateral frontal horns of the lateral ventricles (line arrows) consistent with intraventricular hemorrhage. Bilateral trigones are dilated (stars) consistent with hydrocephalus. There is effacement of all convexity subarachnoid spaces due to increased intracranial pressure. Figure 58-2. Axial head CTA source image through the lateral ventricles. There is irregular contrast enhancement (arrow) in the left basal ganglia just lateral to the superior aspect of the left thalamic hematoma. The lateral ventricles are dilated with intraventricular hemorrhage. Figure 58-3. Axial CTA source image through the hematoma showing a focal peripheral contrast enhancement (arrow)—the so-called spot sign. Figure 58-4. Coronal CTA MIP through the basal ganglia. There is a left basal ganglia collection of vessels-a nidus (vertical white arrow) just laterally to the left thalamic hematoma fed by multiple left lenticulostriate arteries (transverse white arrow) and draining via a large thalamostriate vein (black vertical arrow). There is an isolated large arterial branch, a thalamoperforator, traced to the left posterior communicating artery within the left thalamic hematoma with a small rounded end corresponding to the "spot sign" (line arrow) possibly a microaneurysm. A right transfrontal external ventricular drain is present (star).

DIFFERENTIAL DIAGNOSIS N/A.

DIAGNOSIS Left thalamic hematoma with spot sign (associated basal ganglia arteriovenous malformation [AVM]).

DISCUSSION The thalamus is a common location for primary intracerebral hematoma (PICH) of hypertensive origin. The CT demonstrates the classical hyperdense mass of acute hematoma in the left thalamus with surrounding edema and dissection into the ventricles. Hypertensive hematomas are more common in the elderly. Elderly patients are often considered unlikely to harbor secondary vascular causes for hematoma and they may not be investigated. However, in the young, parenchymal hematoma anywhere should be considered secondary (SICH) and investigated for treatable causes such as AVM, aneurysm, cerebral cavernous malformation (CCM), neoplasm, coagulopathy, or infection. CTA in this situation demonstrates an AVM in the adjacent left basal ganglia. A "spot sign" is also demonstrated

in the hematoma. The classical "spot sign" is a 1- to 2-mm hyperdense focus on CTA source images usually located peripherally within the hematoma. The spot sign has been associated with hematoma expansion which is very predictive of neurologic deterioration in primary ICH. Hematoma expansion is an independent predictor of mortality and morbidity. About 30% of PICH undergo expansion. Enlargement of the spot sign on post-contrast CT following a CTA has been suggested as representing active extravasation which is also predictive of hematoma expansion. It is interesting that the spot sign in this hematoma is located peripherally within the hematoma at the end of a single thalamoperforator which does not appear to have any link to the basal ganglia AVM. "Spot sign mimics" have been described in SICH due to neoplastic calcification, micro AVM, pseudoaneurysms, and aneurysms. About 20% of SICH undergo expansion.

Question for Further Thought

1. What is the basis of the "spot sign"?

Reporting Responsibilities

Acute hematoma requires direct reporting. The complications should be categorized and reported accordingly.

What the Treating Physician Needs to Know

- Size and location of the parenchymal hematoma
- Complications such as intraventricular hemorrhage (IVH), subarachnoid hemorrhage (SAH), mass effect, and hydrocephalus
- Enumeration of arterial feeders and venous outflow on CTA to the AVM
- Presence of the spot sign or extravasation if visible
- If follow up, is there expansion of the hematoma?
- All hematoma in the young should be aggressively investigated

Answer

1. It is not clear whether the "spot sign" represents a primary or a secondary phenomenon in primary ICH. Presence of a primary phenomenon such as pseudoaneurysm, amyloid-related microaneurysms, and Charcot-Bouchard aneurysms in hypertension has been debated for years. The peripheral location of the "spot sign" in most PICH may suggest a secondary phenomenon such as vascular injury; torn or stretched vessel. "Spot sign" mimics have been demonstrated in secondary ICH.

CLINICAL HISTORY *1-day-old baby with in-utero diagnosis of a complex left temporal lobe mass.*

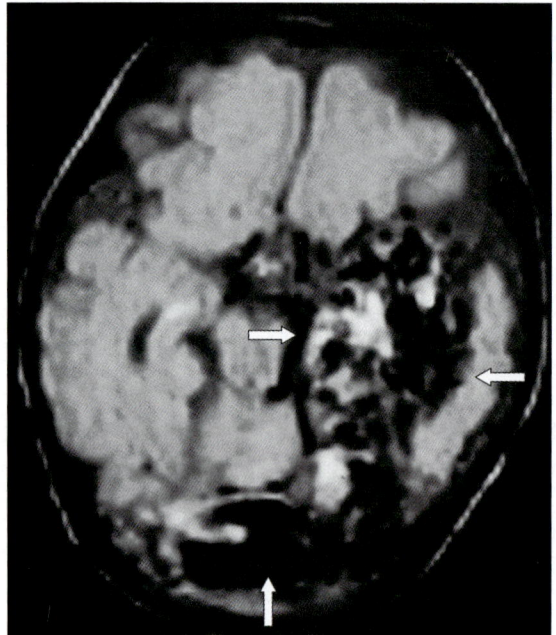

FIGURE 59-1

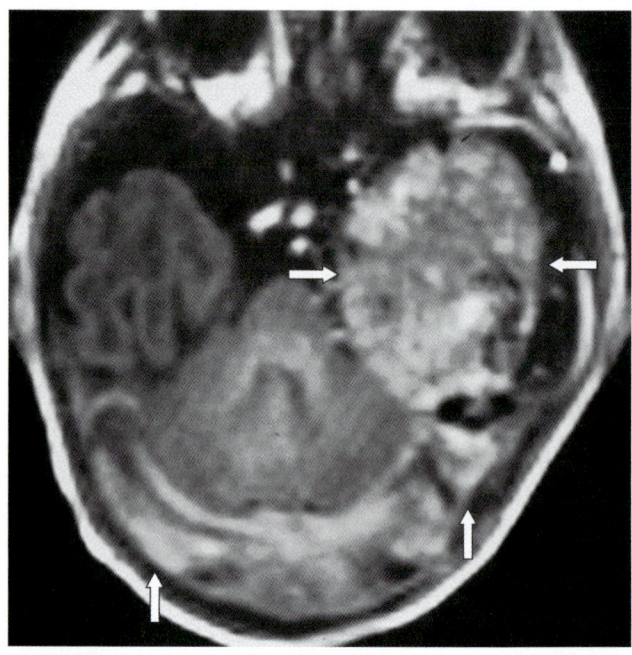

FIGURE 59-2

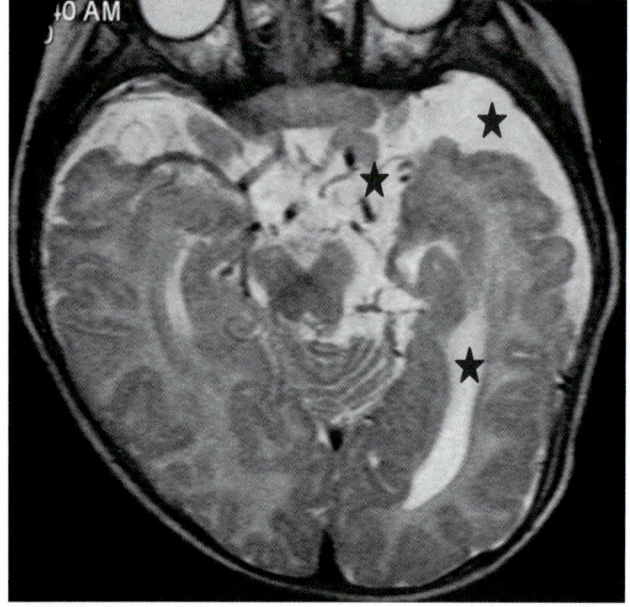

FIGURE 59-3

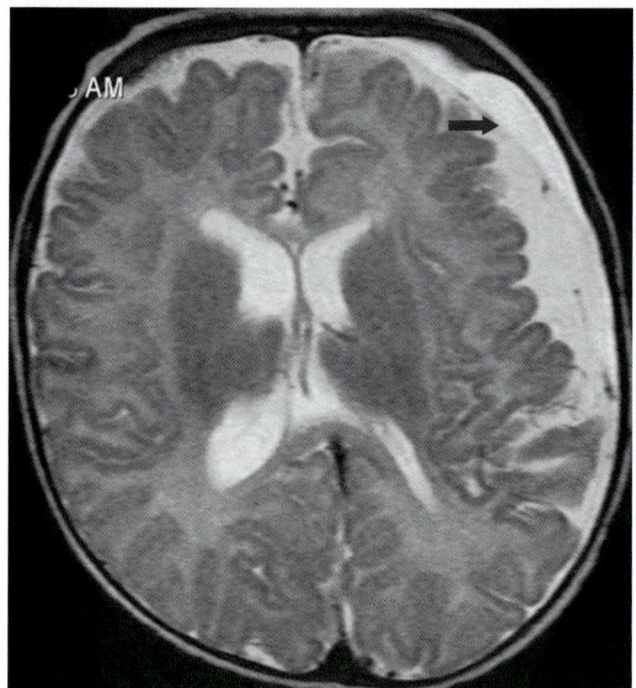

FIGURE 59-4

FINDINGS Case previously published BJR 2006; 79: e140-e144.

Figure 59-1. Axial FLAIR through the midbrain. There is a large collection of tubular signal voids measuring about 5 cm in maximum dimension in the left temporal lobe (transverse arrows). There is mild mass effect on the midbrain. This tangle of blood vessels drains into the large torcula (vertical arrow). There is hyperintense brain parenchyma interspersed within the mass presumably gliosis. Figure 59-2. Axial T1WI through the temporal lobes.

There is a large, ovoid, and heterogeneous left temporal lobe well-defined mass (transverse arrows). The bilateral transverse sinuses are large (vertical arrows). Figures 59-3. Follow-up axial T2WI through the midbrain at age of 4 months. There is complete disappearance of the left temporal lobe mass with widening of the cerebrospinal fluid (CSF) spaces (black stars) surrounding the left temporal lobe consistent with volume loss. Figure 59-4. Axial T2WI through the lateral ventricles. There is a crescentic hyperintense left frontal extraaxial collection (black arrow).

DIFFERENTIAL DIAGNOSIS Dural arteriovenous fistula (DAVF), arteriovenous malformation (AVM), glioma.

DIAGNOSIS Spontaneous thrombosis of AVM.

DISCUSSION An AVM is composed of a tangle of vessels called the nidus with one or more arterial feeders and one or more venous outflow. The nidus is what differentiates an AVM from the other vascular malformations particularly DAVF. One of the less well-known aspects of AVM is why a small percentage can disappear completely without a trace. AVM is described as congenital, and we are not sure whether they grow once formed but spontaneous regression is a well-known rare feature. Clinical presentations of AVM include headache, seizures, focal neurologic deficit, and altered mental status when complicated by hemorrhage. The reasons for complete thrombosis are not well understood. These have included seizure activity, parenchymal and subarachnoid hemorrhages, arterial feeder stenosis,

and venous outflow occlusion, embolic phenomenon from arterial feeders or aneurysms, and hypercoagulable states. There is no evidence of significant encephalomalacia in this patient to suggest underlying significant prior hematoma, and there was no significant clinical event between the two studies to suggest seizure activities. The presence of a left frontal subdural collection may suggest a prior subdural hematoma, but it may well represent an effusion complicating the volume loss.

Question for Further Thought
1. Can a thrombosed AVM reopen?

Reporting Responsibilities
Discovery of an AVM and follow-up evaluation findings deserve direct reporting because of possible catastrophic complications. Spontaneous thrombosis which occurs in 1% to 3% of all AVMs is a rarity and deserves immediate reporting to prevent unnecessary invasive studies.

What the Treating Physician Needs to Know
- Location, size, arterial feeders, venous outflow, and associated parenchymal changes
- Any complications following the spontaneous thrombosis

Answer
1. Yes, there has been a reported recanalization of a previously asymptomatic thrombosed AVM. Because of this, it is recommended that such thrombosed AVM should be followed up for at least 3 years to ensure permanent thrombosis.

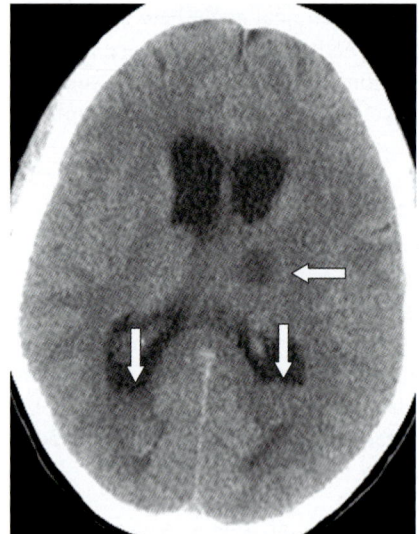

FIGURE 60-1

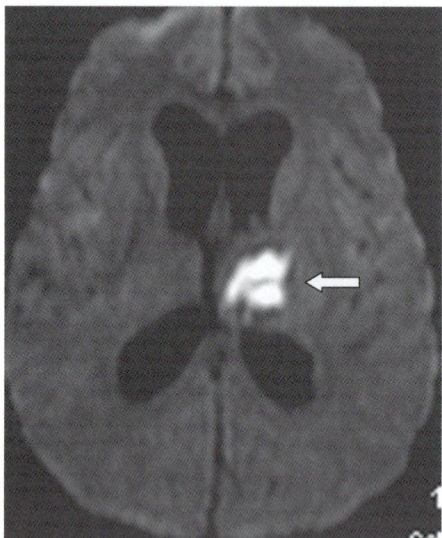

FIGURE 60-2

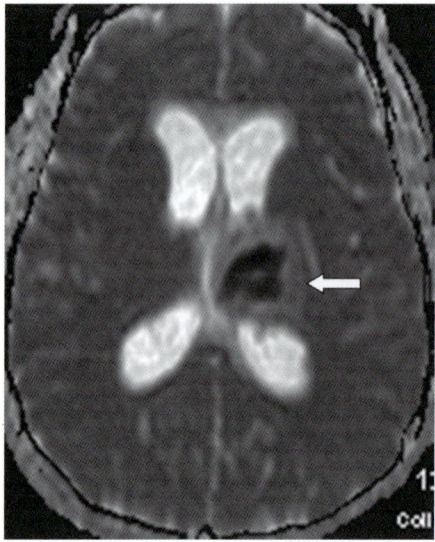
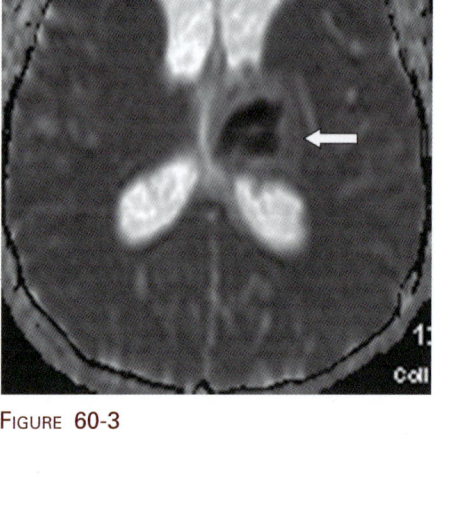

FIGURE 60-3

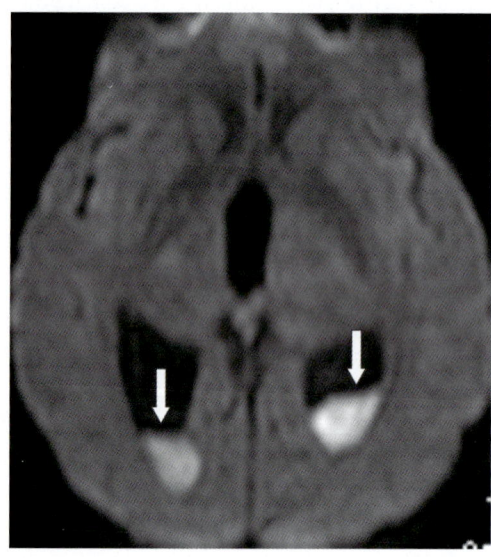

FIGURE 60-4

FINDINGS Figure 60-1. Axial NCCT of the head through the thalami. There is a well-defined small hypodensity in the left thalamus (arrow). There are fluid-fluid levels in the trigones bilaterally consistent with debris (vertical arrows). There is ventriculomegaly. Effacement of convexity subarachnoid spaces is present due to raised intracranial pressure. Figures 60-2 and 60-3. Corresponding axial DWI and ADC map through the thalami. There is a left thalamic focal restricted diffusion (arrows) with surrounding small edema consistent with an abscess. Figure 60-4. Axial DWI

through the trigones. There is bilateral intraventricular restricted diffusion with fluid-fluid levels in the trigones consistent with cellular debris (arrows). Figure 60-5. Axial FLAIR through the third ventricle. There is a left thalamic well-circumscribed hyperintensity (transverse arrow) corresponding to the changes seen in Figures 60-1 to 60-3. There are fluid-fluid levels in the trigones (vertical arrows). The precipitate is hyperintense. There is hydrocephalus with periventricular edema. Figure 60-6. Postcontrast coronal T1WI. There is a left thalamic smooth

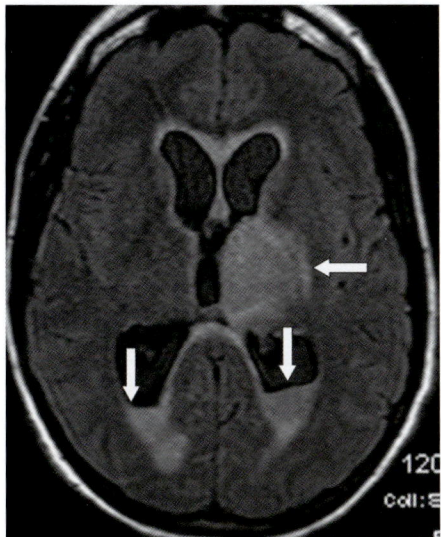

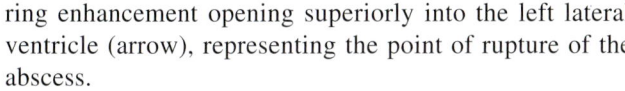

FIGURE 60-5

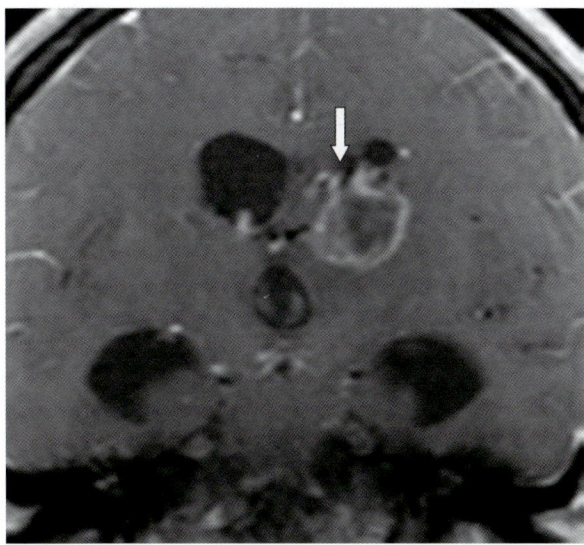

FIGURE 60-6

ring enhancement opening superiorly into the left lateral ventricle (arrow), representing the point of rupture of the abscess.

DIFFERENTIAL DIAGNOSIS Pyogenic abscess, tuberculous abscess, fungal abscess, necrotic tumor.

DIAGNOSIS Left thalamic pyogenic abscess with ventriculitis.

DISCUSSION A brain pyogenic abscess is typically a well-defined cystic lesion with surrounding hypodense vasogenic edema on NCCT. Following contrast administration, there is usually a smooth ring enhancement separating the cystic lesion from the surrounding edema. The mass effect depends on the size of the abscess and its surrounding edema. Most pyogenic abscesses are located in the white–gray matter junction. MRI is the preferred examination for evaluating this condition. An abscess is round with central restricted diffusion and surrounding vasogenic edema. It is hypointense on T1WI and hyperintense on T2WI. There is a smooth thin ring contrast enhancement separating the abscess from the edema. There is a mass effect, and the degree of herniation depends on the size and the amount of surrounding edema. An abscess is more frequently supratentorial in location distributed almost evenly between all cerebral lobes. It is solitary in over 50% of cases. It could be difficult to differentiate a pyogenic abscess from a fungal or tuberculous abscess. Fungal abscess tends to have a rather irregular thick contrast-enhancing wall with internal projections, while the tuberculous abscess wall is smooth, multilobulated, or crenated. Fungal abscess may show internal hypointensity or heterogeneity on spin echo sequences with peripheral restricted diffusion. MRS has been shown to demonstrate presence of lipid and lactate in pyogenic,

tuberculous and fungal abscesses and the presence of various amino acids only in pyogenic abscesses. Tumoral cavities generally do not restrict diffusion centrally, but lipids and lactate peaks could be present on MRS. Abscesses close to the ventricles could rupture into the ventricle producing ventriculitis. In up to 30% of adult cases and up to 90% of neonatal cases, ventriculitis and meningitis could complicate cerebral abscess. Hydrocephalus is a known complication of meningitis and ventriculitis. The cellular debris within the ventricles usually restricts diffusion. There may or may not be ependymal enhancement. Follow-up MRI in this patient eventually showed ependymal enhancement and subdural empyema.

Pyogenic brain abscess is usually hematogenous in origin. Direct inoculation of the brain is always a possibility during surgical interventions. The common presentations include headache, fever, focal neurologic deficit, and altered mental status. Definitive diagnosis requires CSF examination or stereotactic guided drainage with culture. The CSF is usually cloudy or turbid with pleocytosis, low glucose, and high protein. Treatment is with appropriate antibiotics. CSF diversion may be necessary for the treatment of hydrocephalus and ventriculitis.

Question for Further Thought

1. How safe is a lumbar puncture (LP) in the presence of a significant mass effect from an abscess?

Reporting Responsibilities

An abscess is an emergency requiring direct reporting. Presence of hydrocephalus or ventriculitis or significant mass effect such as subfalcine, transtentorial, uncal, or transforaminal herniation should be appropriately stated and communicated as such.

What the Treating Physician Needs to Know

- MRI is preferable to CT in the evaluation of the patient suspected of a brain abscess
- Location and number if more than one
- Is LP safe? Significant mass effect may contraindicate LP
- It could be impossible to determine the offending organism by imaging

Answer

1. LP could be detrimental in the presence of intracranial mass effect or raised intracranial pressure resulting in herniation as it may worsen the herniation. In this case, CSF was obtained through an external ventricular drain, while the abscess was stereotactically drained under CT guidance.

61

CLINICAL HISTORY   *59-year-old male native of Mexico was admitted with decreased level of consciousness, weight loss of approximately 40 pounds, and persistent low-grade fever, night sweats, and fatigue.*

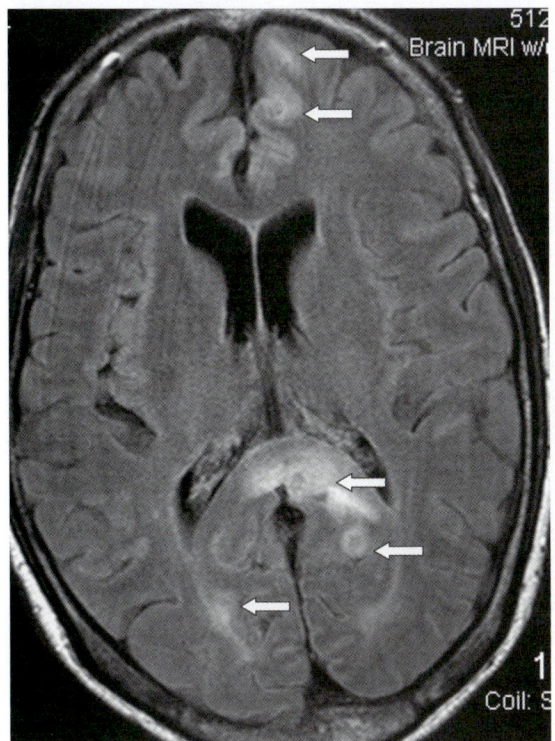

FIGURE 61-1

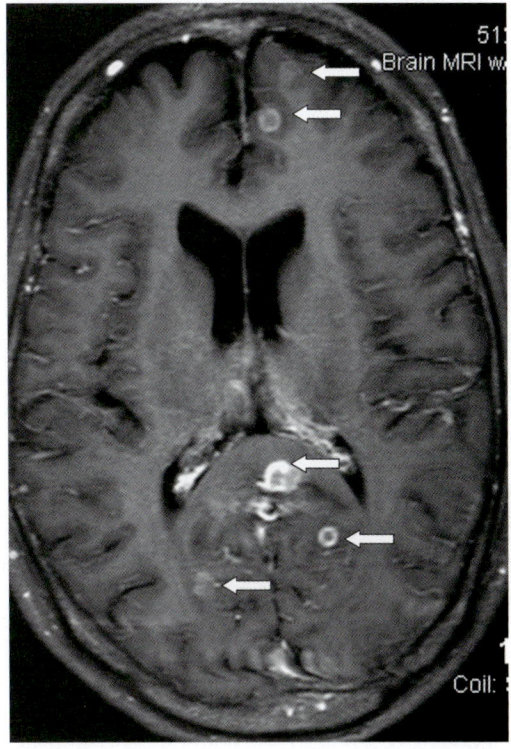

FIGURE 61-2

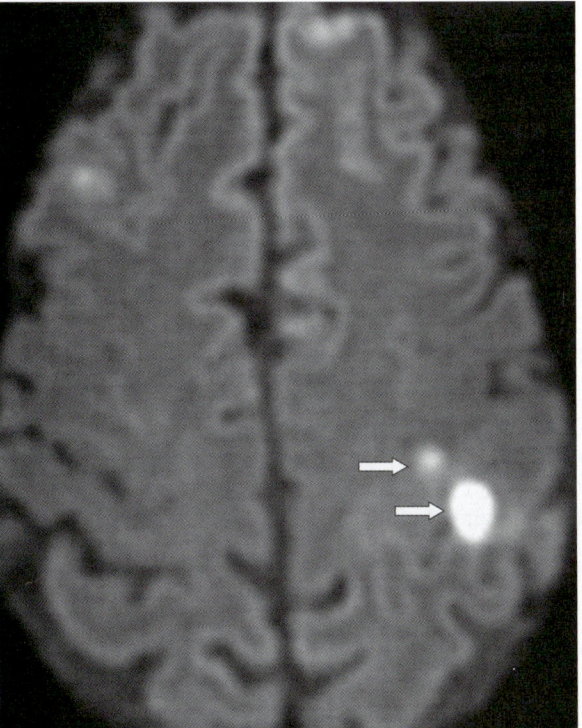

FIGURE 61-3

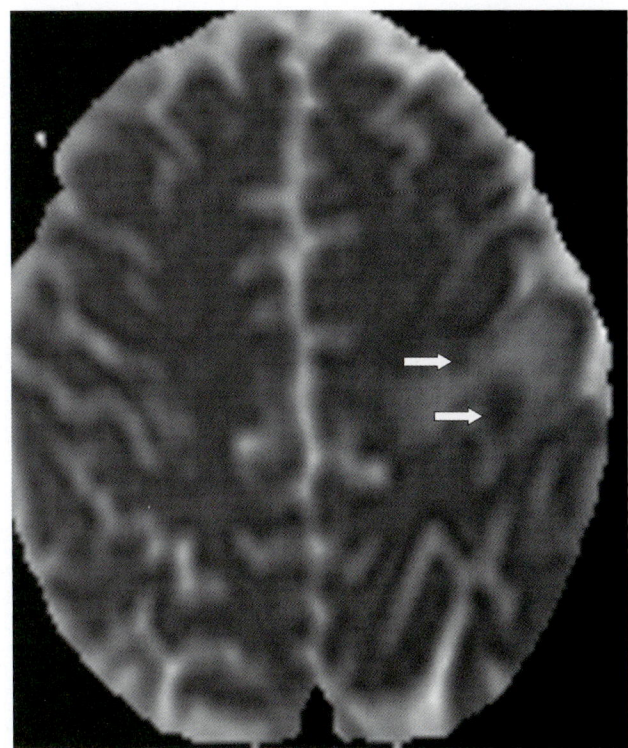

FIGURE 61-4

129

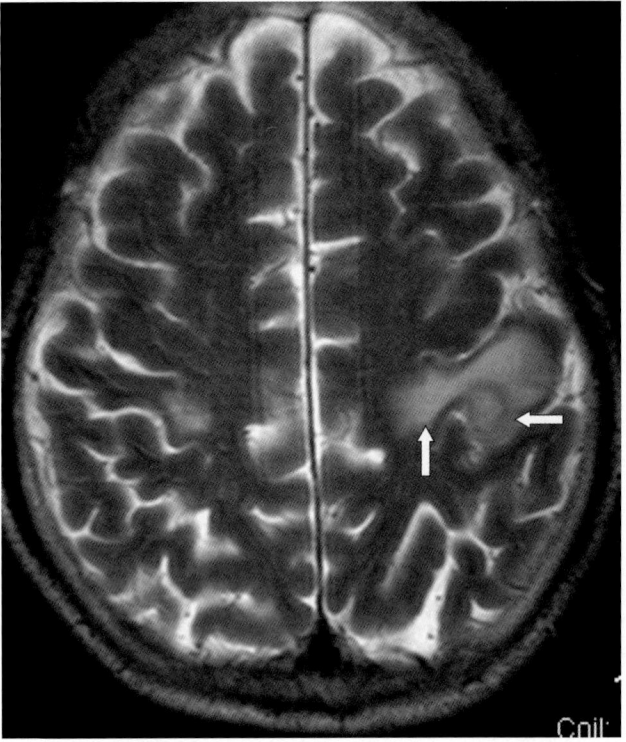

FIGURE 61-5

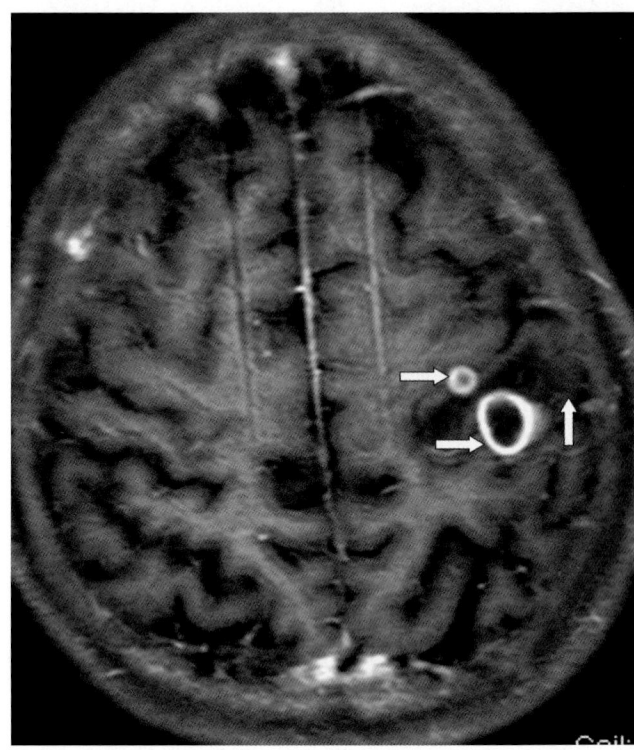

FIGURE 61-6

FINDINGS Figures 61-1 and 61-2. Axial FLAIR and post-contrast T1WI MRI through the splenium of the corpus callosum showing multiple ring-enhancing small lesions measuring about 1 cm or less in size in the left parasagittal frontal lobe, left splenium, and in bilateral occipital lobes (arrows). Lesions are surrounded by very minimal hyperintensity on the FLAIR except in areas where they coalesce as in the splenium where the surrounding T2 hyperintensity is large. Lesions are mostly cortical and/or subcortical in location. Figures 61-3, 61-4, 61-5, and 61-6. Axial DWI with corresponding ADC map, T2WI, and post-contrast T1WI through the superior centrum semiovale. There are more multifocal cortical subcortical lesions with central diffusion restriction in bilateral frontal lobes. The two posterior left frontal lobe lesions (transverse arrows) show smooth thick ring enhancement in Figure 61-6 with surrounding vasogenic edema (vertical arrows in figures 5 and 6). The larger left posterior frontal lobe lesion measures about 1.6 cm with a hyperintense core and hypointense rim on the T2WI (Figure 61-5 transverse arrow). There are many more lesions in the brainstem, cerebellum, and cerebrum (not shown). There is very minimal leptomeningial enhancement.

DIFFERENTIAL DIAGNOSIS Tuberculomata/abscess, metastases, neurocysticercosis, chronic pyogenic abscesses, toxoplasmosis.

DIAGNOSIS Tuberculomata and tuberculous (TB) abscess.

DISCUSSION Tuberculomata and TB brain abscesses are space-occupying lesions 0.4–1 cm and over 1 cm in size, respectively. CT of TB granulomata may show nonspecific hypodensities, while the larger abscesses may show a smooth isodense ring surrounding a hypodense core. These lesions tend to show smooth ring enhancement following contrast administration. TB shows restricted diffusion on DWI particularly the larger abscesses with the smaller lesions being poorly defined. There is a hypointense smooth ring with a central hyperintense core on T2WI. The rim tends to be hyperintense on FLAIR with smooth enhancement following contrast administration. Presence of leptomeningeal enhancement suggests meningitis particularly at the base of the brain and the large fissures. Tuberculomata and TB abscesses could be single or multiple, but more often the tuberculomata are multiple. There is usually considerable vasogenic edema surrounding the larger abscesses. The larger abscesses often show a crenated appearance with a heterogeneous core on T2WI. The crenated rim may distinguish TB from pyogenic abscess where the ring is almost always smooth. Metastatic rings are usually irregular and generally do not restrict diffusion centrally. Calcifications may be present in neurocysticercosis with minimal edema. Toxoplasmosis tends to show the concentric target pattern on T2WI and the eccentric target sign on post-contrast images.

Clinical presentation is usually with fever or low-grade temperature, malaise, headache, nausea, vomiting, especially in cases of meningitis. Seizures, focal neurologic deficits, and altered mental status are other symptoms. CSF evaluation usually shows elevated white cells with lymphocytic predominance, high protein, and low glucose. Diagnosis was made by brain biopsy and drainage of the large lesion. Bronchoalveolar lavage culture was positive for acid fast bacilli (AFB) after 6 weeks. Corticosteroid treatment in addition to quadruple drug regimen (isoniazid (INH) + pyrazinamide (PZA) + ethambutol (EMB) + rifampicin (RIF)) usually reduces tuberculoma size and perilesional edema leading to symptomatic improvement and seizure control. Surgical therapy for intracranial tuberculoma is considered only when a positive diagnosis is not possible by other means, medical therapy fails, or when decompression is necessary.

Question for Further Thought

1. How common is tuberculoma and TB brain abscess?

Reporting Responsibilities

Direct reporting is always necessary if an abscess or multifocal lesions are present. Presence of herniation, significant edema, leptomeningeal enhancement, and hydrocephalus should be reported as these may influence management decisions. If bland infarcts are present they should be emphasized as these usually indicate vascular complication that is more common with meningitis.

What the Treating Physician Needs to Know

- Number and location of lesions to allow decision regarding management choices
- Complications such as hydrocephalus or herniations that may require surgical intervention
- Is lumbar puncture (LP) safe? Significant herniation may preclude an LP
- Patients started on anti-TB medication can have a paradoxical reaction with worsening of the symptoms and expansion of the tuberculoma

Answer

1. *Mycobacterium tuberculosis* is the second cause of death worldwide, accounting for approximately 9 million deaths each year. In the United States, the majority of cases are diagnosed in the homeless, intravenous drug abusers, patients with AIDS, foreign-born persons (especially from countries with high-prevalence of TB), prison inmates, migrant farm workers, and alcoholics. Intracranial tuberculomas develop in up to 1% of patients with active tuberculosis and up to 28% of those with TB meningitis.

CLINICAL HISTORY *Young female presenting with seizures.*

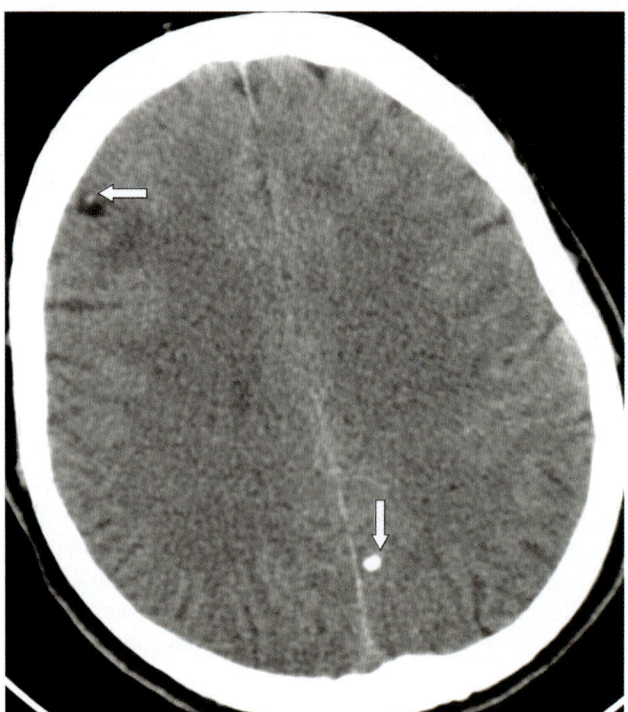

FIGURE 62-1
Courtesy of Annette Douglas, MD.

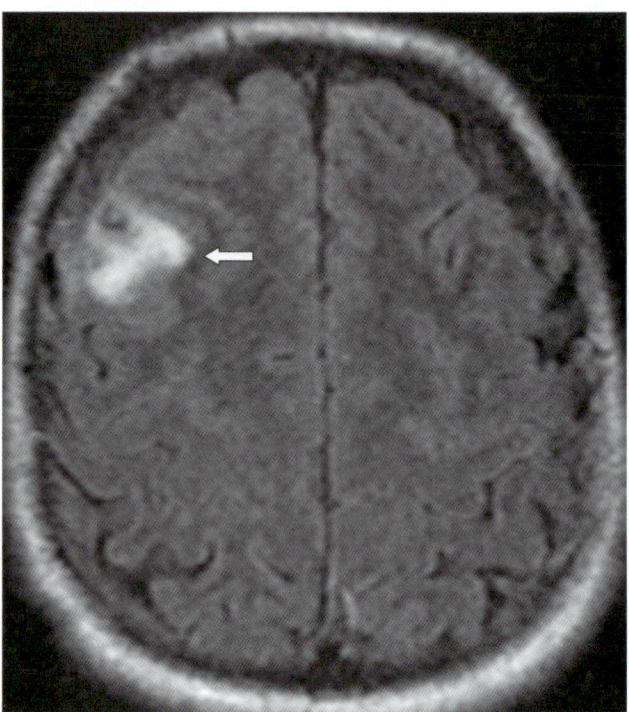

FIGURE 62-2
Courtesy of Annette Douglas, MD.

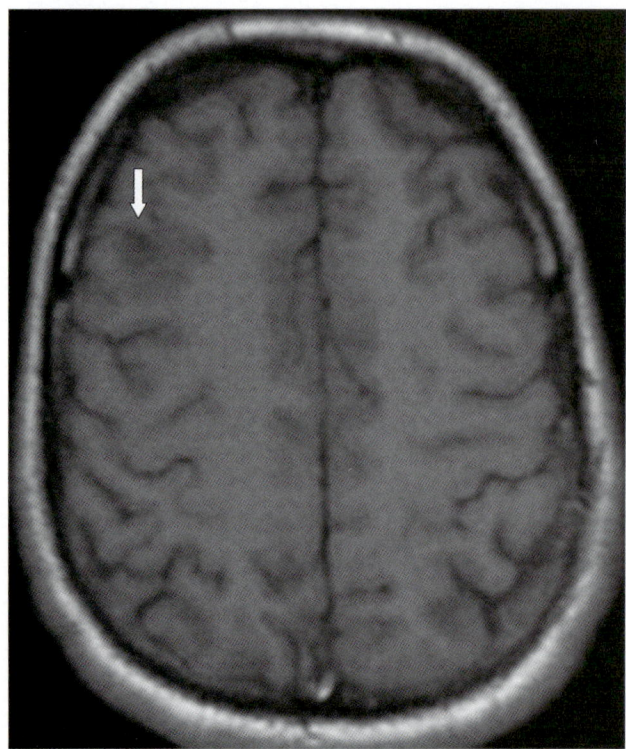

FIGURE 62-3
Courtesy of Annette Douglas, MD.

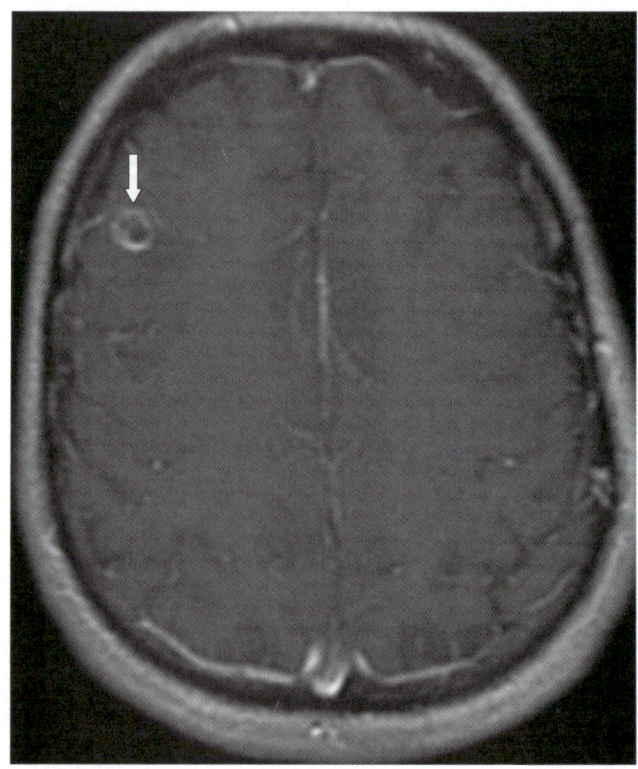

FIGURE 62-4
Courtesy of Annette Douglas, MD.

FINDINGS Figure 62-1. Axial NCCT through centrum semiovale. There is a small right frontal lateral cortical cyst with an eccentric tiny calcification (transverse arrow). There is a subtle hypodensity on its medial aspect. A small cortical calcification is present in the left parasagittal parietal lobe (vertical arrow). Figure 62-2. Axial FLAIR MRI through the same level. There is a tiny hypointense ring with a central hyperintensity surrounded by a well-defined lobulated hyperintensity (arrow) consistent with vasogenic edema. There is mild effacement of local sulci. Figures 62-3 and 62-4. Axial pre- and post-contrast T1WI through same level. There is a smooth ring contrast enhancement within the hypointense lesion (arrow).

DIFFERENTIAL DIAGNOSIS Pleomorphic xanthoastrocytoma (PXA), neurocysticercosis (NCC), metastasis, cerebral cavernous malformation (CCM).

DIAGNOSIS NCC vesicular/colloidal.

DISCUSSION This is a transition between the vesicular and colloidal stage of NCC involution. The tiny calcification is the scolex usually present in the nonreactive vesicular stage. The surrounding edema and contrast enhancement are consistent with host reaction associated with colloidal degeneration, the most reactive stage of the four stages of NCC and represents the so-called acute encephalitic phase. There is an intense reaction of the host to leakage of the cysticercus antigen as it degenerates, resulting in breakdown of the blood–brain barrier with surrounding contrast enhancement and edema. There could be a single cyst or multiple cysts. The entire brain could be riddled with similar lesions. MRI offers the best characterization of the lesions and their surrounding reactions. In this patient there is a second small calcified left parietal focus consistent with the calcified final stage of the involution. Perilesional edema is uncommon in CCM unless they have recently bled. Multiplicity of lesions is uncommon in PXA. Meningeal attachment and scalloping of inner table are common in PXA. Metastases rarely show calcifications.

Cysticercosis is the most common cause of epilepsy in the world. It is most prevalent in the poor countries of the world but increasingly diagnosed in the developed world as a result of globalization. The seizures are due to the intense inflammation resulting in perilesional edema associated with the colloidal and granular nodular stages but seizures have been known to occur also in the calcified nodular stage. The calcified lesions are common in asymptomatic patients in the endemic parts of the world such as in Latin America. Other presenting symptoms could include headache, neurologic deficit, and mental status changes. Diagnosis is usually confirmed by ELISA or electroimmunotransfer blot assay (EITB) with a specificity of about 100%. NCC is treated with antiparasitic medication albendazole with praziquantel as an alternative along with antiseizure and anti-inflammatory therapy. Intense inflammation is usually associated with dying parasite.

Question for Further Thought

1. Where can you find NCC in the CNS?

Reporting Responsibilities

Colloidal stage of cysticercosis is an emergent state that should be reported directly to the referring physician. Location, number, presence of mass effect, and the amount of edema should all be noted. Presence of other stages of the disease and complications should be reported.

What the Treating Physician Needs to Know

- Location of lesions
- Presence of other stages of the disease
- Presence of complications such as hydrocephalus or meningitis

Answer

1. NCC could be found in the parenchymal, subarachnoid, and intraventricular locations. Parenchymal lesions undergo the four-stage degeneration. There is controversy regarding location of so-called parenchymal cysts. A large autopsy series found that most of these cysts are situated in the crypts of the sulci or in perivascular spaces rather than in the brain parenchyma. The literature, however, maintains that parenchymal disease exists. Intraventricular and subarachnoid NCC does not undergo the stages of degeneration. They remain cystic, can rupture, or obstruct the CSF pathway. Intraventricular cyst can be demonstrated to shift position within the ventricular system on MRI. Subarachnoid cysts could be the most difficult to diagnose. If they are large enough, they could be confused with arachnoid cyst. Large basal cistern and perisylvian cysts also known as racemose NCC tend to have multiple cysts that are associated with intense reaction and contrast enhancement and can result in arachnoiditis with consequent communicating hydrocephalus. Spinal involvement is not uncommon but should be suspected in basal disease.

CLINICAL HISTORY   *63-year-old male with liver transplantation 4 years prior was admitted for mental status changes and headache.*

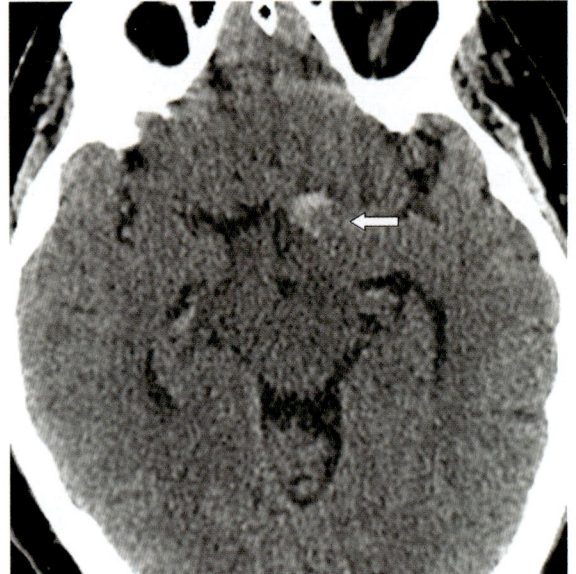

FIGURE 63-1

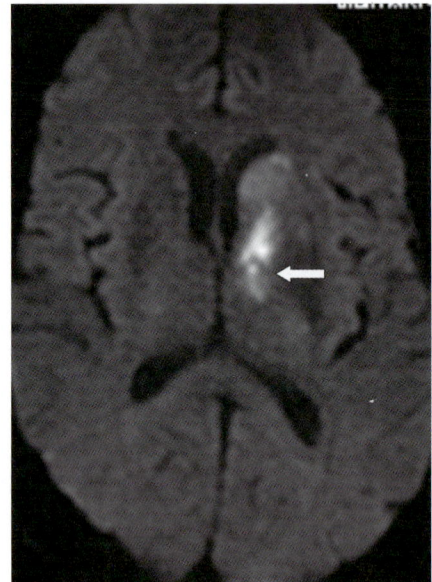

FIGURE 63-2

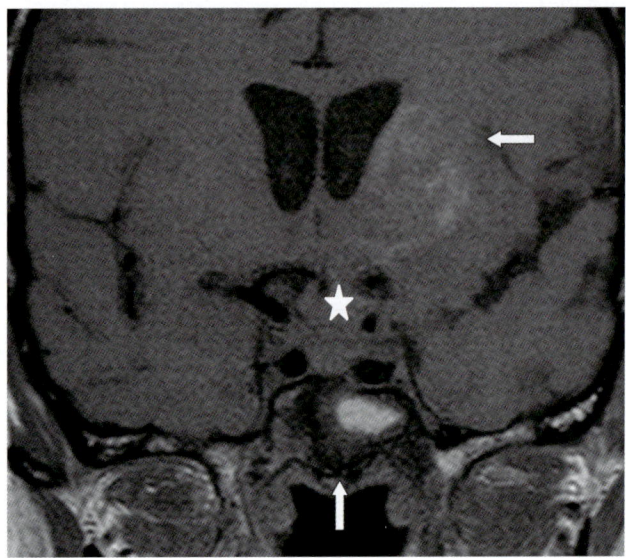

FIGURE 63-3

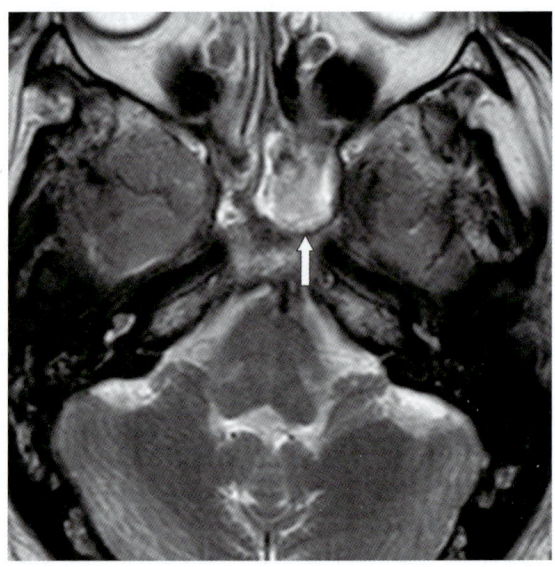

FIGURE 63-4

FINDINGS   Figure 63-1. Axial NCCT of the head. There is a small focus of hyperdensity (blood) in the anterior left suprasellar cistern in the vicinity of the left internal carotid artery (ICA) (arrow), and the rest of the suprasellar cistern is isodense to brain presumably due to inflammatory tissue. Figure 63-2. DWI through the level of the basal ganglia. There is restricted diffusion in the left basal ganglia and thalamus (arrow) and elsewhere in the left cerebral

hemisphere (not shown). Figure 63-3. Coronal non-contrast T1WI through the level of the sphenoid sinus. There is hyperintense sphenoid sinus opacification with surrounding hypointense material (vertical arrow). The sella turcica and suprasellar cerebrospinal fluid (CSF) are isointense with the brain (star) consistent with "granulation/inflammatory tissue" replacing the suprasellar CSF. There is patchy left basal ganglia hyperintensity consistent with hemorrhagic infarcts

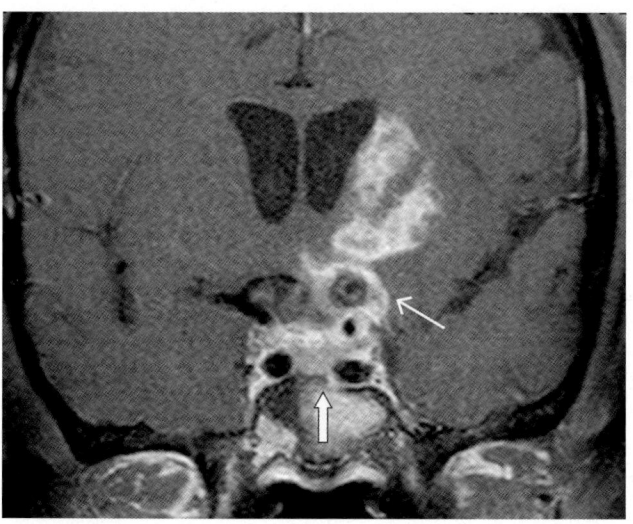

FIGURE **63-5**

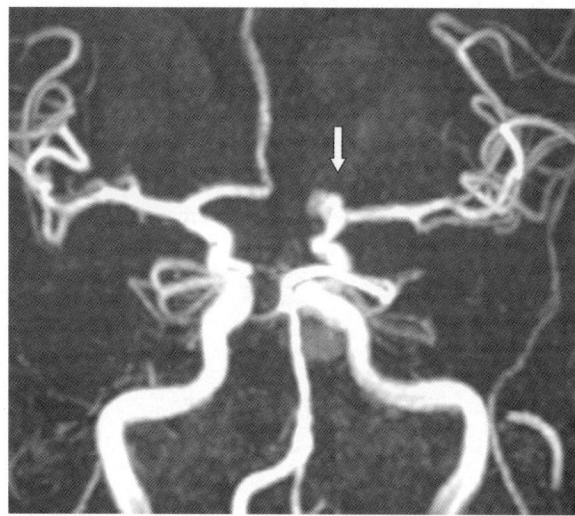

FIGURE **63-6**

(transverse arrow). Figure 63-4. Axial T2WI through the sphenoid sinus. There is mixed signal intensity within the sphenoid sinus (vertical arrow), either blood or fungus infection. Figure 63-5. Coronal post-contrast T1WI through the levels of the suprasellar cistern and basal ganglia. There is diffuse contrast enhancement extending from the sphenoid sinus through the sella turcica and suprasellar cistern (inflammation) into the left basal ganglia (subacute infarct). There is a defect in the floor of the sella turcica (vertical arrow) suggesting route of infection to the cranial cavity. There is a target-like hypointensity in the region of the left ICA terminus suggesting an aneurysm (transverse arrow). Figure 63-6. 3D TOF MRA. There is a lobulated aneurysm of the left ICA terminus with occlusion of the left anterior cerebral artery (ACA).

DIFFERENTIAL DIAGNOSIS subarachnoid hemorrhage, fungal infection, left internal carotid aneurysm, basal meningitis.

DIAGNOSIS Mycotic aneurysm (MA) of the left internal carotid terminus due to transdural fungal invasion from the sphenoid sinus.

DISCUSSION This left ICA MA is due to transdural spread of sphenoid sinus *Aspergillus* spp. infection via the sella turcica into the suprasellar cistern. Like every aneurysm, there is an outpouch from the left ICA terminus. This developed over a period of weeks. The suprasellar subarachnoid hemorrhage (SAH) was due to rupture of the aneurysm with subsequent intraventricular hemorrhage (IVH) (not shown). Left hemispheric infarcts are a product of distal embolization and/or occlusion of small vessels due to the infection. SAH, intracerebral hemorrhage (ICH), and IVH are complications of a ruptured aneurysm. MA represents an abnormal focal arterial dilatation due to degeneration of the arterial wall secondary to contiguous spread of an infection resulting in proximal MA, bloodstream infection, or septic embolization resulting in distal MA. Bacteria (*Streptococci* spp., *Staphylococci* spp.), fungi (*Aspergillus* spp., *Candida* spp., *Coccidioides*, agents of mucormycosis), parasites, and viruses have been implicated as etiologic agents. CTA and MRA are equally effective in demonstrating MA.

MA accounts for 0.7% to 6.5% of all intracranial aneurysms. Infective endocarditis, cavernous sinus thrombophlebitis, sinusitis, otitis media, mastoiditis, meningitis, and orbital cellulitis are the common causes of MA. Intracranial MAs are usually silent. The patient might develop signs and symptoms later in the course of the disease due to aneurysm enlargement, SAH, or ICH. The most common symptoms are fever, headache, seizures, focal neurologic deficits, or mental status changes. Unruptured MAs carry a 30% mortality, while rupture is associated with much higher mortality up to 80%. These patients require long-term antibiotic therapy. Aggressive treatment is recommended in the immunocompromised patient. There are specific indications for endovascular and surgical treatment of MA. Left nasal endoscopy with left total ethmoidectomy and left sphenoidotomy was performed in this patient revealing acute and chronic inflammation with fungal hyphae suggestive for *Aspergillus*. The patient was treated with oral and intravenous antifungal medication.

Question for Further Thought

1. How do we monitor MA to assess the response to treatment?

Reporting Responsibilities

MA is an emergent condition deserving of direct reporting. The number and locations of other aneurysms should be noted. Presence of infarcts, SAH, IVH, ICH, distal vascular occlusions, and arterial spasms should be documented. Hydrocephalus may require emergent ventricular drainage and should be directly communicated.

What the Treating Physician Needs to Know

- Location, number, and size of aneurysms on initial and follow-up imaging
- Complications such as SAH, ICH, infarcts, hydrocephalus on initial and follow-up study. These will affect management decisions

- Presence of inciting pathology such as sinus infection or underlying cardiac disease

Answer

1. CTA and MRA are equally effective in monitoring the progress of MA. CTA appears to be more effective for small distal MA. There is no consensus as to whether this should be done weekly or monthly.

CLINICAL HISTORY *48-year-old female with chronic lymphocytic leukemia and disseminated varicella-zoster virus infection presenting with altered mental status.*

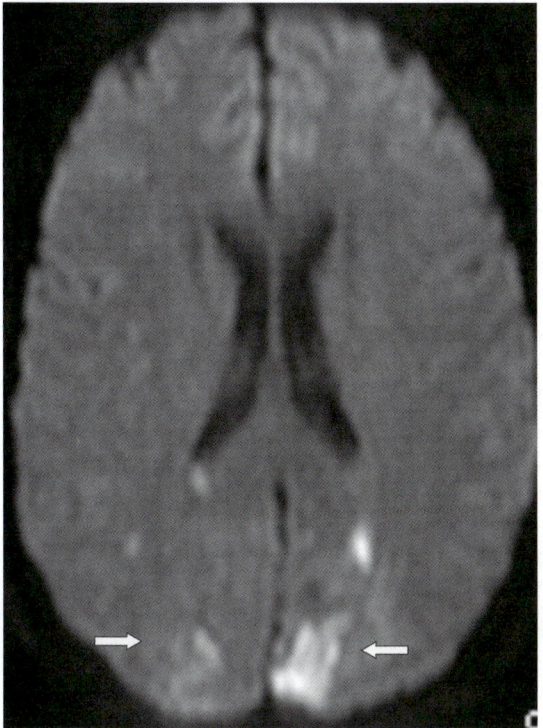

FIGURE 64-1

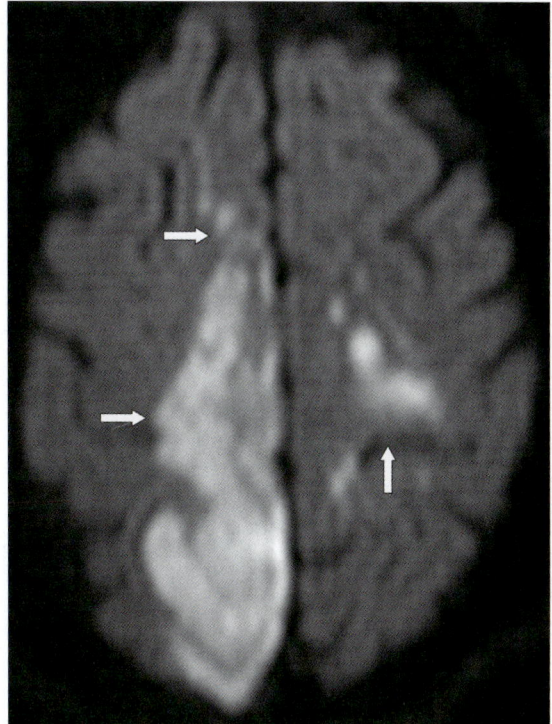

FIGURE 64-2

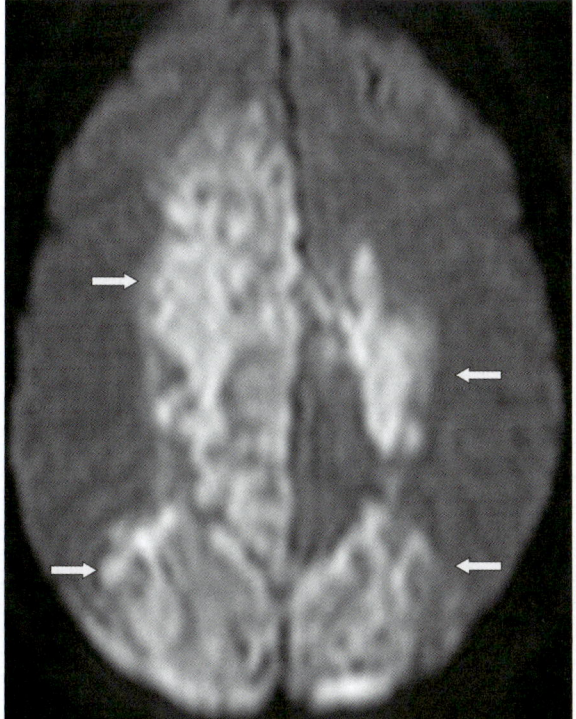

FIGURE 64-3

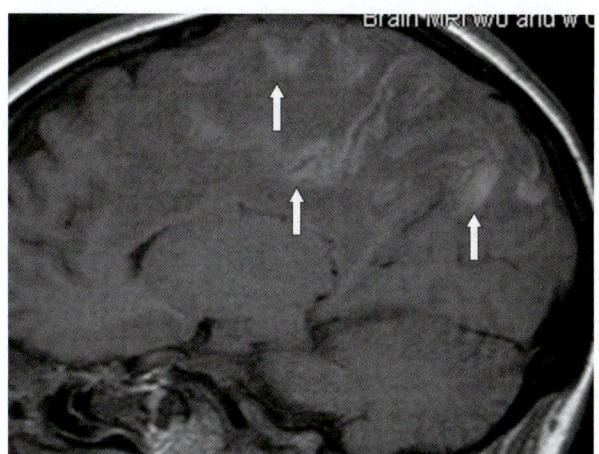

FIGURE 64-4

FINDINGS Figures 64-1 and 64-2. Axial DWI through the levels of the lateral ventricles and the vertex, respectively. Multifocal bilateral areas of restricted diffusion in multiple vascular territories, bilateral posterior cerebral artery (PCA) (figure 1 arrows), right anterior cerebral artery (ACA) (figure 64-2 transverse arrows), and left watershed region (figure 64-2 vertical arrow). Figure 64-3. Axial DWI follow-up through the vertex. There is progression of bilateral cerebral areas of restricted diffusion (arrows). Similar progression of

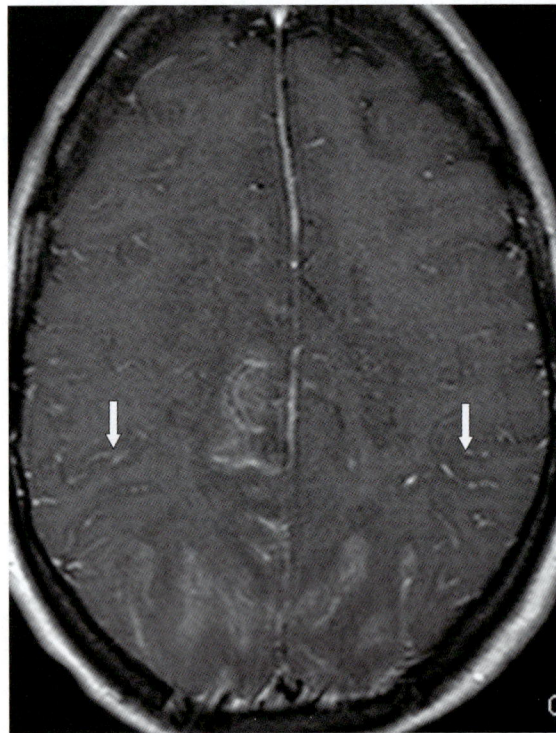

FIGURE **64-5**

T2 hyperintensities was present on FLAIR/T2WI (not shown) in bilateral ACA and PCA territories. Figure 64-4. Right parasagittal non-contrast T1WI on follow-up. There is gyriform hyperintensity in the right frontoparietal lobes (arrows) consistent with hemorrhagic infarcts. Figure 64-5. Axial postcontrast T1WI through the level of the centrum semiovale. There is bilateral leptomeningeal enhancement (arrows) superimposed on the underlying gyriform hyperintensity of subacute hemorrhage in bilateral frontoparietal lobes.

DIFFERENTIAL DIAGNOSIS Multifocal infarcts, embolic infarcts, varicella-zoster virus encephalitis (VZVE).

DIAGNOSIS Varicella-zoster virus encephalitis (VZVE).

DISCUSSION VZVE presents as multifocal and multiterritorial areas of diffusion restriction on DWI with corresponding T2 hyperintensity consistent with infarctions. Lesions are hypointense on T1WI. Hemorrhagic conversion is common. When contrast enhancement occurs, it is patchy. The initial lesions in this patient did not contrast enhance and were not hemorrhagic. Follow-up study showed hemorrhagic conversion and leptomeningeal enhancement. White matter (WM) and gray matter (GM) may be affected showing typical patterns of T2 hyperintensity associated with infarcts. Cerebellitis with diffuse cerebellar T2 hyperintensity is the commonest presentation in children. It may not be possible to distinguish embolic or multifocal infarcts from lesions of VZVE. The presence of recent vaccination or history of chickenpox or the the presence of zoster rash and prodromal symptoms help in this regard.

Apart from meningitis and encephalitis, VZV also causes Ramsay Hunt syndrome, Bell's palsy, acute disseminated encephalomyelitis (ADEM), and myelitis. In the adult immunocompetent patients, VZVE presents as large vessel vasculopathy (granulomatous arteritis) with large bland or hemorrhagic infarctions, while in the immunocompromised patients, small vessel vasculopathy results in small ovoid GM–WM junction mixed ischemic or demyelinative lesions. Ventriculitis/periventriculitis is rare but makes up the third pattern of encephalitis. Myelitis presentations include loss of pain/temperature or position/vibration sense, Brown-Séquard syndrome, sphincter disturbances, and sensory abnormalities.

VZV infection occurs in all ages and shows no gender preference. Encephalitis tends to present more commonly in children as acute cerebellar ataxia (ataxia, tremor, vomiting, and headache 1–3 weeks after chickenpox). The typical zoster dermatomal rash may not be present, but could precede or occur after the encephalitis by a long period. Treatment is usually with anti-viral.

Question for Further Thought

1. What is the route of entry of the virus to the central nervous system (CNS)?

Reporting Responsibilities

Presence of restricted diffusion indicates an acute event which could be ongoing and requires direct reporting. The multifocality of lesions with the appropriate history should alert the radiologist to the diagnosis with the other differentials mentioned. A mixed pattern of encephalitis could suggest the diagnosis. Cerebellitis in a child should raise the suspicion of VZV infection. MRA or CTA may show occlusion of large vessels and should be recommended. ICA occlusion occurs in herpes zoster ophthalmicus and loss of signal void in the ICA may be a pointer to that diagnosis.

What the Treating Physician Needs to Know

- Location of lesions for purposes of biopsy if it becomes necessary
- Presence of multifocal infarcts is not specific. Embolic phenomenon should be excluded
- The history is key to the diagnosis. Unfortunately the typical rash could be absent, and that should not prevent suspicion of the diagnosis
- Is there a mixed pattern of encephalitis? Small and large vessel patterns of infarcts and/or ventriculitis/periventriculitis should also raise suspicion of VZVE
- Are there other imaging methods to confirm diagnosis? CTA or MRA could be useful in defining the vasculopathy

Answer

1. The virus gains entry into the CNS via neurons. Virus could remain dormant in the dorsal root ganglion for a long time before subsequently invading the CNS through the axons or the vasculature.

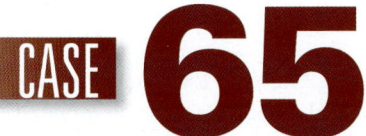

CASE 65

CLINICAL HISTORY *54-year-old male with AIDS on antiretrovirals presenting with tremors, jerking movement of limbs, and dropping objects.*

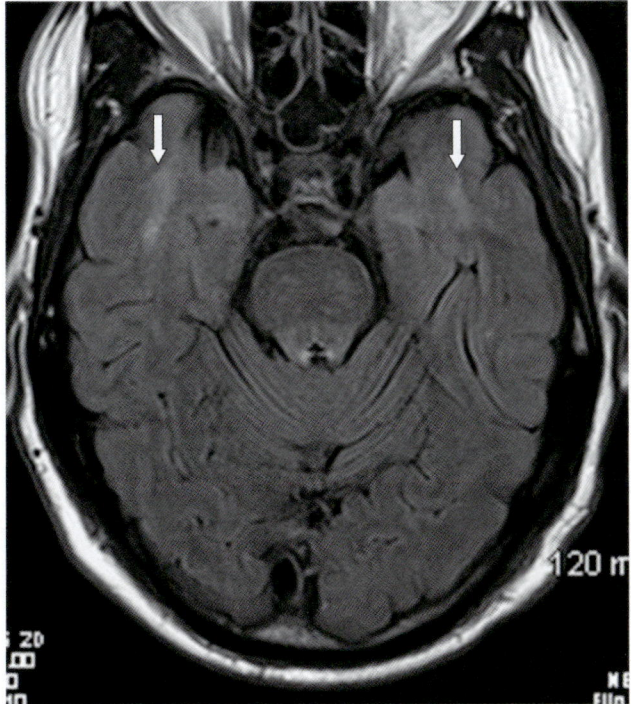

FIGURE 65-1

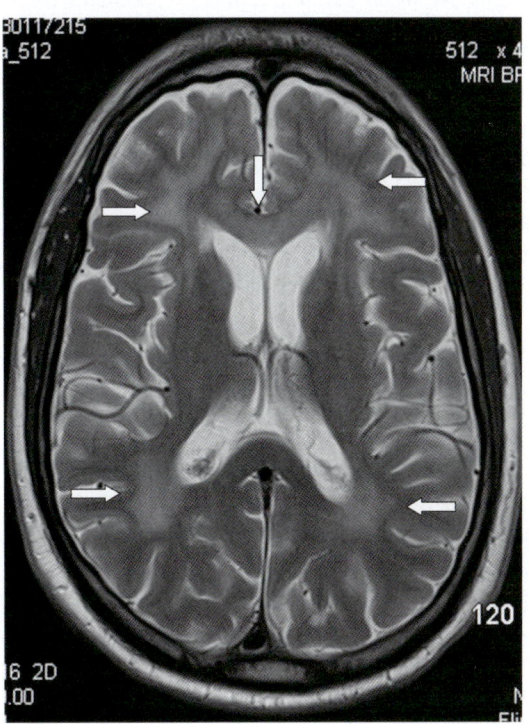

FIGURE 65-2

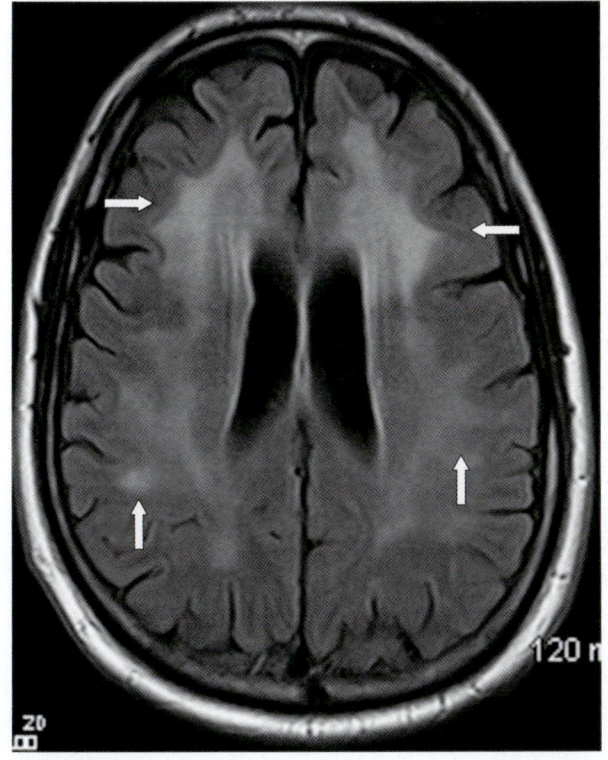

FIGURE 65-3

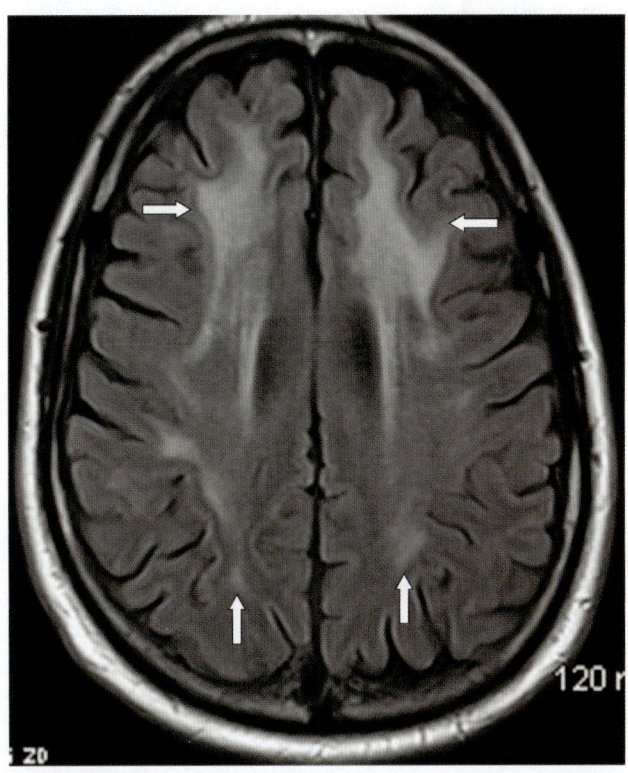

FIGURE 65-4

FINDINGS Figure 65-1. Axial FLAIR through the temporal lobes. There is bilateral anterior temporal lobes white matter (WM) hyperintensity (arrows). Figure 65-2. Axial T2WI through the basal ganglia. There is confluent bilateral symmetrical WM hyperintensity around the frontal and occipital horns extending from the ventricular walls to the subcortical regions (arrows). The frontal WM hyperintensity extend across the genu and anterior body of the corpus callosum (vertical arrow). This T2WI captures the degree of brain volume loss which is mild in this case. Figures 65-3 and 65-4. Axial FLAIR through the corona radiata and centrum semiovale, respectively. There is predominant symmetrical bilateral frontal lobes confluent WM hyperintensity extending from ventricular wall to subcortical regions (transverse arrows). The lesions are more subcortical, smudgy, and not as confluent in the parietal and occipital WM with relative sparing of the deep WM (vertical arrows). It is noted that there is no mass effect, and the post-contrast images (not shown) do not show areas of contrast enhancement.

DIFFERENTIAL DIAGNOSIS Chronic small vessel ischemic changes, progressive multifocal leukoencephalopathy (PML), HIV encephalopathy (HIVE), leukodystrophy, Binswanger's disease.

DIAGNOSIS HIVE.

DISCUSSION Imaging features of HIVE consist of diffuse, confluent, or smudgy WM changes that are predominantly frontal with involvement of the genu of the corpus callosum but occur elsewhere in the corona radiata and centrum semiovale. These lesions are hypointense on T1WI and hyperintense on FLAIR and T2WI. They generally extend from ventricular walls to subcortical WM in the frontal lobes and around the occipital horns but are predominantly subcortical elsewhere. They are more often symmetrical without mass effect or contrast enhancement. Unilateral lesions have been reported. Basal ganglia calcifications are seen in adults but more common in children. There is varying degrees of brain volume loss affecting both cortical and subcortical regions resulting in enlargement of the ventricles and sulci. Caudate nucleus atrophy is common. MRS shows low N-acetyl aspartate (NAA) peak with elevated myoinositol not only in the WM but also in the GM. Presence of lactate peak has also been noted, and this disappears following successful treatment of the encephalopathy. CT shows corresponding non-contrast-enhancing confluent hypodensity in similar locations as in MRI along with global brain volume loss. PML is usually subcortical and not necessarily bilateral. PML may contrast enhance with a T1WI cortical hyperintensity in immune reconstitution inflammatory syndrome (IRIS). Chronic small vessel ischemic changes are usually monotonous small WM changes which may be confluent in severe cases. Binswanger disease tends to be globally confluent and not necessarily frontal predominant.

HIVE usually presents with a combination of cognitive deficit, movement disorders such as tremors, gait instability and weakness, depressive symptoms, and behavioral changes. HIVE is the result of direct HIV infection of the brain macrophages and/or microglial cells. On autopsy of AIDS patients with HIVE, demyelination, microglial nodules, multinucleated giant cells, and perivascular infiltration are described. Diagnosis is based on neuropsychological testing of suspected individuals and exclusion of alternate conditions. Cerebrospinal fluid (CSF) studies are helpful in the diagnosis and excluding mimics such as cryptococcosis, toxoplasmosis, PML, or syphilis. Highly active antiretroviral therapy (HAART) is the primary treatment of choice, and its benefit is well documented.

Question for Further Thought
1. What are the risk factors for HIVE?

Reporting Responsibilities
Routine reporting is sufficient in this case. It should be clearly distinguished from opportunistic infections that are common in patients with AIDS, and most of such lesions tend to contrast enhance in either the parenchyma or meninges.

What the Treating Physician Needs to Know
• Pattern of WM lesions and degree of volume loss
• Other associated abnormalities
• Exclusion of opportunistic infections and neoplastic changes

Answer
Risk factors for HIVE include older age at seroconversion, female gender, duration of HIV infection, presence of a prior AIDS-defining diagnosis, low CD4+, and low nadir CD4 count. These risk factors suggest that severe and prolonged immunosuppression may have long-lasting effects on neuropsychiatric performance regardless of subsequent viral suppression. Other factors such as high plasma HIV-RNA load, anemia, low weight, presence of hepatitis C virus, and substance abuse are associated with increase in the prevalence of neurocognitive deficits and dementia.

CLINICAL HISTORY *15-year-old female who first developed vertigo and imbalance with complete improvement. Six weeks later she presented with lower extremity numbness and weakness, bowel and bladder dysfunction.*

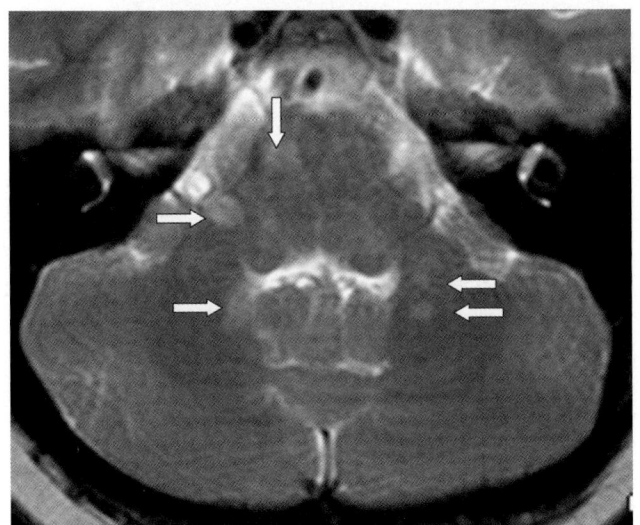

FIGURE 66-1

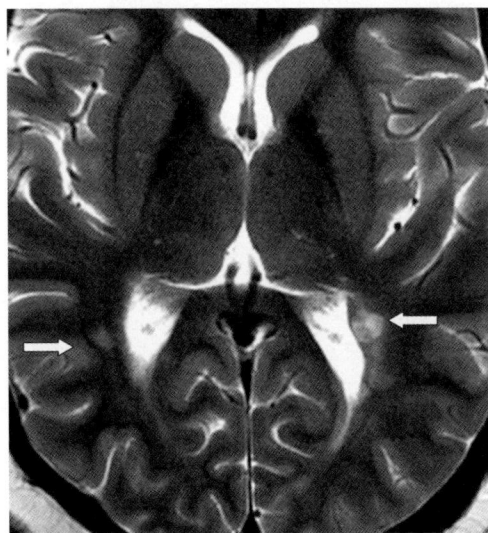

FIGURE 66-2

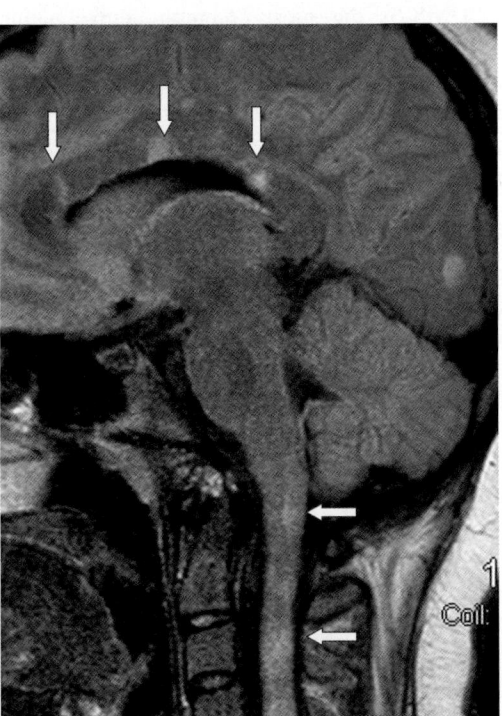

FIGURE 66-3

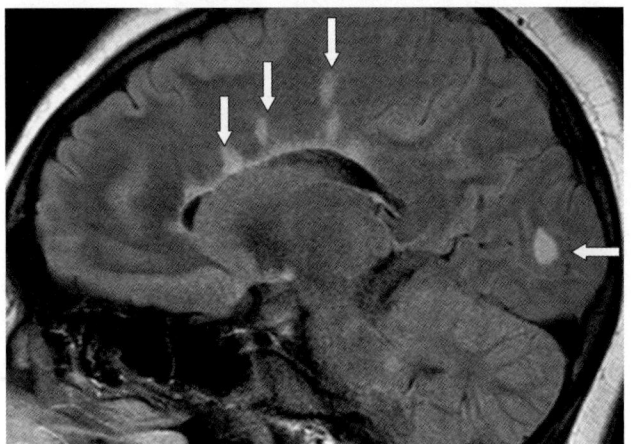

FIGURE 66-4

FINDINGS Figure 66-1. Axial MR T2WI through the lower brainstem. There are multifocal brainstem, bilateral brachium pontis, and cerebellar hyperintense lesions (arrows). Figure 66-2. Axial T2WI through the trigones of the lateral ventricles. There are bilateral peritrigonal hyperintense lesions (arrows). Figure 66-3. Sagittal FLAIR through the corpus callosum showing multifocal corpus callosal hyperintense

lesions of varying shapes and sizes abutting the callososeptal interface (vertical arrows). There are also multiple cervical spinal cord hyperintense lesions (transverse arrows). Figure 66-4. Parasagittal FLAIR showing multiple ovoid periventricular and deep WM lesions (so-called Dawson fingers, vertical arrows). There is an occipital subcortical lesion (transverse arrow). Figure 66-5. Axial FLAIR through the upper corona radiata showing multiple subcortical lesions (arrows). Multiple periventricular and deep white matter (WM) lesions are also demonstrated. Lesions are of varying shapes and sizes. Figure 66-6. Axial T1WI through the centrum semiovale. There are deep WM multifocal hypointense lesions, the so-called T1-weighted black holes (transverse arrows). Figure 66-7. Axial post-contrast T1WI through the same level. There are multiple contrast-enhancing lesions

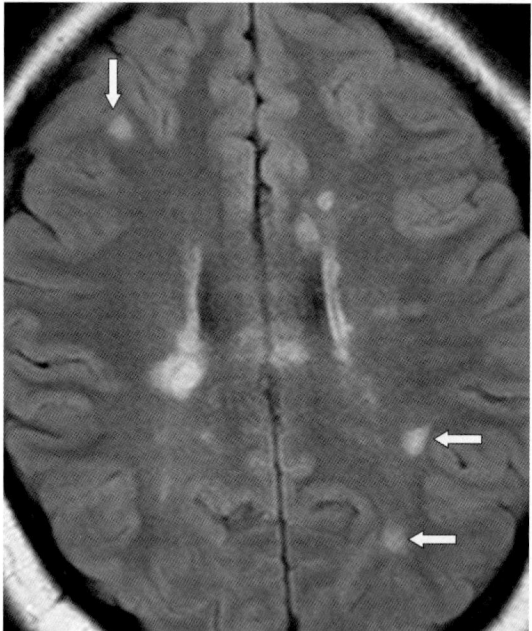

FIGURE 66-5

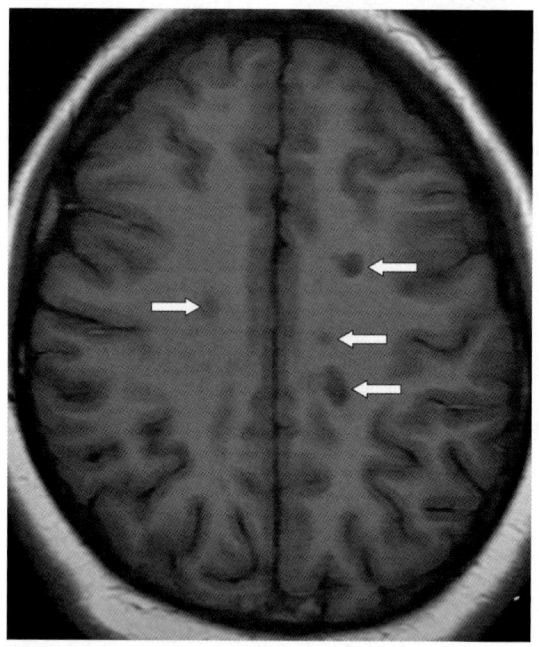

FIGURE 66-6

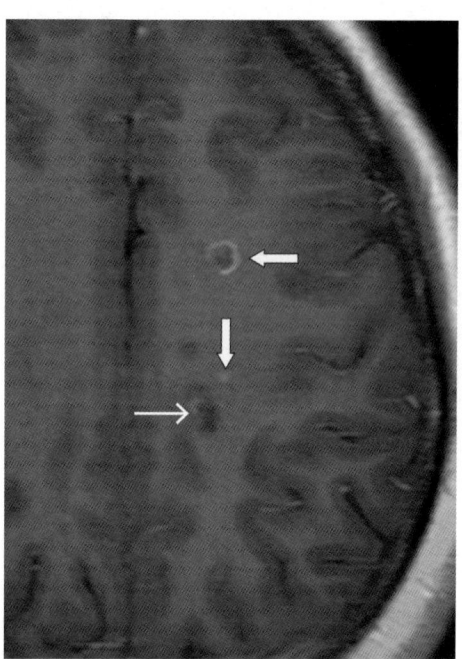

FIGURE 66-7

of the incomplete ring (transverse arrow), punctate (vertical arrow), and a small arc enhancement (line transverse arrow) in the left centrum semiovale.

DIFFERENTIAL DIAGNOSIS Multiple sclerosis (MS), vasculitis, sarcoidosis, Susac syndrome, acute disseminated encephalomyelitis (ADEM).

DIAGNOSIS Multiple sclerosis (MS).

DISCUSSION MS is the most common demyelinating inflammatory disease involving the WM of the central nervous system (CNS). It remains a clinical diagnosis supported by MRI and laboratory findings. MRI is the examination of choice for the evaluation of the suspected MS patient presenting with the so-called clinically isolated syndrome (CIS) in whom MRI lesions suggestive of demyelination are found in about 50% to 70%. Typical MRI lesions are T2 hyperintense WM lesions of varying shapes and sizes found in the periventricular, deep, and subcortical WM of the cerebrum, brainstem, brachium pontis, and cerebellum. Presence of lesions in the corpus callosum (CC) and the spinal cord lends strong support to the diagnosis of MS. CC lesions typical of MS abut the callososeptal interface; pattern not seen in vasculitis or sarcoidosis or Susac syndrome. Most of these lesions are round, ovoid, flame shaped, linear, or punctate. Large lesions more than 2 cm in size are classified as tumefactive. Smudgy or confluent WM T2 hyperintensity is also found in the MS brain. MR spectroscopy and DTI have shown abnormality in the apparent normal WM in MS patients. Increasingly, deep and cortical gray matter (GM) involvement is being reported. GM lesions are more common in ADEM. This case illustrates the various patterns of contrast enhancement in MS, which includes the nodular type in about 68%; incomplete thin ring, which is almost pathognomonic for MS in about 23%; and arc and other patterns in about 9%. Leptomeningeal enhancement is generally absent in MS but present in its mimics. Contrast enhancement is the hallmark of active/acute lesion. Up to 80% of contrast-enhancing lesions have T1-weighted hypointensity, so-called black holes. Less than 40% of the black holes become permanent. The number of black holes correlates well with the degree of disability. Steroid treatment may modify the pattern of contrast enhancement. Contrast enhancement usually resolves within 6 weeks.

MS is a disease of the temperate climate and is more common in women than men. Pediatric involvement is present in about 5% of MS population. Its presentation or exacerbation may include features such as optic neuritis in as many as 50%, transverse myelitis, brainstem symptoms such as vertigo, diplopia, imbalance, Bell's palsy, and less frequently focal neurologic deficit. These lesions may wax and wane. Supportive laboratory findings include cerebrospinal fluid (CSF) and vestibular evoked potential (VEP) findings. CSF studies in this patient revealed no pleocytosis or abnormal protein but an increase in IgG index and synthesis and positive oligoclonal bands. The presence of oligoclonal bands in the CSF is not diagnostic of MS but supportive of demyelination. A comprehensive blood workup was done to rule out MS mimics in this patient.

Question for Further Thought

1. What are the various types of MS?

Reporting Responsibilities

Routine reporting is sufficient. An ideal MRI report for MS should contain the number of lesions unless they are "too numerous to count," the size of the lesions, the shape of the lesions, the borders of the lesions, and the pattern of enhancement and presence or absence of leptomeningeal enhancement. "Periventricular lesions" are to be reserved for the ones clearly abutting the ventricles. Location of the infratentorial lesions should be described. Presence of "black holes" or at least a description that the T2 lesions are associated with T1 hypointensities should be acknowledged. The term such as "nonspecific" should be avoided in the context of clear abnormalities in the spinal cord. The degree of volume loss should be reported.

What the Treating Physician Needs to Know

- Location, number, pattern, and contrast enhancement of lesions on initial MRI
- Presence of new lesions, both contrast and non contrast enhancing, and their location on follow-up studies
- Pattern of volume loss and presence of black holes on T1WI
- Criteria for diagnosis of MS keep changing; hence, a full description of positive and negative findings is always helpful to the referring physician

Answer

1. MS is characterized clinically into four categories. Relapsing–remitting MS (RRMS) is characterized by relapses and remissions and more common in women than men (3:1). Secondary progressive MS (SPMS) is characterized by secondary slow progression of RRMS with and without superimposed relapses. Primary progressive MS (PPMS) is characterized by at least 1 year of progression of spastic mono- or paraparesis or ataxia. Progressive relapsing MS (PRMS) is characterized by at least 1 year of progression of the neurologic deficit with superimposed relapses. The diagnosis of relapsing type of MS is done by fulfilling the criteria of dissemination in time (DIT) and dissemination in space (DIS). The presence of enhancing and non-enhancing lesions on the same MRI is enough to fulfill the criteria for DIT. The presence of at least one lesion in two of the four typical MRI locations for demyelination is enough to fulfill the criterion of DIS. These typical locations are periventricular, juxtacortical, infratentorial, and spinal cord.

CLINICAL HISTORY *28-year-old right-handed female with initial presentation of right-sided occipital and neck pain, forgetfulness, and subsequent decreased visual acuity and left hemianopsia.*

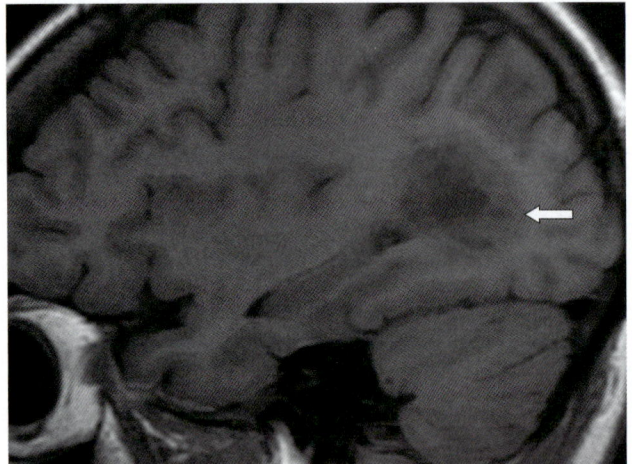

FIGURE 67-1

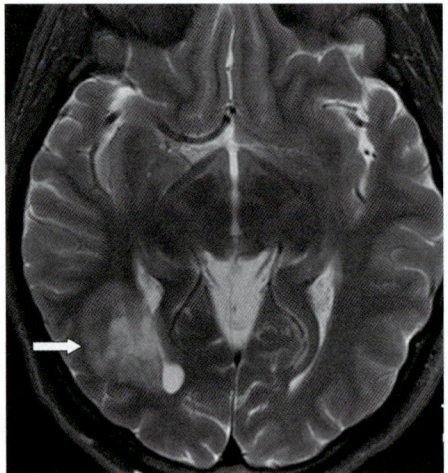

FIGURE 67-2

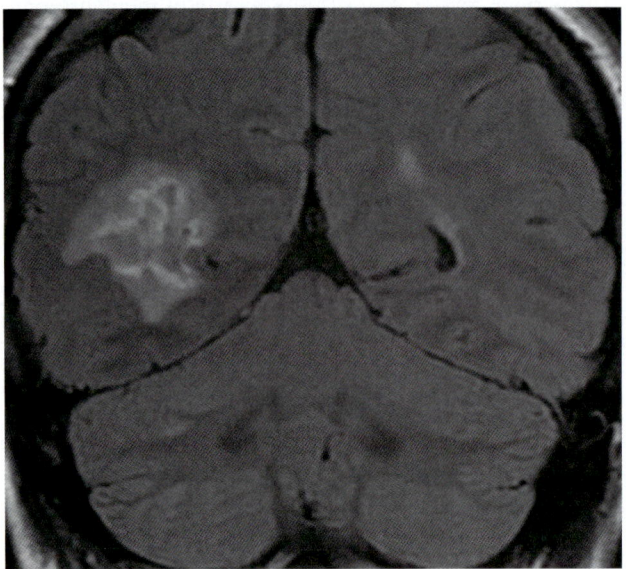

FIGURE 67-3

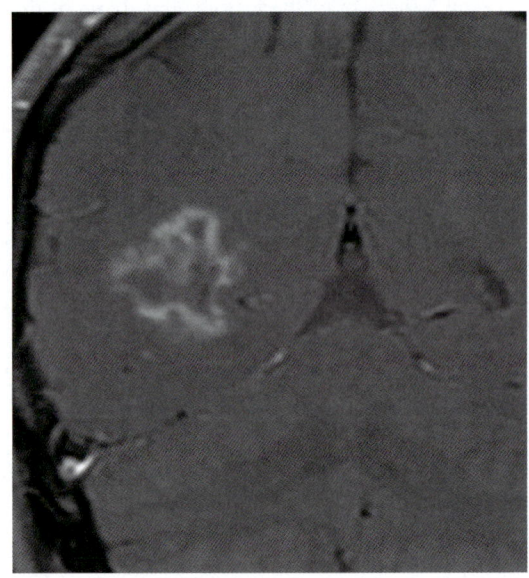

FIGURE 67-4

FINDINGS Figure 67-1. Right parasagittal T1WI MRI of the brain showing a heterogeneous hypointense lesion in the right occipito-temporo-parietal white matter (WM) with very minimal mass effect (arrow). Figure 67-2. Axial T2WI through the mass. The mass (arrow) is lateral to the right trigone and occipital horn showing shades of hyperintensity from central almost cerebrospinal fluid (CSF) intensity to less hyperintense variegated heterogeneous periphery. There is no significant mass effect. Figure 67-3. Coronal FLAIR through the lesion showing a three-layer pattern of isointense irregular core with surrounding irregular crinkled hyperintensity and a periphery of smudgy medium hyperintensity presumably edema. Figure 67-4. Coronal

post-contrast T1WI. There is a 3.3 cm × 2 cm irregular thick crinkled avid enhancement corresponding to the middle layer in Figure 67-3 surrounding an irregular iso/hypointense core. The peripheral portion is isointense with the surrounding brain. The axial post-contrast images (not shown) show some discontinuity in the enhancing portion. There were a few non-contrast-enhancing periventricular focal T2 hyperintensity elsewhere in the bilateral cerebral WM (not shown).

DIFFERENTIAL DIAGNOSIS Tumefactive multiple sclerosis (TMS), astrocytoma, granuloma, progressive multifocal leucoencephalopathy (PML).

DIAGNOSIS TMS.

DISCUSSION TMS as opposed to tumefactive demyelinating lesion (TDL) occurs in the contest of multiple sclerosis (MS) in which case the diagnosis of MS is established with the dissemination in time and space criteria as well as other criteria satisfied. A tumefactive demyelination could also progress to MS after satisfying the usual criteria. TMS is described as large well-demarcated mass-like WM lesions larger than 2 cm with little mass effect and edema. The other MRI characteristics include hypointensity on T1WI and hyperintensity on FLAIR and T2WI with a variety of contrast-enhancing patterns including incomplete ring, arc, or nodular contrast enhancement as seen in other MS plaques. The central nonenhancing core of the incomplete ring is thought to represent a more chronic phase of the demyelination. TMS lesions are usually single but multiple lesions are reported. The size makes confusion with other neoplastic/inflammatory lesions such as glioblastoma (GB), lymphoma, abscess, and PML possible. However, the pattern of enhancement and surrounding edema and the location tend to cast doubt on the differentials. There may be areas of restricted diffusion and decreased perfusion, thus separating TMS from some of its mimics. Dilated vascular structures within tumefactive lesions have been reported in T2-echoplanar MR perfusion. Balo concentric sclerosis, another form of demyelinating process, usually presents with many concentric rings of alternating zones of demyelinated and myelinated WM somewhat dissimilar to this present case.

TMS is more common in women and because of its mass-like configuration may present with symptoms of mass lesions such as headache, focal neurologic deficit, and aphasia. Her CSF was positive for oligoclonal bands along with high glucose. Serology was negative for multiple other diseases. These lesions are supposed to respond very rapidly to steroid therapy with resolution of the lesions and their mass effect. However, in this patient, despite initial treatment with intravenous corticosteroid and subsequent oral steroid therapy, the lesion was unrelenting and showed progression with new lesions elsewhere in the brain on several follow-up MRI.

Question for Further Thought

1. What other lesions can be confused or coexist with TMS?

Reporting Responsibilities

Since the diagnosis is almost always in doubt, direct reporting is appropriate. Hint of high-grade malignancy should be stressed. Advanced imaging such as perfusion and MR spectroscopy (MRS) may be helpful in this regard and can be recommended. Presence of leptomeningeal enhancement may suggest alternative diagnosis.

What the Treating Physician Needs to Know

- Location is important regarding planning for biopsy
- Is there any significant mass effect? Is lumbar puncture (LP) safe?
- Presence of other WM lesions that might suggest MS
- Any leptomeningeal enhancement?

Answer

1. TMS like other TDLs has been described rarely in association with astrocytoma. Solitary TMS lesion has preceded the appearance of lymphoma and therefore longitudinal monitoring of single TDL is warranted. Histologic diagnosis of TDL may be misinterpreted as a neoplasm given its hypercellular nature and the frequent presence of atypical reactive astrocytes and mitotic figures. These features pose a potential trap for the pathologist.

CLINICAL HISTORY *21-year-old female with dizziness, ataxia, and left-sided hearing loss.*

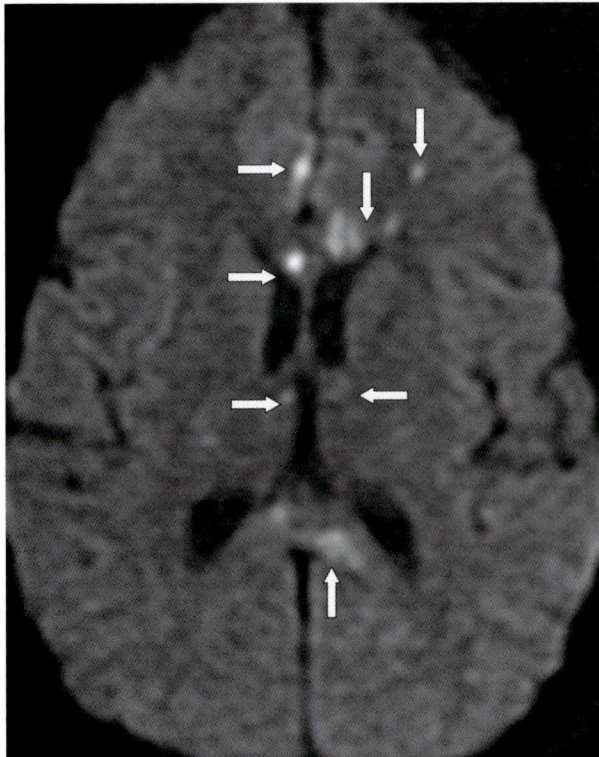

FIGURE 68-1

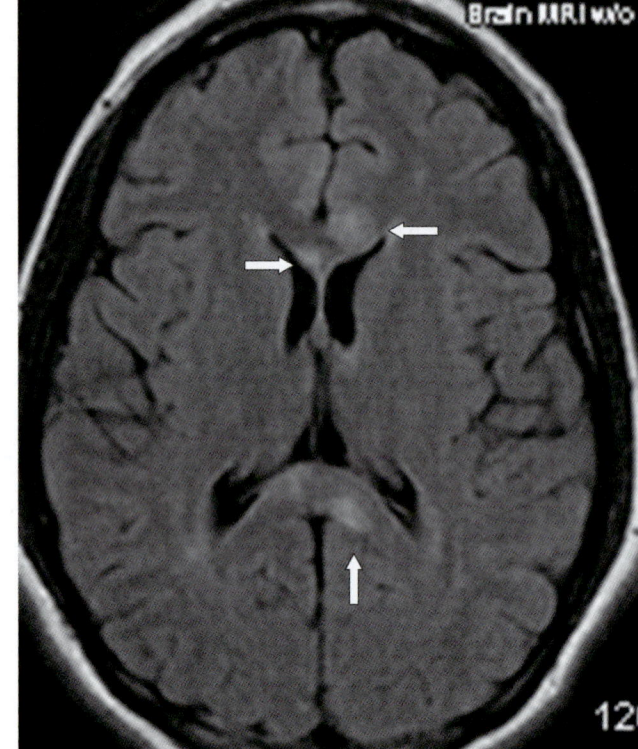

FIGURE 68-2

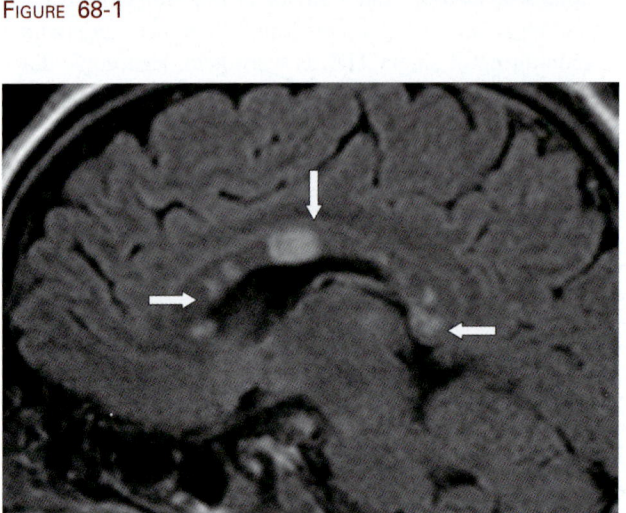

FIGURE 68-3

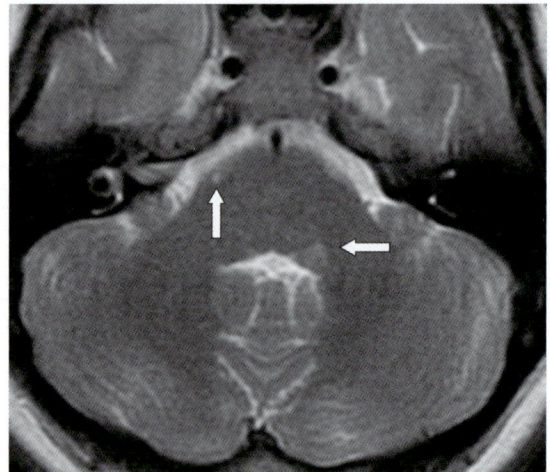

FIGURE 68-4

FINDINGS Figures 68-1 and 68-2. Axial DWI and FLAIR MRI through the corpus callosum (CC). There are multifocal CC, bilateral periventricular and subcortical hyperintense lesions with subtle lesions in the anterior thalamus bilaterally, and right cingulate cortex (arrows). Figure 68-3. Sagittal FLAIR MRI through the CC showing multiple round hyperintense lesions in the genu, body, and splenium of the CC (arrows) with no significant callososeptal interface hyperintensity. The so-called snowball lesion (vertical arrow) is a large round focal hyperintensity in the CC. Figure 68-4. Axial T2WI through the brachium pontis. There is a medial left brachium pontis focal hyperintensity adjacent to the fourth ventricle (transverse arrow) and a small lesion anteriorly in the basis pontis on the right (vertical arrow).

There were no obvious areas of restricted diffusion on these images. Post-contrast images (not shown) did not reveal any abnormal contrast enhancement.

DIFFERENTIAL DIAGNOSIS Susac syndrome (SS), vasculitis, multiple sclerosis (MS), acute disseminated encephalomyelitis (ADEM).

DIAGNOSIS Susac syndrome (SS).

DISCUSSION Imaging findings in SS consist of multifocal T2 hyperintensities in both white matter (WM) and the deep and cortical gray matter (GM) of the brain. The involvement of the corona radiata and centrum semiovale and the CC is present in all patients and the lesions are best seen on the FLAIR. Brachium pontis, brainstem, and cerebellar hemispheres are involved in between 30% and 52% of patients. Lesions in the CC preferentially affect the central region and are round resulting in "snowball" lesions, in contrast to the callososeptal interface lesions found in MS. "Dawson fingers," the ovoid periventricular (perivenular) lesions characteristic of MS, are not common in SS. The deep GM of the basal ganglia and thalami is affected (similar to ADEM and vasculitis but in contrast to MS) in up to 70% of patients. Contrast-enhancing lesions in both GM and WM could be seen in up to 70% of affected population. A very small percentage of the lesions may restrict diffusion. Leptomeningeal enhancement is present in about 30% of SS patients and distinguishes SS from MS or ADEM where leptomeningeal enhancement does not often occur. An extensive blood and cerebrospinal fluid (CSF) workup is required to rule out other vascular, neoplastic, toxic, and infectious diseases.

The etiology of SS is not definitely known but it is believed to be a microangiopathy with microinfarcts possibly immune mediated and multisystemic in presentation. It is characterized by the triad of microangiopathy of the brain, eye, and ear, resulting in encephalopathy, severe headache, behavioral changes, mental status changes, and confusion along with visual impairment and sensorineural hearing loss (SNHL). It is more common in women than men and more commonly occurs between the third and sixth decades of life. All the three elements of the syndrome may not be present initially; hence, imaging may be the pointer to the correct diagnosis. SS is confirmed by demonstrating branch retinal artery occlusion (BRAO) by fluorescein angiogram. BRAO is usually not painful in contrast to optic neuritis in MS. The SNHL is sometimes associated with vertigo, tinnitus, and nystagmus. The treatment of SS involves treatment of exacerbations with high-dose corticosteroids and IVIG. Long-term immunosuppressants may be required. The disease tends to stabilize within 2 to 4 years with varying degrees of residual impairment.

Question for Further Thought

1. Is a brain biopsy necessary to make the diagnosis of SS?

Reporting Responsibilities

This is usually not an acute situation and routine reporting may be sufficient. In the presence of MRI findings suggestive of MS in a patient with encephalopathy, SS should be in the differential. Leptomeningeal enhancement and basal ganglia involvement are uncommon in MS and should be highlighted. Imaging of the spinal cord is clinically warranted.

What the Treating Physician Needs to Know

- Detailed description of lesions
- Presence of leptomeningeal enhancement may prompt CSF evaluation
- CSF may occasionally show elevated IgG index or synthesis rate with oligoclonal band
- SS is an uncommon disorder and may not be on the radar of the radiologist who is not privy to all the information. A report of possible MS on the MRI in an encephalopathic patient should result in clinical evaluation for SS

Answer

1. In the presence of the clinical triad of encephalopathy, hearing loss, and visual impairment, a brain biopsy is not warranted. In comatose patients who cannot cooperate with an eye or ear examination, a biopsy may be indicated to tailor treatment and differentiate SS from ADEM or other forms of vasculopathy. Biopsy tends to show perivascular inflammation and microinfarctions without vessel wall necrosis.

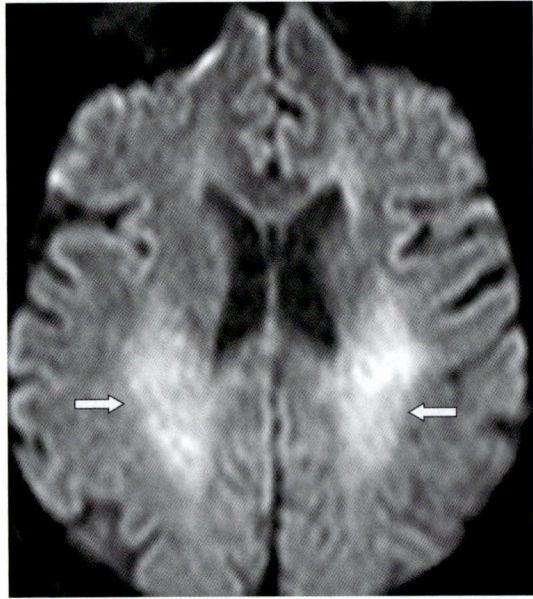

FIGURE 69-1

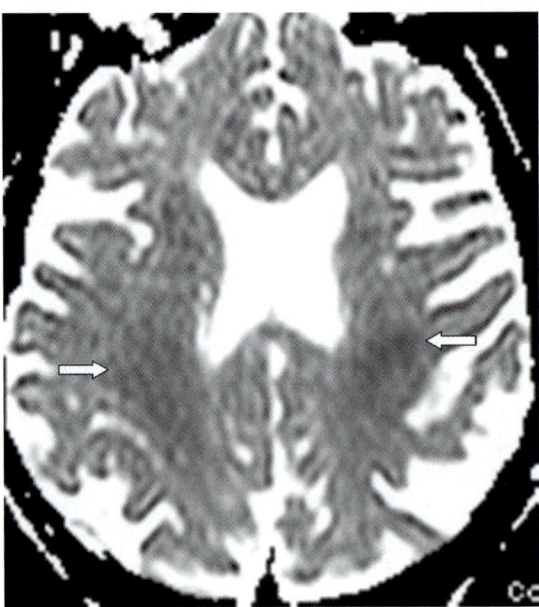

FIGURE 69-2

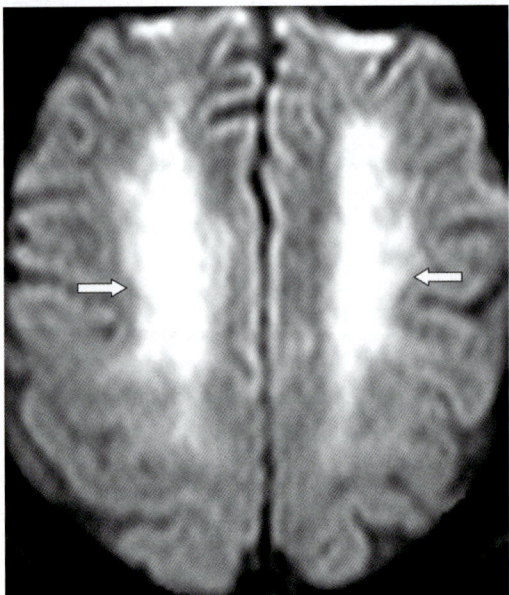

FIGURE 69-3

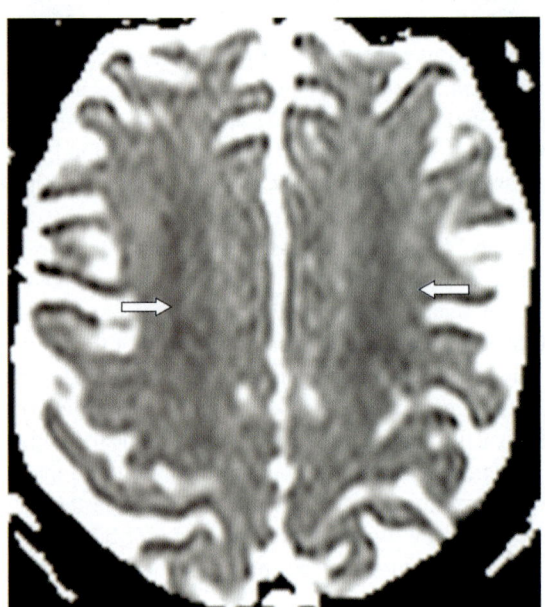

FIGURE 69-4

FINDINGS Figures 69-1 to 69-4. Axial MR DWI and corresponding ADC maps through the corona radiata (Figures 69-1 and 69-2) and the centrum semiovale (Figures 69-3 and 69-4) demonstrating bilateral mainly posterior smudgy or confluent white matter (WM) restricted diffusion in the posterior corona radiata and smudgy/confluent restricted diffusion throughout the entire WM of the bilateral centrum semiovale (arrows). There is sparing of the subcortical U fibers. Figures 69-5 and 69-6. Axial FLAIR images through the corona radiata

and centrum semiovale, respectively, showing smudgy T2 hyperintensity in bilateral corona radiata and centrum semiovale. MRI done 5 days before this set (not shown) did not demonstrate any significant WM diffusion restriction. There was no contrast enhancement.

DIFFERENTIAL DIAGNOSIS Toxic leukoencephalopathy, delayed WM hypoxic ischemic encephalopathy (HIE) (delayed posthypoxic leukoencephalopathy, DPHL), leukodystrophy, acute disseminated encephalomyelitis (ADEM).

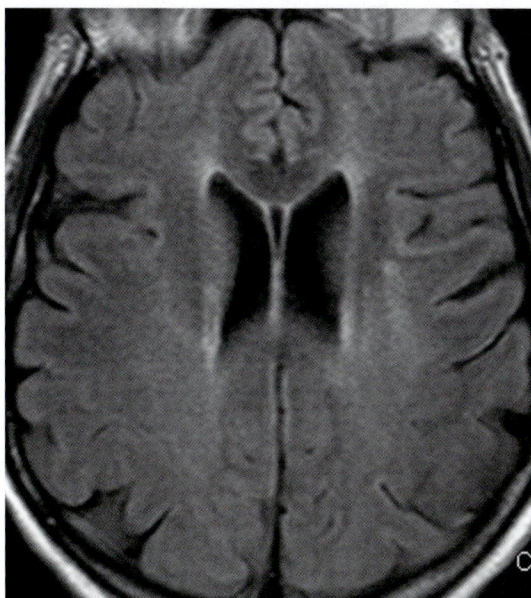

FIGURE 69-5

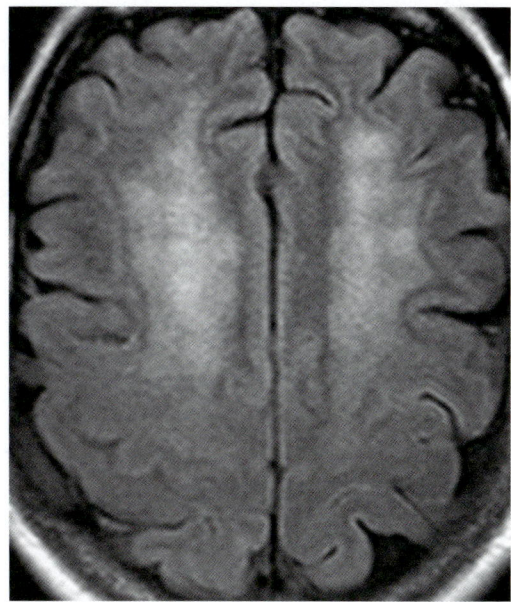

FIGURE 69-6

DIAGNOSIS Delayed posthypoxic leukoencephalopathy (DPHL).

DISCUSSION The classical imaging findings of DPHL are bilateral symmetrical WM confluent restricted diffusion with similar T2 hyperintensity in the cerebral hemispheres days or weeks following a hypoxic event. Initial imaging at the time of initial insult is often normal. Depending on the cause of the initial insult, cerebellar and internal capsular lesions may also be present particularly in heroin-related hypoxic changes known as 'chasing the dragon'. The deep or superficial gray matter (GM) is usually spared but imaging changes in these structures have been reported. The WM changes are reversible along with excellent clinical recovery over the long term. It may be difficult to exclude the differential diagnoses at imaging without the benefit of the history. The syndrome of delayed neurologic deterioration with cerebral demyelination has been reported in the setting of carbon monoxide (CO) poisoning. The basal ganglia are usually involved in CO poisoning. However, this syndrome is now more commonly seen in the context of drug overdose with heroin or benzodiazepine and in other situations that lead to severe hypoxia.

A month prior to her current admission this patient was found unresponsive. She was found to be in cardiogenic shock with shocked liver and acute renal failure. She was treated, improved close to her baseline, and was sent home. She reportedly started feeding dirt to the family pet and wore her underwear on the outside of her pants. She was not able to ambulate without support as she was weak and unsteady. She was readmitted 2 weeks following her initial discharge with mental status change. Neuropsychiatric behavior is a prominent feature of DPHL. Seizure may also be a feature of this disorder.

It is well known that anoxic or hypoxic injury produces acute neurologic deficits with changes visible in the deep or cortical GM. GM is very susceptible to hypoxia. It is less well known that severe neurologic consequences may be delayed for days or weeks after the injury and that the corresponding imaging findings may be delayed even later and confined to the WM. The temporal separation between the injury and the neuropsychiatric consequences and/or imaging findings presents a diagnostic challenge. It has been reported that 3% of victims of acute CO intoxication have delayed neurologic sequelae 2 to 40 days (mean 2.4 days) after the initial injury. The delay is caused by the selective necrosis of myelin-producing glia cells in the border zones of the WM. Underlying pathology may include WM vacuolation, gliosis, and spongiform changes.

The rarity of this condition seems to suggest unidentified individual susceptibilities to hypoxic neuronal injury. An extensive workup for inflammatory, infectious, paraneoplastic, vascular, metabolic, and inherited leukodystrophies was undertaken and yielded no positive answer in this patient. Increased myelin basic protein (MBP) in the cerebrospinal fluid (CSF) and abnormal imaging were the only abnormalities found. Management is generally supportive and the long-term prognosis is good.

Questions for Further Thought

1. Is DPHL always preceded by unresponsiveness?
2. What is the difference between HIE and DPHL?

Reporting Responsibilities

The restricted diffusion demands prompt and direct reporting. The predominant WM location of lesions should evoke ischemic or toxic leukoencephalopathy. High index of suspicion is necessary in this rather uncommon presentation of a common problem.

What the Treating Physician Needs to Know

- Absence of complications such as brain swelling and herniations
- CSF evaluation is necessary and LP is safe in the absence of mass effect
- Most patients improve within 3 to 6 months. The likelihood of recovery is inversely related to the patient's age.

Answers

1. DPHL is always preceded by unresponsiveness except in cases associated with CO poisoning.
2. DPHL is a rare complication of HIE occurring in 2.75% of patients with CO poisoning. While HIE mostly affect GM, DPHL is mostly a WM disease. It is not well understood why only a small subset of HIE develop DPHL.

CLINICAL HISTORY *52-year-old female was admitted with generalized tonic–clonic seizures and confusion 3 months following a diagnosis of syndrome of inappropriate antidiuretic hormone SIADH.*

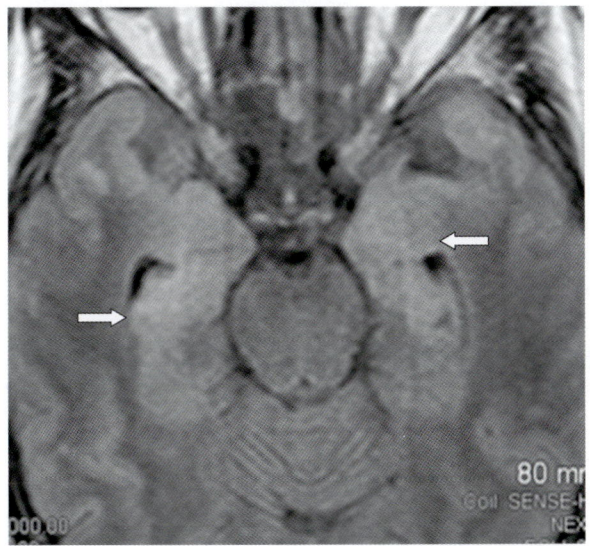

FIGURE 70-1

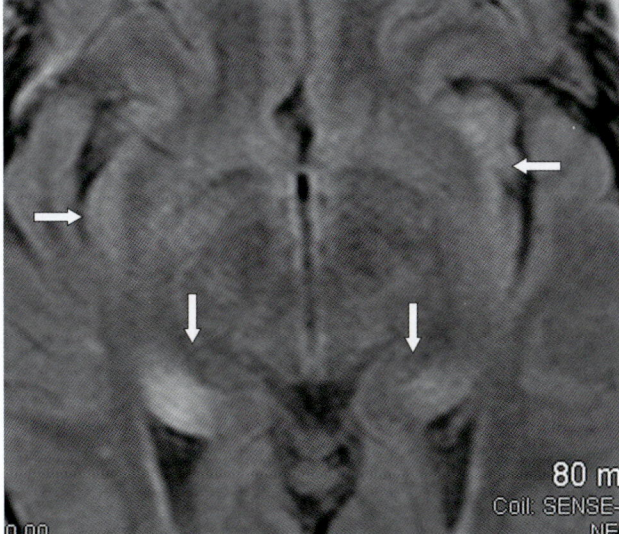

FIGURE 70-2

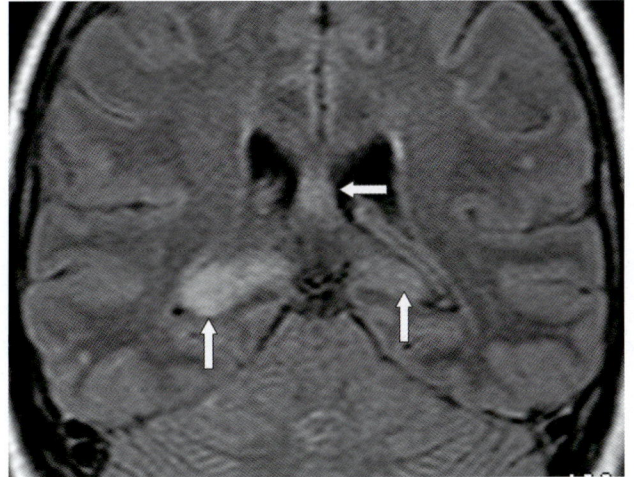

FIGURE 70-3

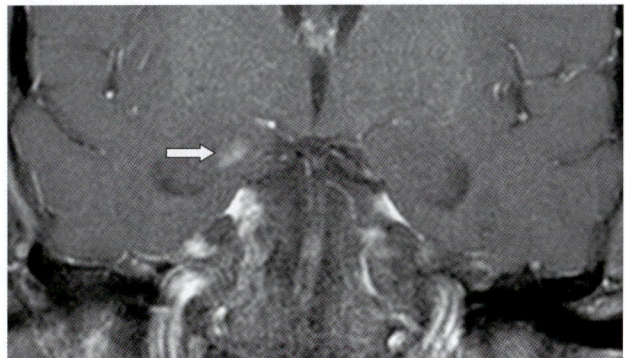

FIGURE 70-4

FINDINGS Figure 70-1. Axial MR FLAIR through the temporal lobes. There is bilateral almost symmetrical mesiotemporal smudgy hyperintensity (arrows). Figure 70-2. Axial FLAIR through the hippocampi. There is asymmetric bilateral hippocampal hyperintensity (vertical arrows) and hyperintense insula cortex bilaterally (transverse arrows). Figure 70-3. Coronal FLAIR through hippocampi. There is bilateral asymmetric hippocampal hyperintensity larger on the right than the left (vertical arrows). The transverse arrow points to the hyperintense fornix. Figure 70-4. Coronal post-contrast T1WI through the temporal lobes showing a small right mesiotemporal lobe contrast enhancement (transverse arrow).

DIFFERENTIAL DIAGNOSIS Limbic encephalitis (paraneoplastic), herpes simplex encephalitis (HSE) and human herpes virus 6 (HHV6) encephalitis, seizure-related changes, gliomatosis.

DIAGNOSIS Paraneoplastic limbic encephalitis (PLE).

DISCUSSION MRI is the examination of choice in the evaluation of a patient suspected of PLE. CT is fairly insensitive to the changes as it may be difficult to appreciate the hypodensity of the temporal lobes. The classical MRI finding in PLE is bilateral mesiotemporal lobes smudgy T2 hyperintensity with or without significant mass effect which is best demonstrated on the FLAIR images. These changes could be significantly subtle on T2WI. Corresponding hypointensity could be present on T1WI. Other sites that could show T2 hyperintensities are the hippocampus, the column of fornix, insula, and the subfrontal orbital gyrus regions. Diffusion restriction is not usually a feature of PLE but may be present in seizure-related changes. Contrast enhancement present in this case is a rare finding and has been reported in only a few cases. MRI may not be positive in some cases of PLE and a high index of suspicion should be kept if the clinical picture is suggestive and no other etiology is found. There is suggestion that positron emission tomography (PET) imaging may show temporal lobe lesions in this subset. It may be difficult to differentiate PLE from other causes of mesiotemporal T2 hyperintensity such as HSE, HHV6, gliomatosis, and seizure-related changes. The gold standard for excluding HSE and HHV6 infection is cerebrospinal fluid (CSF) polymerase chain reaction (PCR) which has a sensitivity of over 95% for HSE. HSE and HHV6 are treatable diseases with high mortality if treatment is delayed. Volume loss is the final pathway of a healed PLE. Gliomatosis will not show volume loss on follow-up.

PLE is an autoimmune disorder that is associated with onconeuronal antibodies to intracellular and cell surface antigens in the neuropil. The tumor-associated antibodies in PLE include anti-VGKC, NMDA-R, AMPA-R, HU, Ma2, amphiphysin, and CV2/CRMP5 antibodies. It may take up to 5 years for the discovery of associated tumor. The classic clinical manifestations of PLE include rapid onset of mood dysfunction, hallucinations, seizures, and short-term memory loss. CSF study in this patient showed minimal pleocytosis, normal protein, and matching oligoclonal band (OGB) in the serum and CSF. Herpes virus panel and other extensive infectious and inflammatory workup were negative. A 24-hour video electroencephalogram (EEG) demonstrated mild-to-moderate diffuse cerebral dysfunction, intermittent poorly formed bifrontal epileptiform activity, and multifocal seizures, arising out of the left hemisphere and the left temporal region.

Questions for Further Thought

1. How does SIADH fit in the clinical picture of PLE?
2. What are the other supportive laboratory findings in PLE?

Reporting Responsibilities

Direct reporting is important in view of the differential of herpes encephalitis since delay in treatment of HSE could be catastrophic. Mass effect if present should be reported.

What the Treating Physician Needs to Know

- Presence of significant mass effect since lumbar puncture (LP) is always indicated in this situation
- There are no other imaging methods to confirm the diagnosis
- Techniques for cancer screening include CT chest, abdomen, and pelvis or body FDG-PET as well as assay for the tumor-associated antibodies. Such tumors may include ovarian, breast, testicular, small cell lung, and lymphoma

Answers

1. PLE can be associated with hypothalamic–pituitary dysfunction that could result in SIADH.
2. CSF typically shows lymphocytic pleocytosis, high protein, and frequent elevation of IgG index and synthesis. A normal CSF study except for the presence of OGB is also possible. Assay for the various paraneoplastic antibodies is important. EEG is abnormal showing generalized or focal slowing or epileptiform discharges in the temporal lobes. The constellation of findings on clinical examination, CSF study, EEG, and MRI should guide the clinician to the right diagnosis.

CLINICAL HISTORY *15-year-old male with T-cell lymphoblastic lymphoma. Three months after initiation of methotrexate treatment, the patient developed a headache with a progressive right-sided brachiofacial weakness and dysarthria.*

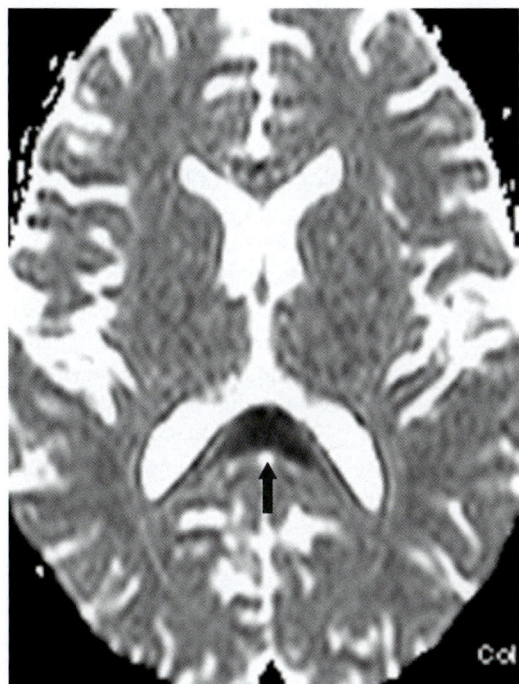

FIGURE 71-1

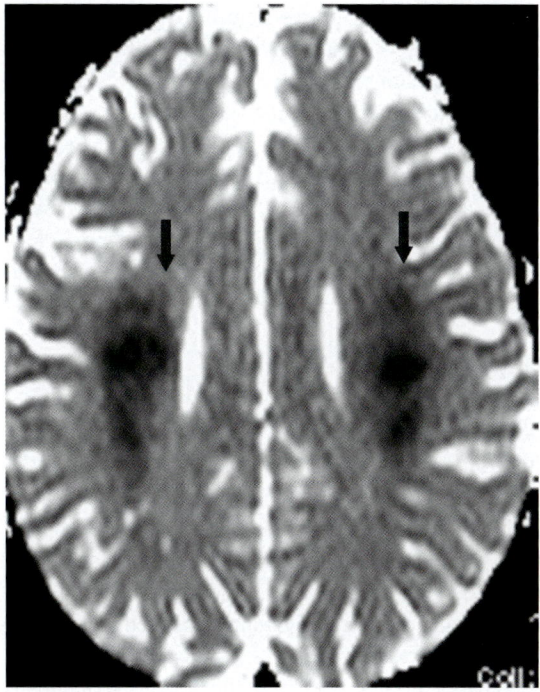

FIGURE 71-2

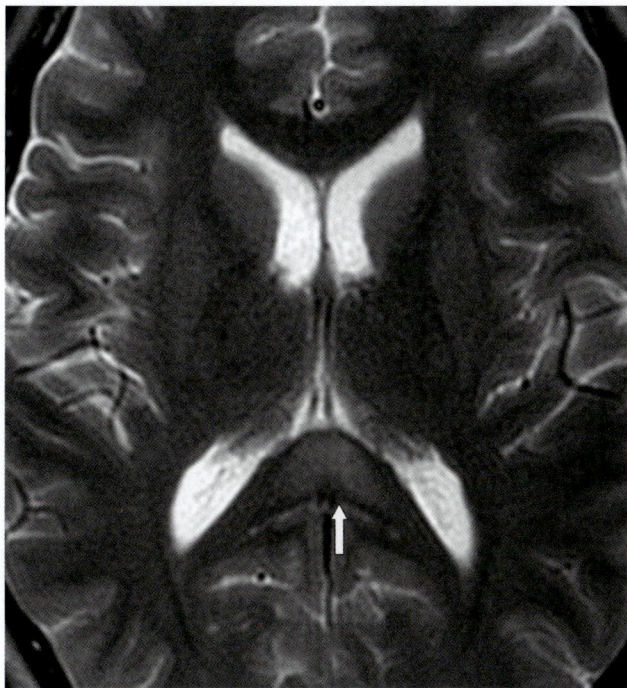

FIGURE 71-3

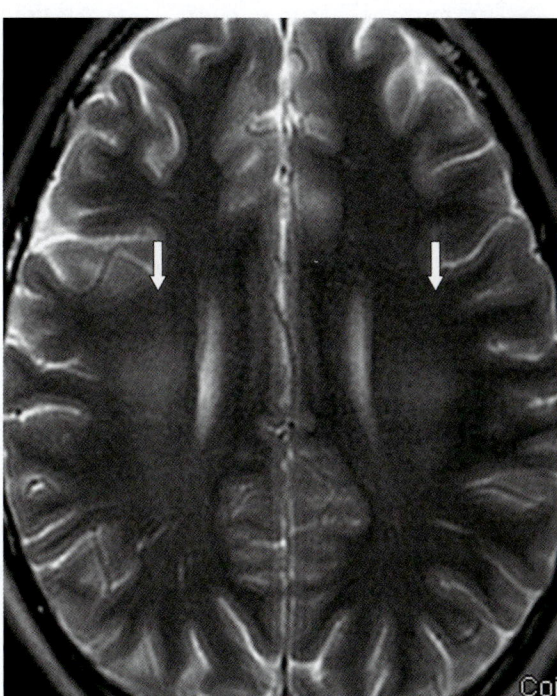

FIGURE 71-4

FINDINGS Figure 71-1. Axial ADC map through the splenium of corpus callosum. There is focal restricted diffusion of the splenium (arrow). Figure 71-2. Axial ADC map through the corona radiata. There are bilateral symmetrical white matter (WM) areas of restricted diffusion (arrows). Figures 71-3 and 71-4. Axial T2WI through the splenium and the corona radiata, respectively. There are confluent hyperintensity in the splenium and bilateral WM (arrows).

DIFFERENTIAL DIAGNOSIS Toxic encephalopathy, methotrexate leukoencephalopathy (MTX LE), posterior reversible encephalopathy syndrome (PRES), delayed post-hypoxic leukoencephalopathy (DPHL) hypoglycemia, hypoxic ischemic encephalopathy (HIE).

DIAGNOSIS MTX LE.

DISCUSSION The MRI findings in MTX LE include bilateral symmetrical diffusion restriction in the cerebral WM mostly in the corona radiata and centrum semiovale with corresponding hyperintensity on FLAIR and T2WI. The T2 hyperintensity may lag behind the DWI changes. Basal ganglia involvement has also been reported. WM lesions are usually smudgy and diffuse and occur more frequently than basal ganglia lesions. Basal ganglia lesions could resemble changes of HIE. Unilateral lesions and lesions isolated to the corpus callosum or specific areas (anterior or posterior) of the centrum semiovale (CSO) have been reported. There is usually no mass effect and contrast enhancement has not been a feature. Lack of cortical and subcortical involvement differentiates MTX LE from PRES. DPHL could resemble MTX LE. These DWI changes are transient and resolution of lesions occurs in a mater of days or weeks. Clinical improvement is the norm. Persistence of small residual T2 changes has been reported as late as 39 months following the event. Reintroduction of MTX may be associated with recurrence in up to 56%. Lower MTX dosage might prevent recurrence.

MTX is an important component in the treatment of acute lymphocytic leukemia (ALL). Time of occurrence of MTX LE from the time of MTX administration is variable and most of the reported cases have been within 1 or 2 weeks following administration of MTX but could be as long as 127 months. The clinical presentation of MTX LE includes headache, mental status changes, stroke-like symptoms, choreoathetosis, and seizures. Symptoms may fluctuate. Patients are generally adolescents with no gender preference. The incidence of acute neurotoxicity associated with treatment of ALL with a variety of drugs including MTX is about 5% to 18%. The pathophysiology of MTX toxicity is not definitely

known and there are different theories. MTX competitively inhibits the enzyme dihydrofolate reductase (DHFR) that is required for the synthesis of tetrahydrofolate, an important precursor for purine base synthesis. The likely depletion of brain folate stores as a result of this interaction may be responsible for the neurotoxicity. MTX also promotes release of adenosine from fibroblasts and endothelial cells. High levels of adenosine dilate blood vessels and promote release of neurotransmitters that may slow the rate of neuron discharge and may play a part in the pathophysiology of MTX neurotoxicity. Increased concentration of homocysteine, an excitotoxic neurotransmitter, is also present. Increased homocysteine is thought to cause small vessel vasculopathy which conceivably could promote the changes seen on MRI. The pathology of MTX LE includes variable changes of demyelination, loss of oligodendroglia, focal or diffuse areas of WM necrosis, mineralizing microangiopathy, and glial damage that could be widespread throughout the CNS. Management of MTX LE has included high-dose folinic acid, aminophylline, and leucovorin with mixed result. MTX was stopped in this patient and he improved.

Question for Further Thought

1. Is MTX the only chemotherapeutic agent known to cause LE?

Reporting Responsibilities

Restricted diffusion usually indicates cytotoxic edema suggesting infarction. The history is important in arriving at the diagnosis. Direct reporting is necessary so that prompt management could begin. Although the entity is called MTX LE, gray matter could be affected and this may explain the presence of choreoathetosis in some patients. Presence of gray matter involvement may mimic HIE.

What the Treating Physician Needs to Know

- Is there evidence of true ischemia?
- MTX LE has been seen with all forms of MTX administration and at different dosages. The risk, however, is higher with high-dose treatment, intrathecal administration, and cranial irradiation
- The clinical recovery of MTX LE (days) is faster than the MRI recovery (months)

Answer

1. No. Other chemotherapeutic agents used in combination have been associated with LE and these include vincristine, melphalan, cyclophosphamide, BCNU, adriamycin, procarbazine, bleomycine, cisplatin, and nitrogen mustards.

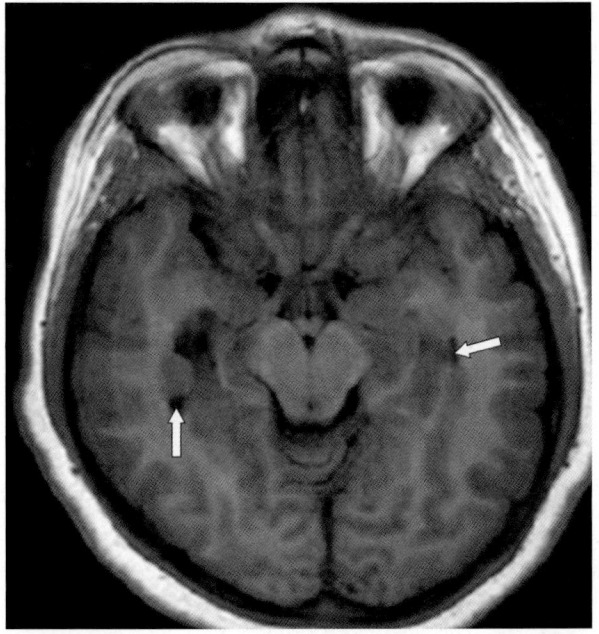

FIGURE 72-1.

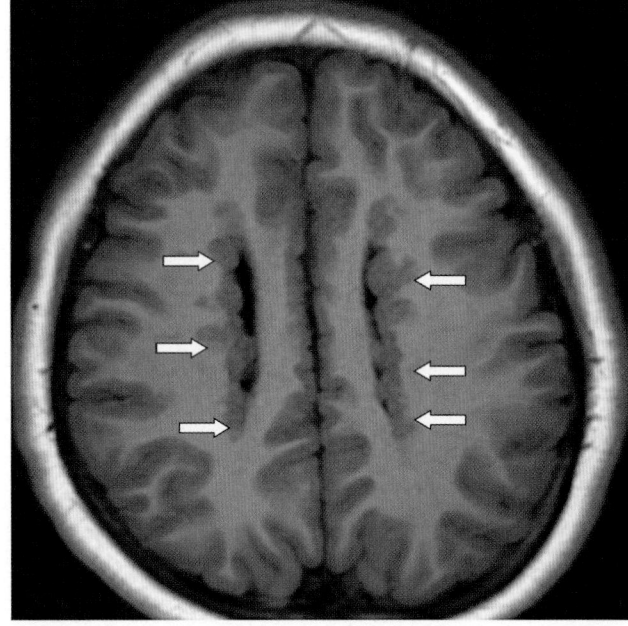

FIGURE 72-2.

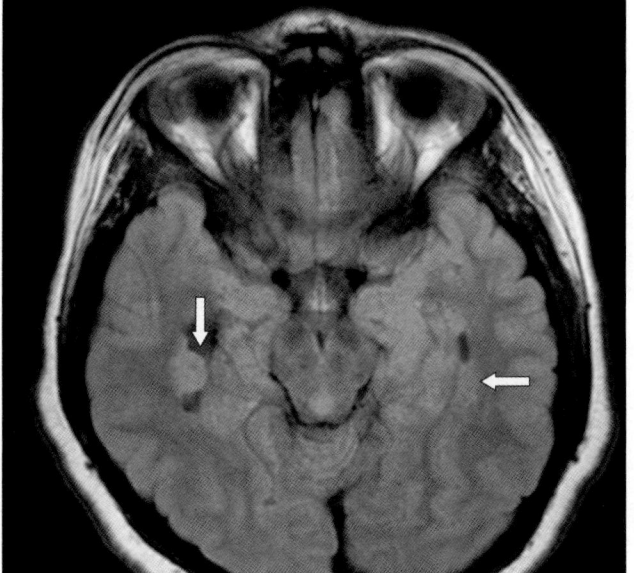

FIGURE 72-3.

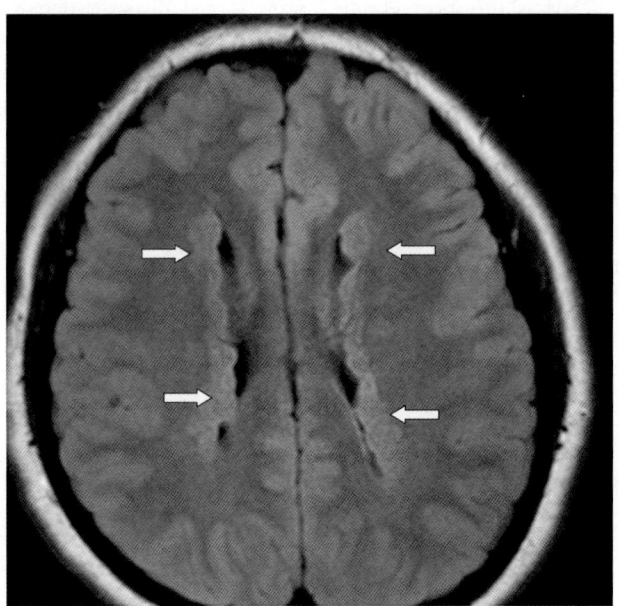

FIGURE 72-4.

FINDINGS Figure 72-1. Axial T1WI through the temporal horns. There is a subependymal nodule isointense with cortical gray matter (GM) projecting into the right temporal horn (vertical arrow). Similar but less defined nodules surround the left temporal horn (transverse arrow). Figure 72-2. Axial T1WI through the body of the lateral ventricles. There are multiple bilateral symmetrical contiguous subependymal nodules isointense with cortical GM projecting into the lateral ventricles (arrows). Figures 72-3 and 72-4. Axial FLAIR through the temporal horns and body of the lateral ventricles, respectively. There are multiple symmetrical isointense (to GM) contiguous subependymal nodules projecting into the temporal horns and body of the lateral ventricles (arrows).

DIFFERENTIAL DIAGNOSIS Heterotopic GM, tuberous sclerosis complex, toxoplasmosis, subependymoma.

DIAGNOSIS Periventricular nodular GM heterotopia (PNH).

DISCUSSION Both CT and MRI are capable of demonstrating the changes of PNH but MRI best depicts the classical findings. Classically, these are round or ovoid subependymal nodules that follow GM density on CT and GM intensity on all MRI sequences. These nodules could be single or multiple, matted or confluent, of varying sizes and usually project into the ventricles. They are more common around the trigones but are found all around the lateral ventricles. PNH does not contrast enhance. This case represents the bilateral and symmetrical PNH, in which multiple and contiguous nodules symmetrically line the entire ventricular walls. PNH is usually associated with other malformations such as Chiari II malformation, Dandy-Walker malformation, agenesis of the corpus callosum, pachygyria, schizencephaly, polymicrogyria, and cerebellar dysplasia. It is always important to look out for these other associated anomalies. Differential diagnosis may include tuberous sclerosis complex (TSC) and toxoplasmosis except that PNH does not calcify. Subependymoma does not usually contrast enhance like PNH. A small subependymoma could therefore mimic PNH. The histology could mimic gangliocytoma.

PNH is the most common migrational disorder due to failed migration of proliferated neuronal and glial tissues from the germinal matrix around the ventricles resulting in abnormal locations of disorganized neuronal tissue in the subependymal region. These tissues are devoid of the final organization exhibited by the cortical neurons. Five types of PNH have been identified. These are (1) bilateral and symmetrical, (2) bilateral single-noduled, (3) bilateral and asymmetrical, (4) unilateral, and (5) unilateral with extension to the cortex. It is likely that genetic factors play a major role in the bilaterally affected patients. The bilateral and symmetrical cases are characterized by a female predominance, associated with the FLIN1 gene, positive family history for epilepsy, and familial occurrence, while the unilateral ones are mostly sporadic. Women with subependymal heterotopia typically present with partial epilepsy during the second decade of life with physical and neurologic development up to that point being typically normal. Men with subependymal heterotopia vary in their clinical presentation depending on whether they have the X-linked or autosomal form. Men with the X-linked form more commonly have associated central nervous system (CNS) and visceral anomalies with typical abnormal development and suffer significant perinatal mortality. Symptomatic men with the autosomal variety have clinical courses similar to symptomatic women.

Question for Further Thought

1. Is there a role for MR spectroscopy in the diagnosis of PNH?

Reporting Responsibilities

Routine reporting is sufficient. Location and type of the heterotopia and other associated congenital abnormalities should be itemized and reported.

What the Treating Physician Needs to Know

- Location of the heterotopia and other associated congenital abnormalities
- Location may not always correspond to seizure focus at electroencephalography (EEG) or magnetoencephalography (MEG)

Answer

1. Usually the MR diagnosis of PNH is not in doubt. MR spectroscopy demonstrates no difference in the spectroscopic pattern of heterotopic GM compared with normal GM. It does not seem to contribute to the diagnosis except that it demonstrates normal GM pattern.

CLINICAL HISTORY *2-year-old male being evaluated for hydrocephalus.*

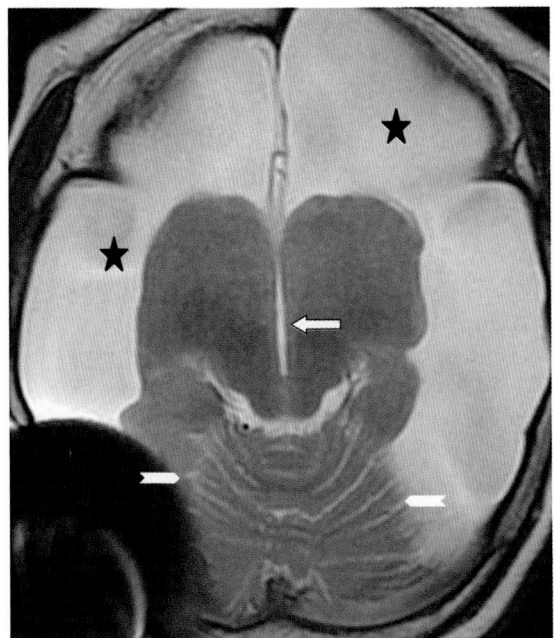

FIGURE 73-1

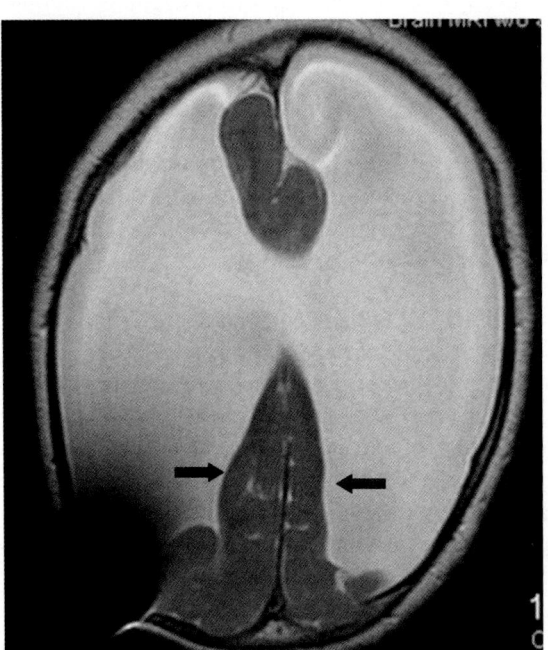

FIGURE 73-2

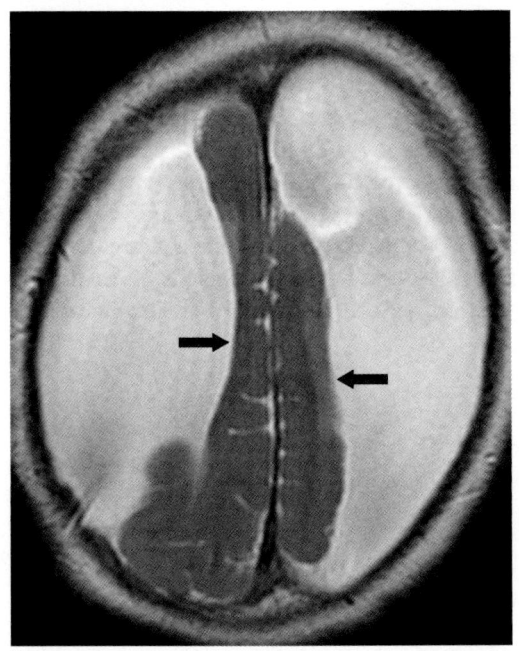

FIGURE 73-3

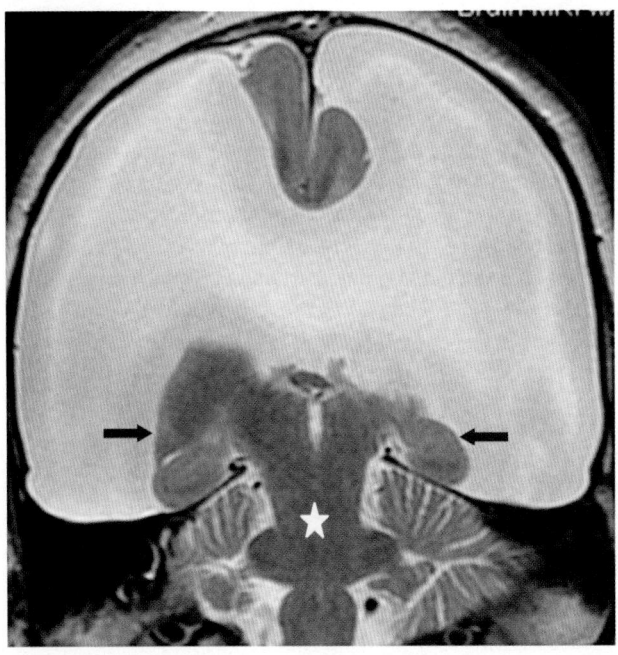

FIGURE 73-4

FINDINGS Figure 73-1. Axial T2WI through the thalami. The frontal lobes are absent and replaced by cerebrospinal fluid (CSF) (stars). There is a slit third ventricle between the thalami (transverse arrow). The superior vermis and cerebellum are normal (chevrons). Figures 73-2 and 73-3. Axial T2WI through the expected levels of the lateral ventricles and the centrum semiovale, respectively. Only small para-falcine strips of frontal parietal lobes are present bilaterally (arrows) with the supratentorial space occupied by CSF. The remnants of the frontal lobes display rounded margins. It is impossible to identify convexity brain mantle. Large signal void artifact posteriorly on the right in Figures 73-1 and 73-2 is from ventriculoperitoneal (VP) shunt valve. Figure 73-4. Coronal T2WI through the middle cranial fossae. Only rudimentary medial temporal lobes are visualized (arrows). Posterior fossa structures are present and grossly normal (stars). The supratentorial space is filled with CSF except for small knobbing of frontal and parietal lobes around the falx cerebri.

DIFFERENTIAL DIAGNOSIS Hydrocephalus, schizencephaly, hydranencephaly, alobar holoprosencephaly.

DIAGNOSIS Hydranencephaly.

DISCUSSION Both CT and MRI are capable of demonstrating all the features of hydranencephaly. There is essentially absent cerebral hemispheres except for small amount of brain tissue along the falx cerebri and posteriorly in the region of the occipital lobes. The entire supratentorial region is full of CSF without identifiable convexity brain mantle. The falx cerebri and interhemispheric fissure are always present. The posterior fossa structures are intact. The thalami are present but the basal ganglia could be rudimentary. There is macrocephaly. Angiographic images in this population usually show severely hypoplastic supraclinoid internal carotid arteries (ICAs). Even in severe hydrocephalus, it is possible to identify thin cerebral mantle on MRI. Large open lip schizencephaly is lined by cortical gray matter (GM). In hydranencephaly, the margin of the rudimentary brain lining the CSF is gliotic. The midline structures of the falx and interhemispheric fissure are not formed in alobar holoprosencephaly. There is usually a brain mantle particularly anteriorly.

Hydranencephaly is a rare congenital abnormality that is diagnosable in utero. The diagnosis can be made by US. It is usually sporadic but has been reported in association with Fowler syndrome, trisomy 13, renal aplastic dysplasia, and polyvalvular developmental heart defect. It has no gender or racial preferences. The pathogenesis is believed to be on the basis of a destructive process involving the cerebral hemispheres probably due to bilateral ICA occlusions and subsequent destruction of the cerebral hemispheres. The posterior circulation is intact hence posterior fossa structures and the occipital lobes are normal. These children present with large heads that easily transluminate. They perish mostly within the first year of life. Attempt is made to control the macrocephaly by shunting.

Question for Further Thought

1. Is it definite that early in utero occlusion of ICA causes hydranencephaly?

Reporting Responsibilities

Direct reporting may be necessary, although prenatal diagnosis may have been made. In any case, it is important to be able to distinguish this entity from its mimics.

What the Treating Physician Needs to Know

- Certainty of the diagnosis and exclusion of the mimics
- Absence of cortical brain mantle distinguishes hydranencephaly from hydrocephalus; hydrocephalus is treatable, while hydranencephaly is not

Answer

1. No, it is not definite but is the most plausible explanation on the basis of experimental occlusion of ICA in monkey fetuses resulting in hydranencephalic changes. Other theories of etiopathogenesis of hydranencephaly include congenital infections such as toxoplasmosis and viral infections resulting in destruction of the cerebral hemispheres, maternal exposure to toxins such as carbon monoxide and butane gas resulting in fetal hypoxic ischemic changes and subsequent brain liquefaction, thromboplastic material from a deceased monochorionic twin resulting in brain destruction, and an extreme form of leukomalacia.

CLINICAL HISTORY *12-year-old male trauma victim.*

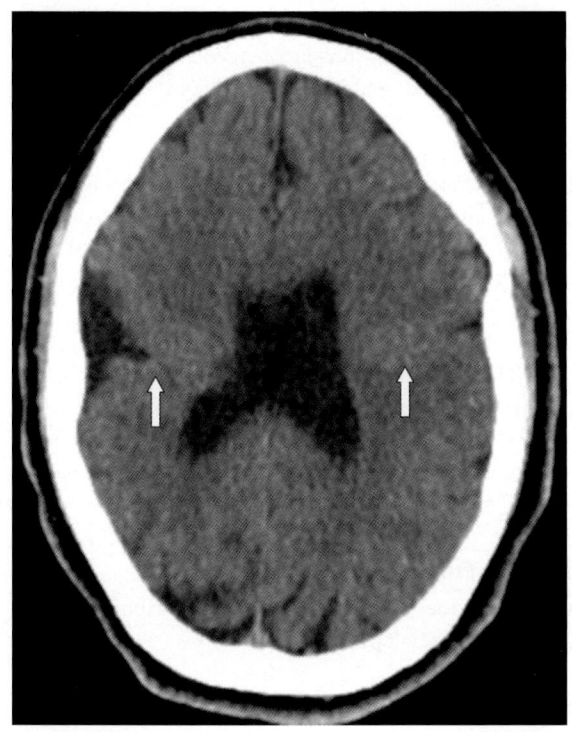

FIGURE 74-1

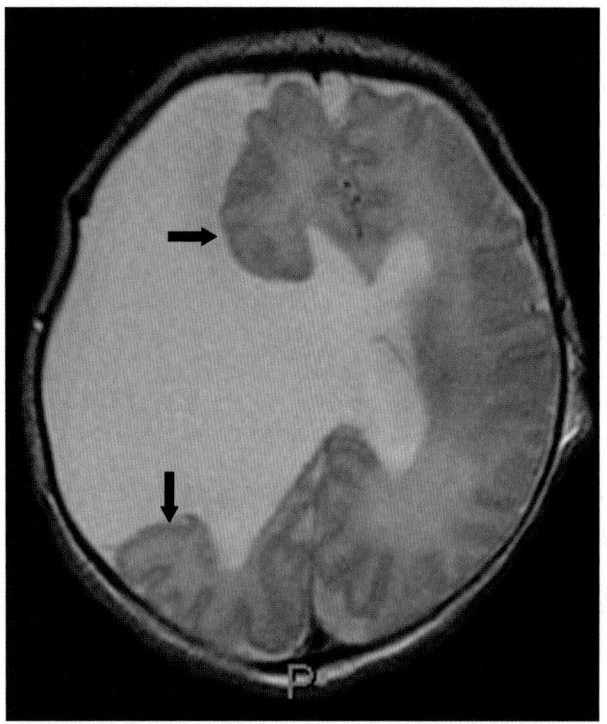

FIGURE 74-2

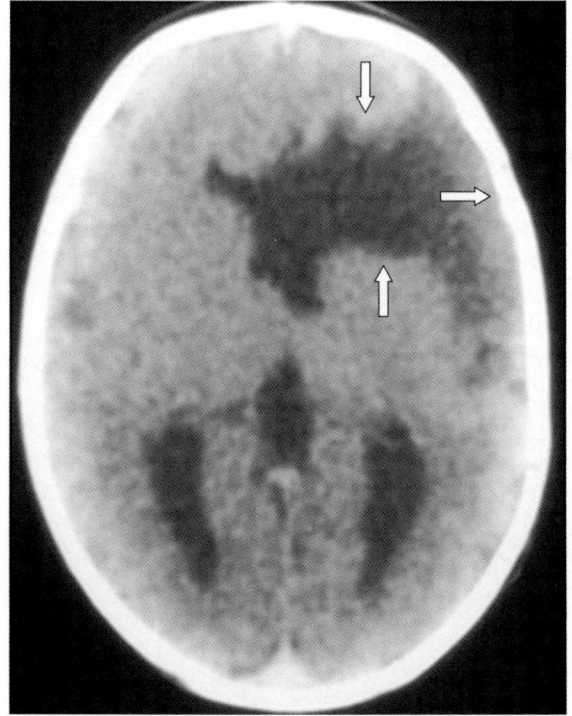

FIGURE 74-3

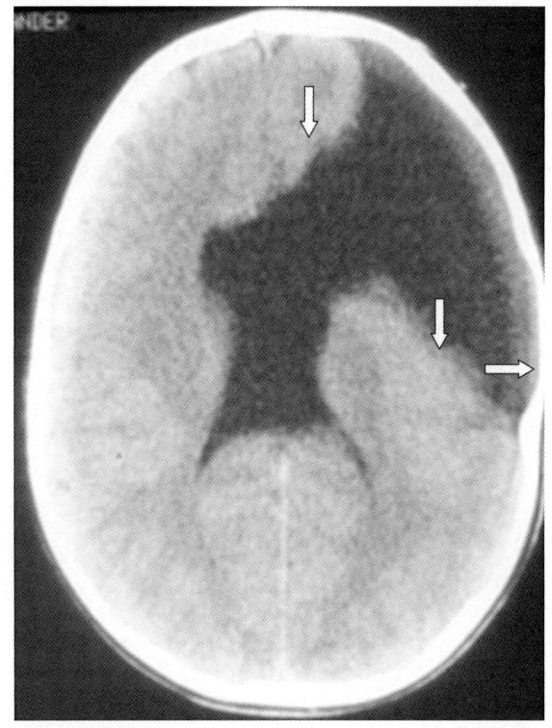

FIGURE 74-4

FINDINGS Figure 74-1. Axial NCCT through the lateral ventricles. There are bilateral suprasylvian coronal clefts lined by cortical gray matter (GM) (arrows). The clefts extend from the subarachnoid space to the lateral ventricular walls. This is consistent with "closed lip" schizencephaly. The ventricles are abnormally shaped with nonvisualization of the septum pellucidum. Figure 74-2. Axial T2WI through the lateral ventricles in a companion patient. There is a wide cleft through the right cerebral hemisphere linking the wide open lateral ventricle to the subarachnoid space. The margin of the cleft is lined by cortical GM (arrows). This is an open lip schizencephaly. The splenium of the corpus callosum and the septum pellucidum are absent. Figures 74-3 and 74-4. Axial NCCT through the lateral ventricles in another companion patient as a baby (Figure 74-3) and as a teenager (Figure 74-4). There is a left frontal open lip schizencephaly lined by GM (vertical arrows) with overlying cranial vault remodeling (transverse arrows). The septum pellucidum is absent.

DIFFERENTIAL DIAGNOSIS Porencephaly, holoprosencephaly, hydranencephaly, arachnoid cyst, schizencephaly.

DIAGNOSIS Schizencephaly.

DISCUSSION Both CT and MRI are capable of demonstrating the changes of schizencephaly, which is basically a cerebral hemisphere cleft that connects the subarachnoid space with the ventricle. This cleft is lined by GM. There are basically two types: the closed lip (type I) and the open lip (type II). In the closed lip, the GM-lined lips are in contact with each other as in Figure 74-1. The lips are widely separated with cerebrospinal fluid (CSF) in between in type II as in Figures 74-2 to 74-4. In utero diagnosis of schizencephaly is possible by both ultrasound and MRI. The closed lip could pose a challenge during in utero diagnosis. In utero ultrasound of the open lip schizencephaly presents a wedge-shaped defect with echogenic cortex lining the cleft. The defect could be unilateral or bilateral, of varying sizes from small to very large and extends from the pial surface to the ventricle wall. The septum pellucidum is usually absent and the thalami are separate in most cases. These changes are also well demonstrated by in utero MRI. MR is more sensitive in detecting small cleft, the GM lining the lips, and the associated migrational malformations. The ventricle wall may be tented pointing to the defect. The other associated findings include absent septum pellucidum in about two-thirds of the cases, absent or focal dysplasia or agenesis of the corpus callosum, migrational malformations, Dandy-Walker malformations, and septooptic dysplasia. The separated thalami differentiate this entity from lobar holoprosencephaly. A porencephalic cyst is usually lined by gliotic tissue rather than GM. Severe bilateral schizencephaly may be difficult to differentiate from hydranencephaly. Arachnoid cyst is an extraaxial CSF containing mass that does not usually communicate with the ventricles.

Schizencephaly is an uncommon disorder of neuronal migration. The clinical presentation depends on the severity of the malformation. Bilateral large lesions are the worst with severe CNS impairment. Presentations include seizures, developmental delay, hemiparesis, quadriplegia, and mental retardation. Treatment is mainly supportive.

Question for Further Thought

1. In what way does in utero diagnosis contribute to management of schizencephaly?

Reporting Responsibilities

Routine reporting is sufficient. Associated anomalies should be itemized for prognostication purpose.

What the Treating Physician Needs to Know

- Severity of malformation and other associated findings
- This is not hydrocephalus but may coexist with hydrocephalus

Answer

1. There is no cure for schizencephaly. Prenatal diagnosis is able to define the severity of the malformation. This could be useful in prognostication. This will help in management of the pregnancy and counseling the parents regarding real expectations once the child is born.

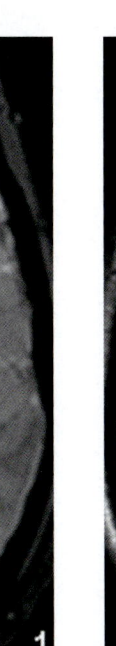

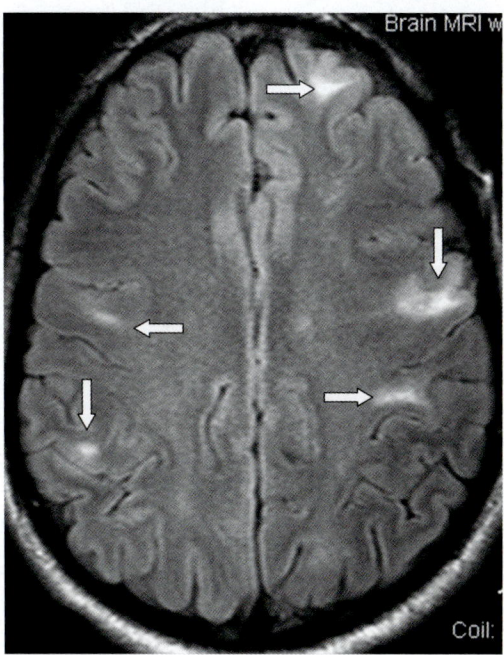

FIGURE 75-1

FIGURE 75-2

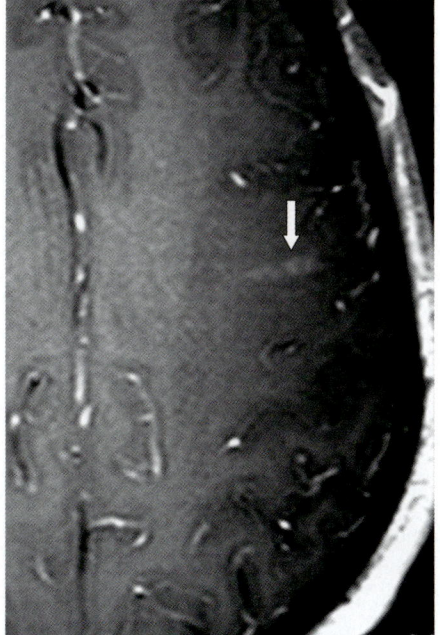

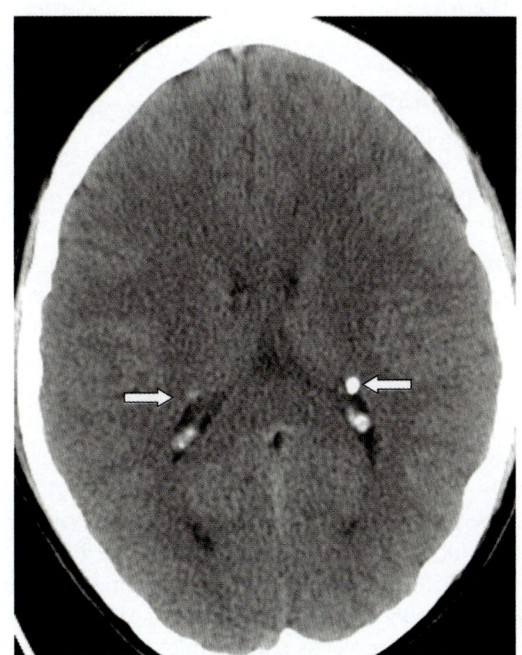

FIGURE 75-3

FIGURE 75-4

FINDINGS Figure 75-1. Axial GRE through the lateral ventricles. There is a left lateral ventricular subependymal round hypointensity (arrow). Figure 75-2. Axial FLAIR image through the level of the centrum semiovale showing multifocal radial white matter hyperintense bands radiating from the subcortical regions in bilateral cerebral hemispheres (arrows). Two left frontal lobe lesions show associated cortical thickening of intermediate intensity. Figure 75-3. Axial post-contrast T1WI through the level of the centrum semiovale. There is a left subcortical flame-shaped contrast enhancement (arrow). Figure 75-4. Axial NCCT through the lateral ventricles. There are bilateral

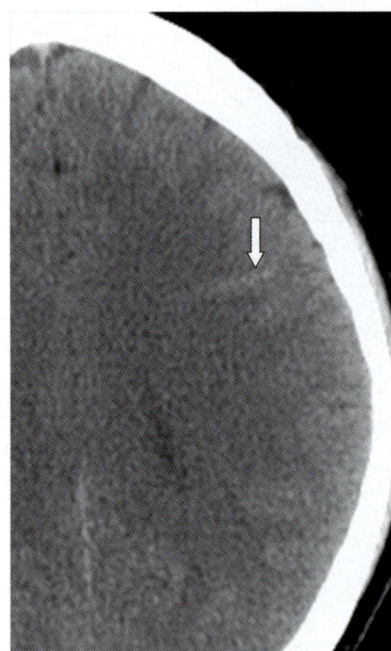

FIGURE 75-5

subependymal hyperdensities consistent with calcifications (arrows). Figure 75-5. Axial NCCT through the left centrum semiovale. There is a thick linear left frontal subcortical hyperintensity consistent with a subcortical tuber (arrow).

DIFFERENTIAL DIAGNOSIS Toxoplasmosis, tuberous sclerosis complex (TSC).

DIAGNOSIS Tuberous sclerosis complex (TSC).

DISCUSSION MRI is the method of choice in the comprehensive evaluation of the brain in TSC. The findings here represent the classical MRI finding in tuberous sclerosis. The GRE is the best MRI sequence for demonstrating the hypointense subependymal calcifications. Subependymal tubers are iso- to hyperintense on other sequences and are seen as mild protrusions into the lateral ventricles. Hemorrhages may behave in a similar fashion but the other findings of subcortical tubers on FLAIR and T2WI suggest otherwise. The subcortical tubers are best demonstrated on the FLAIR and T2WI as multifocal hyperintensities of varying shapes and sizes mostly as subcortical bands radiating to the white matter. Cortical tubers present as cortical thickening and are slightly hyperintense compared with the normal cortical gray matter on FLAIR and T2WI. There is usually no mass effect or surrounding edema. This differentiates tubers from lesions such as multifocal subcortical metastases or hemorrhages.

Tubers tend to be isointense to hypointense on T1WI. About 10% of cortical/subcortical tubers may enhance following intravenous contrast administration. There is a higher incidence of contrast enhancement in subependymal giant cell astrocytoma (SGCA) which occurs in about 1.7% to 26% of patients with TSC. SGCAs are located in the caudothalamic grove region, where they could obstruct the foramen of Monro causing hydrocephalus. The calcifications without the subcortical changes may resemble congenital toxoplasmosis.

Other abnormalities such as hippocampal abnormalities of msiotemporal sclerosis (MTS) and hippocampal malrotation (HIMAL) have been found in a subset of patients with TSC. DTI has been useful in demonstrating additional lesions in white matter (WM) tracts that appear visually normal, indicating a rather more extensive brain involvement that may suggest not only abnormal myelination but may correlate with the extent of the lesion load. CT demonstrates the unmistakable ependymal calcifications which, however, could mimic congenital toxoplasmosis calcifications. However, the associated subcortical tubers and the clinical presentations tend to give the diagnosis a way.

Question for Further Thought

1. What are the clinical manifestations of TSC?

Reporting Responsibilities

Routine reporting is sufficient as this represents chronic changes. However, presence of SGCA with hydrocephalus should trigger direct reporting.

What the Treating Physician Needs to Know

- Location of calcifications and tubers
- Presence of complications such as SGCA and hydrocephalus

Answer

1. TSC is an autosomal dominant neurocutaneous disorder. Neurologic manifestations include seizures, developmental delays, and neuropsychiatric behaviors. There are diagnostic criteria formulated by the National Tuberous Sclerosis Association. There are three categories of TSC: definite, probable, and possible TSC. The common features, however, are the cutaneous lesions of shagreen patch, facial and ungual fibromas, and hypomelanotic macules. Central nervous system (CNS) changes include subependymal nodules and cortical/subcortical tubers and SGCA. Multiple retinal nodular hamartomas, cardiac rhabdomyosarcomas, pulmonary changes, and renal angiomyolipoma are other findings. A family history is also important and genetic testing allows for the DNA sequencing for TSC1 and TSC2 mutations in up to 80% of affected individuals.

CLINICAL HISTORY *A 7-year-old female was initially seen to establish care for known neurofibromatosis. Over the years her lesions grew substantially.*

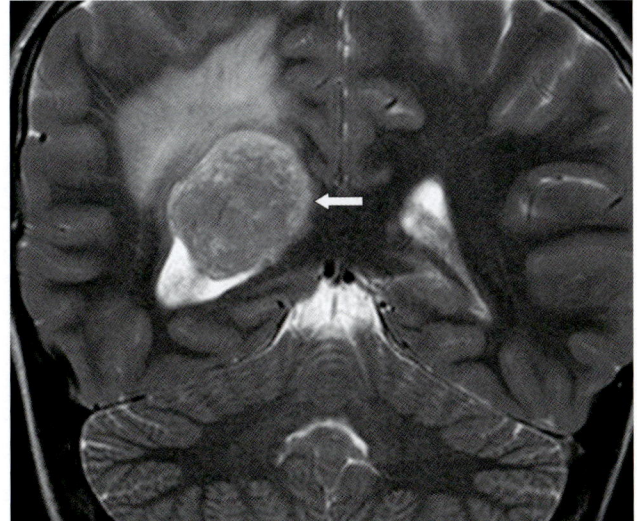

FIGURE 76-1

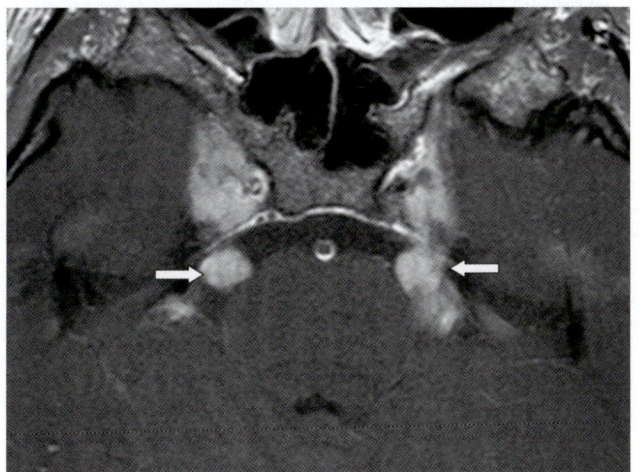

FIGURE 76-2

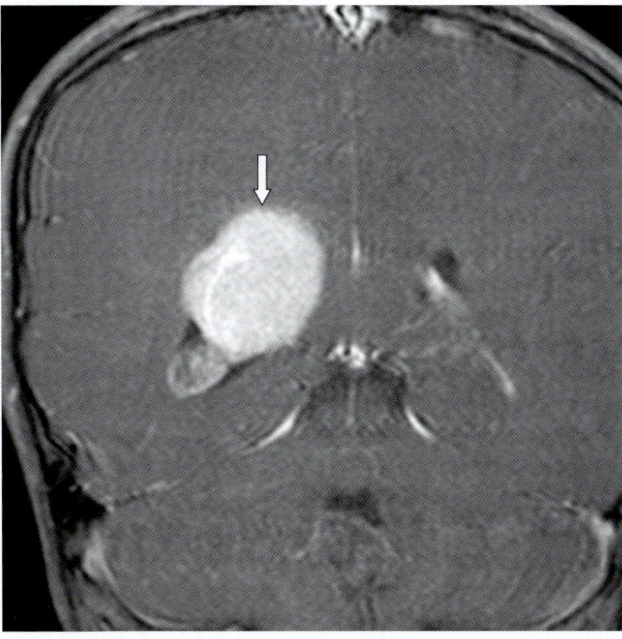

FIGURE 76-3

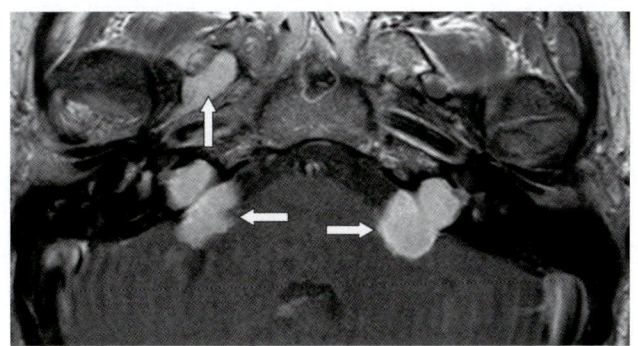

FIGURE 76-4

FINDINGS Figure 76-1. Coronal T2WI through the trigones. There is a 3.9-cm right trigonal isointense (to gray matter [GM]) mass (arrow) with surrounding peritrigonal vasogenic edema superiorly. Figure 76-2. Coronal post-contrast T1WI. The intraventricular mass enhances homogeneously and avidly. This is a surgically proven intraventricular meningioma. Figure 76-3. Axial post-contrast T1WI through the cavernous sinuses. There are bilateral lobulated contrast-enhancing masses along the path of the bilateral trigeminal nerves (transverse arrows). Figure 76-4. Axial post-contrast T1WI through the internal auditory canal (IAC). There are lobulated contrast-enhancing masses in bilateral cerebellopontine angle (CPA) extending into the IACs (transverse arrows). There is a similar contrast-enhancing smooth marginated mass in the region of the right foramen ovale (vertical arrow). Tumors in Figures 76-3 and 76-4

are presumed schwannomas of the trigeminal and vestibular nerves, respectively. Not shown here are right facial nerve and extensive schwannomas of the spinal nerves.

DIFFERENTIAL DIAGNOSIS Neurofibromatosis type 2 (NF2), Neurofibromatosis type 1 (NF1), schwannomatosis.

DIAGNOSIS Neurofibromatosis type 2 (NF2).

DISCUSSION The hallmark of NF2 is bilateral vestibular schwannomas. These could be demonstrated on MRI as avidly contrast enhancing iso- to slightly hypointense masses in the IAC and CPA on T1WI. If they grow substantially, they become lobulated and compress the brachium pontis and the adjoining cerebellum and pons. Intracanalicular extension with widening of the IAC may occur. The mass effect increases as the tumors grow. Schwannomas of other cranial nerves such as facial, trigeminal, and oculomotor nerves are present in about 50% of NF2 population. Meningiomas and ependymomas are common in these patients and they are generally multiple. Intraventricular meningioma is a very rare tumor and presence of intraventricular meningioma in a child should raise the suspicion for neurofibromatosis. MRI with contrast is the most appropriate test for these patients in view of lifelong surveillance for new tumor and tumor growth. The growth of these tumors is usually unpredictable and new tumors spring up all the time. Spinal schwannomas and ependymomas are usually multiple and can grow to enormous sizes. Schwannomatosis usually presents with nonvestibular multifocal schwannomas mostly of the spine and peripheral nerves with a small percentage of intracranial and subcutaneous tissue schwannomas. It does not have any cutaneous stigmata. Most schwannomatosis are sporadic with only about 15% with a family history. NF1 is largely extracranial in its manifestations with cutaneous and peripheral neurofibromas and bone changes predominating. About 15% of NF1 show intracranial manifestations.

NF2 is a rare autosomal dominant disease due to mutation in NF2 tumor suppressor gene (Merlin) on chromosome 22q12. The prevalence is estimated at 1:25,000 births. Family history may be absent in about 50% of NF2. Most NF2 patients present in their second to fourth decades, with a minority of patients presenting in the first decade as in this patient. There is no gender preference. Most will present with vestibular dysfunctions of tinnitus and sensorineural hearing loss. Trigeminal neuralgia, seizures, cataracts, and facial nerve palsy are other common presentations.

Cutaneous schwannomas are common. Neurofibromas are rarely present. Café-au-lait spots are not as common as in NF1. Diagnosis is made on the basis of established criteria that categorize the diagnosis into definite and probable NF2. Genetic testing is necessary to confirm the diagnosis. In view of the unpredictable nature of the many tumors in these patients, it is not possible to treat all tumors. It is recommended that only symptomatic tumors be treated.

Question for Further Thought

1. Is imaging surveillance necessary in NF2?

Reporting Responsibilities

The presence of tumors calls for direct reporting and more so if there is hydrocephalus or compression of eloquent brain regions. Suspicion of NF2 should prompt recommendation for spinal imaging to exclude spinal tumors.

What the Treating Physician Needs to Know

- Location and types of intracranial masses
- Presence of complications such as hydrocephalus, or edema
- Recommendation for spinal imaging
- Growth or quiescence of masses on follow-up imaging

Answer

1. MRI surveillance is recommended in NF2 because of the propensity for multiple and sometimes debilitating intracranial tumors. Both cranial and spine contrast-enhanced MRI are usually used in this population to screen for tumors.

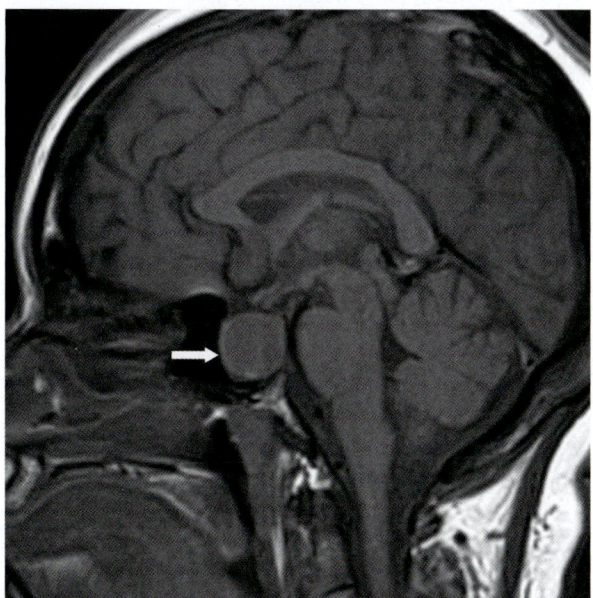

FIGURE 77-1

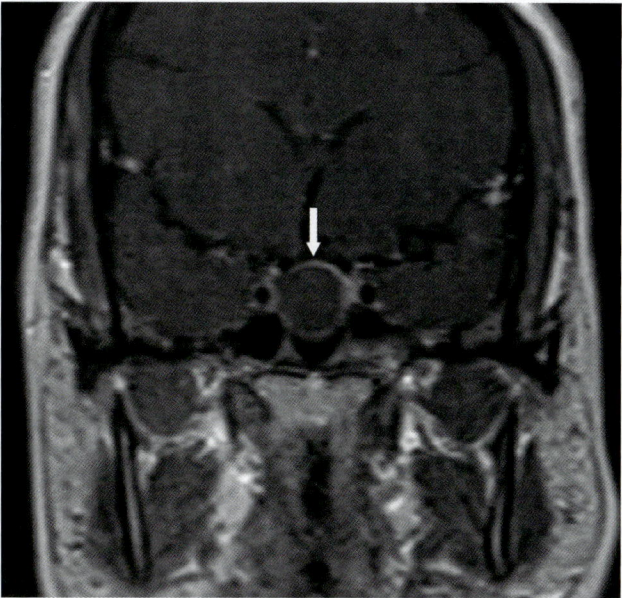

FIGURE 77-2

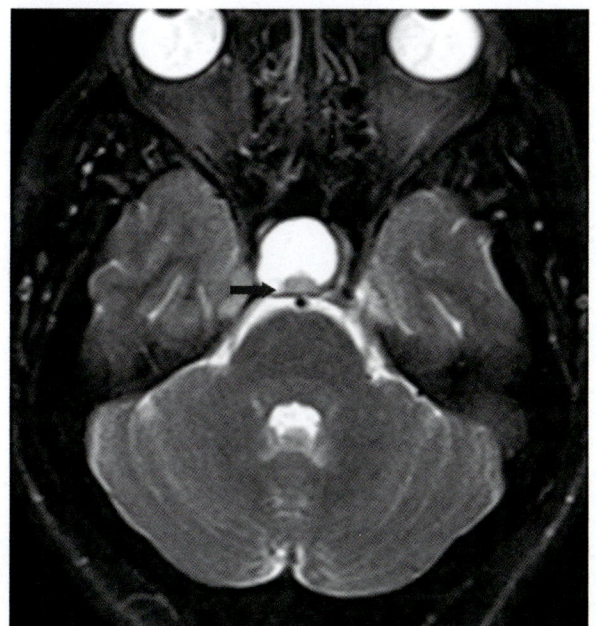

FIGURE 77-3

FINDINGS Figure 77-1. Sagittal T1WI. There is an intrasellar mass that is isointense with the brain (arrow). The hyperintense neurohypophysis is not present. Figure 77-2. Coronal post-contrast T1WI through the sella turcica. The mass does not enhance but its periphery does (arrow) probably due to surrounding normal pituitary tissue. Figure 77-3. Axial T2WI through the sella. There is a posterior mural nodule (arrow) that is typical of this entity and helps differentiate it from other cystic pituitary masses.

DIFFERENTIAL DIAGNOSIS Rathke cleft cyst, cystic pituitary adenoma, craniopharyngioma.

DIAGNOSIS Rathke cleft cyst.

DISCUSSION Typical MRI findings of Rathke cleft cyst include a nonenhancing lesion in the mid-aspect of the pituitary gland. About 50% are hyperintense and 50% are hypointense on pre-contrast T1WI secondary to differences in the mucinous component of the fluid. Characteristic findings include a nonenhancing mural nodule within the cyst and multiple small cysts within the cyst on T2 imaging. They rarely arise in the pituitary stalk.

Rathke cleft cyst (aka pars intermedia cyst) is a result of failure of regression of Rathke cleft, which is the embryologic separation between the adenohypophysis and the neurohypophysis. Rathke cleft is thought to be a remnant of the superior extension of the stomodeum, which is the rostral termination of the aerodigestive tract in the fetus. Rathke cleft cysts are relatively common, found in up to 33% of patients at autopsy. They are generally asymptomatic and found incidentally. Occasionally, they can become large enough to produce symptoms secondary to mass effect with the most common symptoms being headaches, visual field changes, and pituitary dysfunction. Treatment is generally expectant with surgical excision reserved for symptomatic cases.

Questions for Further Thought

1. What is the embryologic function of Rathke cleft?
2. What is the significance of the nonenhancing nodule?

Reporting Responsibilities

Routine reporting is sufficient unless it is large and compressive. Describe the abnormality and its extent. Advise clinician of lack of requirement of follow-up imaging in asymptomatic cases once the diagnosis is achieved.

What the Treating Physician Needs to Know

- Relevant differential diagnosis
- Relative benignity of Rathke cleft cyst

Answers

1. The adenohypophysis forms from the ventral portion of the Rathke cleft. The remaining portion of the cleft forms the pars intermedia that normally regresses.
2. The nonenhancing nodule has been described as a mucin clump on pathologic evaluation. This corresponds with the MRI findings of a nonenhancing nodule that demonstrates T1 hyperintensity on pre- contrast imaging.

CLINICAL HISTORY *Patient presented with long-standing hypopituitarism and recent decreased visual acuity.*

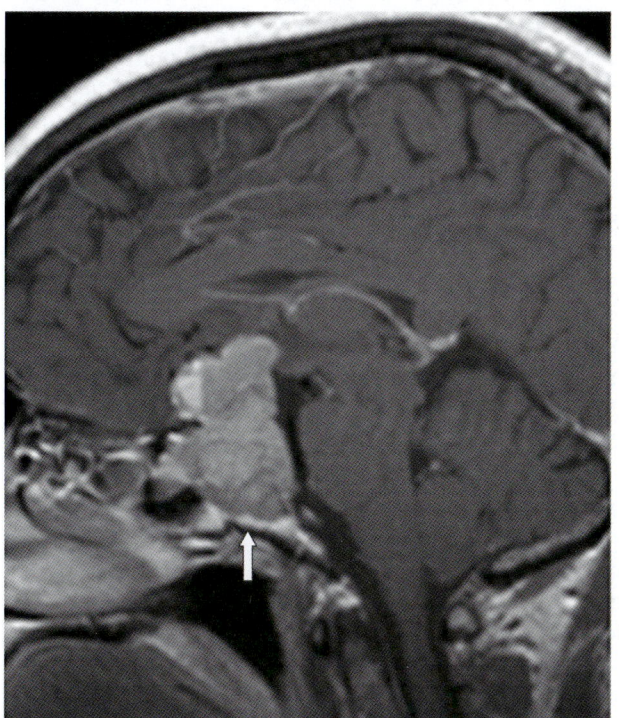

FIGURE 78-1

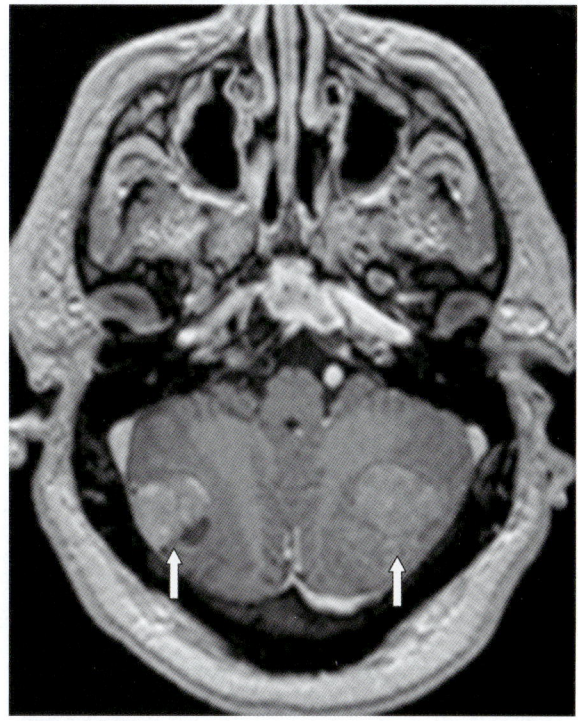

FIGURE 78-2

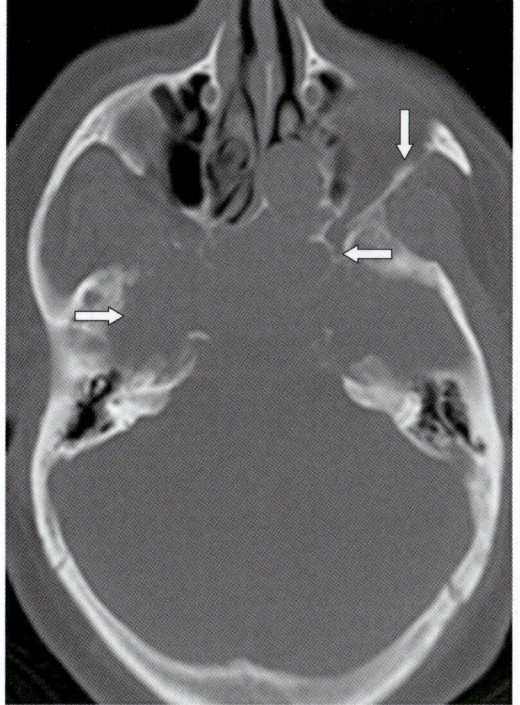

FIGURE 78-3

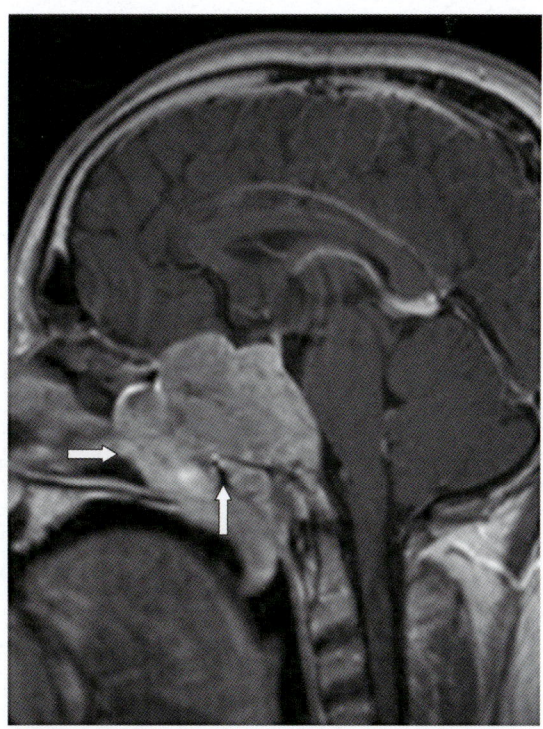

FIGURE 78-4

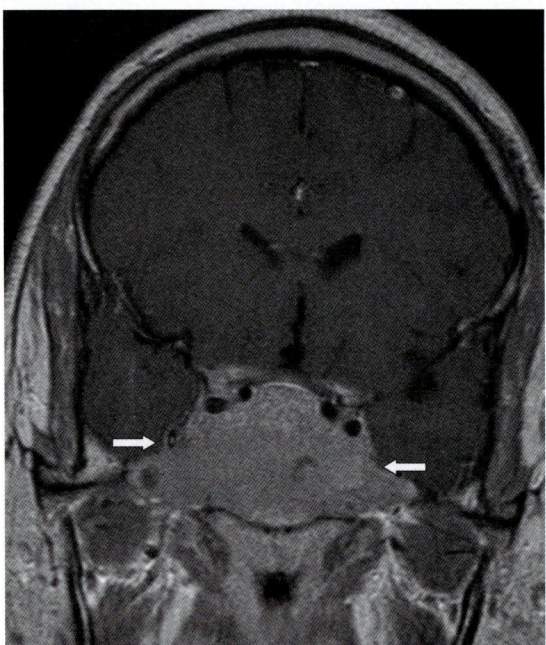

FIGURE 78-5

FINDINGS Figure 78-1. Sagittal post-contrast T1WI. There is a large inhomogeneous sellar mass with suprasellar extension and invasion of the sphenoid sinus (arrow). Figure 78-2. Two months later, a post-contrast axial T1WI shows bilateral cerebellar masses (arrows) that are metastases consistent with metastatic pituitary carcinoma. Figure 78-3. Axial NCCT in a companion case of invasive pituitary adenoma (PA) shows destruction of the central bony skull base (arrows). Figure 78-4. Sagittal post-contrast T1WI in the companion case. There is a large enhancing sellar mass with invasion of the sphenoid sinus and extension into the posterior nasal cavity (arrows). Figure 78-5. Coronal post-contrast T1WI shows invasion of both cavernous sinuses by the sellar mass (arrows).

DIFFERENTIAL DIAGNOSIS Meningioma, metastasis, clival chordoma, chondrosarcoma, plasmacytoma, malignant macroadenoma.

DIAGNOSIS Malignant macroadenoma.

DISCUSSION MRI is the best imaging technique to evaluate malignant PA and depict the tumoral extensions. MRI shows an isointense mass on T1WI with a variable intensity on T2WI and heterogeneous enhancement that invades the central skull base. CT is superior in depicting intratumoral calcifications, expansion of the sella, and disruption of the sella floor. Invasion of the cavernous sinuses best reflects the tumor's aggressiveness, being almost certain when more than 60% of the internal carotid artery (ICA) is encased by the tumor. There is a high probability of cavernous sinus involvement when the venous compartment is obliterated or when the lateral limit of the cavernous ICA is surpassed by the tumor. On the other hand, there is a low probability of cavernous sinus invasion when less than 25% of the intracavernous ICA is encased by the tumor.

PAs show various initial presentations, imaging appearances, and biologic behavior. Although most PAs remain within the sella turcica and have a benign behavior, few may have an aggressive clinical course with progressive growth, resistance to medical treatment, invasion of the adjacent structures (sphenoid bone, cavernous sinus, suprasellar region, sphenoid sinus, and nasopharynx), and recurrence after surgical resection or even rarely progression to pituitary carcinoma, which is defined by the World Health Organization (WHO) as a PA with metastases. The mechanisms underlying this aggressive behavior, despite mostly benign histopathological features, have not yet been fully defined. Nevertheless, aside from the atypical morphologic characteristics and invasive behavior, the WHO classification includes other features suggestive of an aggressive behavior, such as elevated mitotic index, a 3% Ki-67 index, and extensive nuclear staining for p53. Lately, other criteria of aggressiveness and malignancy have been described, including overexpression of endocan in endothelial cells (related to angiogenesis), a reduction in the E-cadherin/catenin expression (in prolactinomas associated with changes in cell-to-cell adhesion and cellular migration), the presence of dysregulated genes (as the overexpression of the hst gene), and DNA abnormalities (basically accumulations of multiple allelic deletions).

The mass was confirmed by biopsy, revealing a pituitary carcinoma. At the 2-month follow-up, the patient had developed ataxia and an abnormal gait. Therapy involves surgical resection to reduce the tumor and decompress the region prior to adjuvant chemo- and/or radiotherapy.

Questions for Further Thought

1. What gender is more affected and which type of secreting adenomas are pituitary carcinomas most frequently related to?
2. Based on imaging, what is the stage or stages that may represent invasion by PA?

Reporting Responsibilities
Direct reporting is essential in malignant tumors. Describe the extension of the invasive PA and involvement of the cavernous sinus, suprasellar structures (such as the optic pathway), and bone. Detect the possibility of craniospinal or systemic metastases, which would point to a pituitary carcinoma with a worst prognosis than invasive macroadenomas.

What the Treating Physician Needs to Know
• Extent of the tumor and invasion of neighboring structures

Answers

1. Pituitary carcinomas are mostly related to adrenocorticotropic hormone (ACTH) or prolactin (PRL)-secreting tumors and are more frequently seen in male patients with pituitary macroadenomas that are resistant to treatment.
2. On the imaging classification, stage III corresponds to a macroadenoma (>1 cm) with enlargement and invasion of the floor of the sella or suprasellar extension, while stage IV defines destruction of the sella.

CLINICAL HISTORY   *Teenage male with precocious sexual development.*

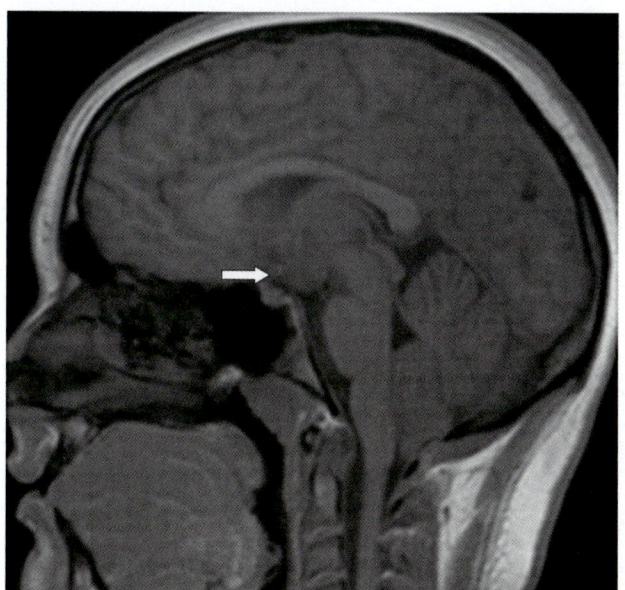

FIGURE 79-1

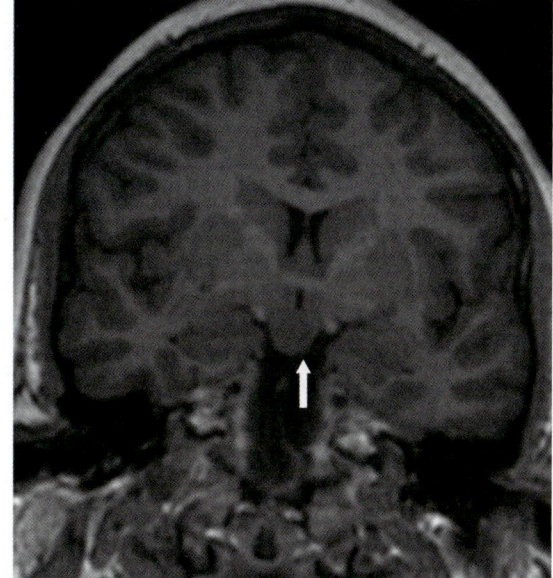

FIGURE 79-2

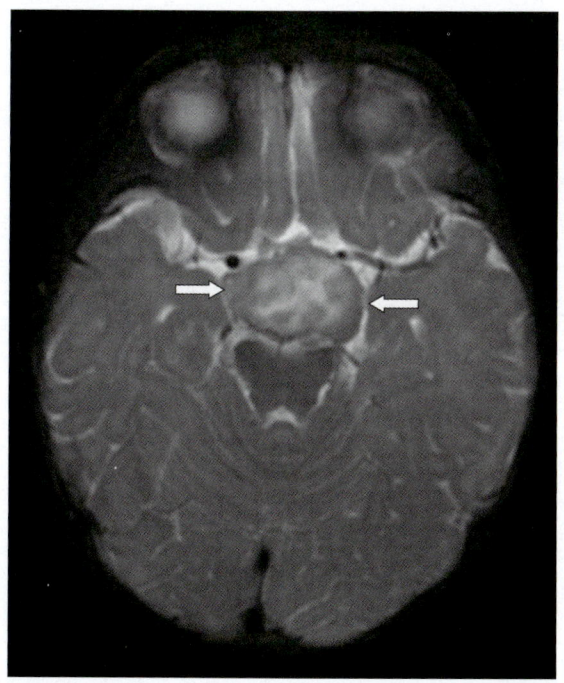

FIGURE 79-3

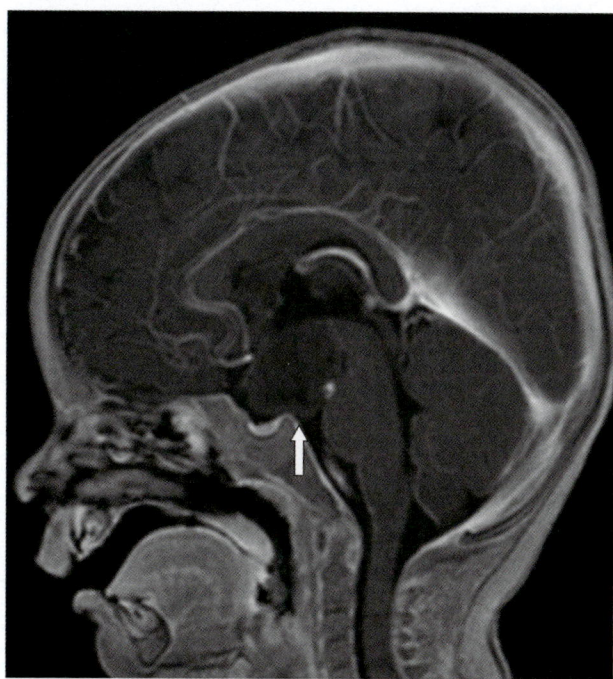

FIGURE 79-4

FINDINGS Figure 79-1. Sagittal non-contrast T1WI. There is a broad-based isointense mass (arrow) in the region of the tuber cinereum. Figure 79-2. Coronal non-contrast T1WI in the same patient shows that the mass has exactly the same signal as the gray matter (GM) (arrow). Figure 79-3. Axial T2WI in a companion case. There is a mass within the suprasellar cistern of heterogeneous intensity containing some central hyperintensities (arrows). Figure 79-4. Sagittal post-contrast T1WI shows the extent of the nonenhancing mass (arrow).

DIFFERENTIAL DIAGNOSIS Hypothalamic-chiasmatic glioma, craniopharyngioma, germinoma, and Langerhans cell histiocytosis, hamartoma of tuber cinereum.

DIAGNOSIS Hamartoma of tuber cinereum (HTC).

DISCUSSION Hamartomas (from the Greek word *hamartia* that means error) arising from the tuber cinereum (Latin for "ash-colored mass"), a part of the hypothalamus located between the mamillary bodies and the pituitary stalk, are rare nonneoplastic congenital heterotopias of GM. Frequently, HTCs are seen as subcentimeter homogeneous sessile (intra-hypothalamic) or pedunculated (parahypothalamic) nonenhancing masses with a similar density or intensity to GM. They are sometimes cystic and generally do not grow when compared on repeated examinations. It has been described in some published series that the variability of iso- to hyperintense signal on T2WI relates directly to the glial content found in hamartomas. Some authors have pointed out that the proton MR spectroscopy findings, consisting of a decrease in NAA/Cr ratio, an increase in the mI, and a probable increase in the Cho/Cr ratio, probably reflect an increased number of dysplastic neurons. Moreover, ictal SPECT and FDG-PET studies demonstrate hypermetabolism localized at the region of the HTC.

Occasionally, HTCs may be considered as giant when they measure over 1 cm in size. Sometimes, truly giant ones are encountered and their signal intensities tend to vary more than that of the more common smaller ones. HTC presents clinically with the classic triad of gelastic seizures, central precocious puberty (oversecretion of gonadotropin-releasing hormone [GnRH]), and developmental delay. Medical treatment is usually administered for the gelastic epilepsy and the precocious puberty associated with hamartomas, although some authors propose a surgical approach in exceptional cases.

Questions for Further Thought

1. With what syndrome is HTC associated?
2. What is the gender preference and age at presentation of HTC?

Reporting Responsibilities

Routine reporting is sufficient in this benign nonneoplastic mass. Describe the location, morphology, and extent of the lesion. Identify and describe any other epileptogenic abnormalities such as focal cortical dysplasias or findings that may suggest mesiotemporal sclerosis. Exclude the possibility of a hypothalamic or optic nerve glioma by the location, lack of enhancement, and absence of growth when compared with prior examinations.

What the Treating Physician Needs to Know

- Localize the seizure-remediable focus or region so that a possible surgical treatment can be determined
- The location and morphology of the lesion, as well as the extent and the relationship with other important structures such as suprasellar structures (optic nerves)

Answers

1. Pallister-Hall syndrome is characterized by HTC, anal atresia, renal anomalies, and limb malformations.
2. Most patients present in the first or second decade of life, with males being more affected than females.

CLINICAL HISTORY *76-year-old patient with a history of bilateral blurred vision of several months now has worsening bilateral diplopia and left pulsatile tinnitus. The right eye is red.*

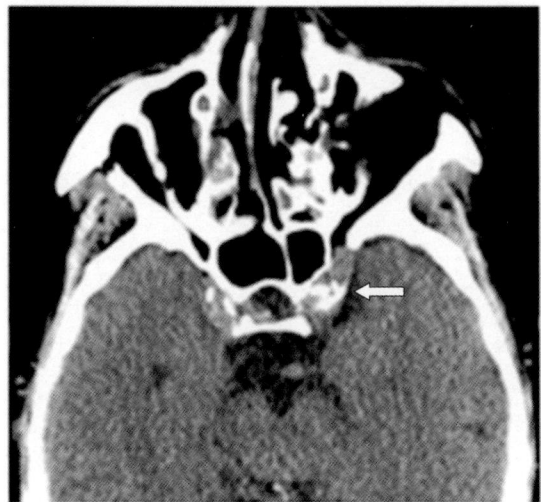

FIGURE 80-1

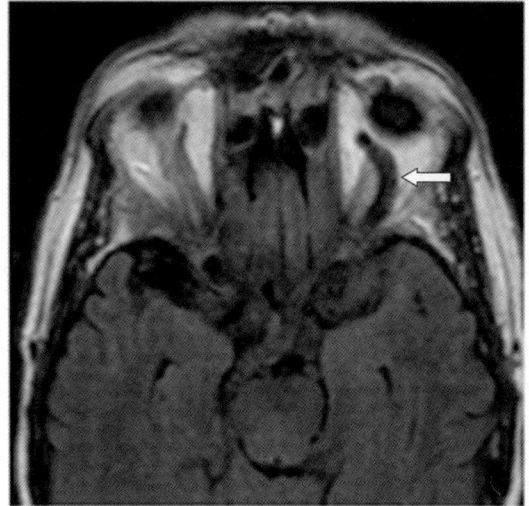

FIGURE 80-2

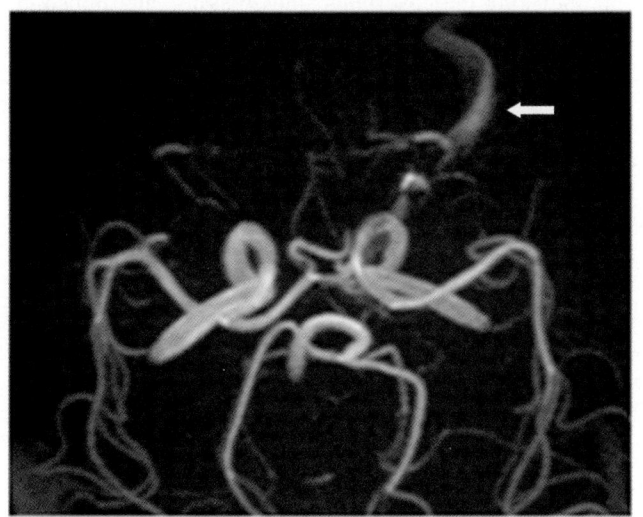

FIGURE 80-3

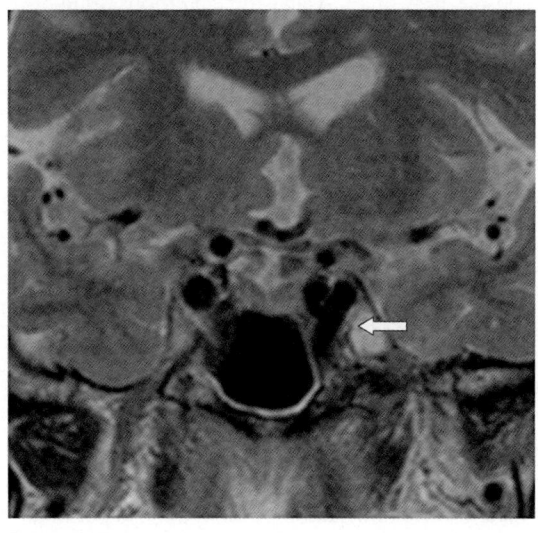

FIGURE 80-4

FINDINGS Figure 80-1. Axial NCCT through the cavernous sinuses. There is a subtle outward bulge of the left cavernous sinus (arrow). Figure 80-2. Axial FLAIR through the orbits. There is an enlarged and tortuous left superior ophthalmic vein (arrow). Figure 80-3. 3D TOF MRA. There is visualization of an enlarged left superior ophthalmic vein (arrow) similar to the arterial structures. Figure 80-4. Coronal T2WI shows an additional "flow void" in the left cavernous sinus (arrow). Figure 80-5. Anteroposterior DSA. There is early opacification of the cavernous sinuses (arrows) during a selective injection of the left internal

carotid artery (ICA). Figure 80-6. Lateral DSA of selective left external carotid artery (ECA). There is ECA feeders from the left middle meningeal artery and sphenopalatine artery (arrows).

DIFFERENTIAL DIAGNOSIS Tolosa-Hunt syndrome, cavernous sinus thrombosis, carotid cavernous sinus fistula, thyroid ophthalmopathy, pseudotumor or retrobulbar masses (such as metastases).

DIAGNOSIS Carotid-cavernous sinus fistula (CCF).

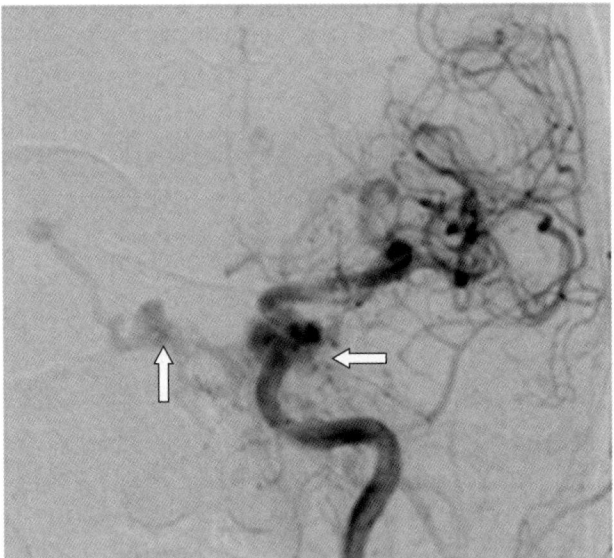

FIGURE 80-5

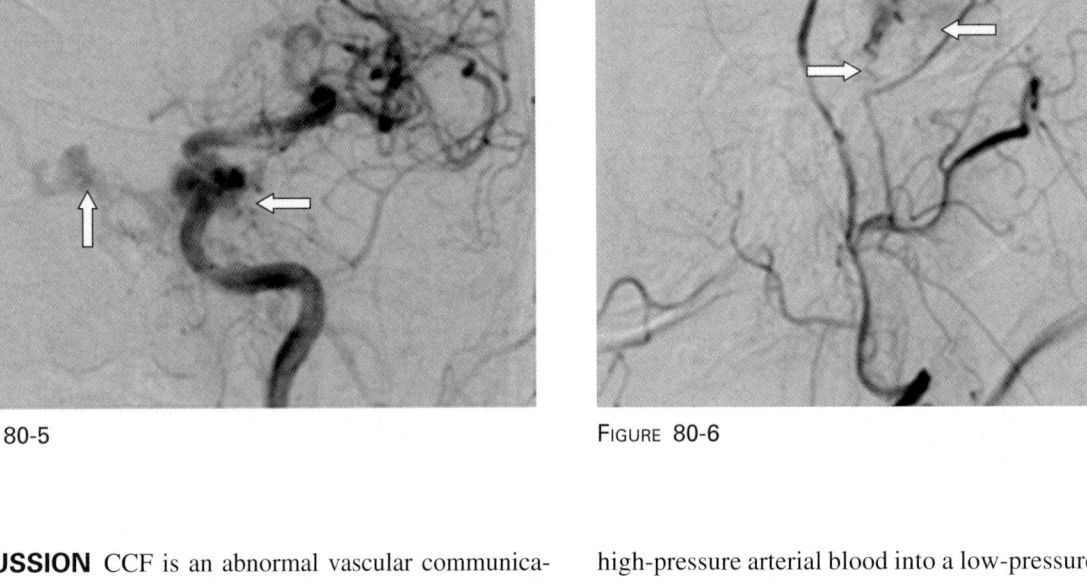

FIGURE 80-6

DISCUSSION CCF is an abnormal vascular communication between the ICA or ECA and the cavernous sinus. CT findings correlate with the underlying physiopathology of CCF and include enlargement and tortuosity of the superior ophthalmic vein, enlargement of the ipsilateral cavernous sinus, thickening of the extraocular muscles and periorbital soft tissues, and proptosis. MRI replicates the CT findings in addition to orbital edema and abnormal flow voids in the affected cavernous sinus. When a high-flow fistula results in retrograde flow into the cortical veins, dilatation of these veins, leptomeningeal thickening, and signs of venous congestion are present and may lead to cerebral edema and hemorrhagic infarctions. Susceptibility weighted imaging clearly shows the multiple, enlarged, and tortuous abnormal cortical veins. Both CTA and MRA are capable of demonstrating the additional vessels or signal voids in the cavernous sinuses and enlargement of arterialized superior ophthalmic vein. DSA is essential for confirmation of the diagnosis, classifying the fistula, and delineating the venous drainage pathways. Enlarged obstructed or thrombosed superior ophthalmic vein along with filling defects could be present in cavernous sinus thrombosis. Enlarged vascular structures are not usual features of the other differential.

CCFs can be classified based on etiology (traumatic or spontaneous), rate of flow (high versus low flow), the anatomy of the fistula (direct or indirect), and number of fistulas (single or multiple). In 1985, Barrow et al. defined four types of CCF (types A–D). Type A is direct and high-flow communication between the ICA and the cavernous sinus, and the rest (B–D) are indirect and low-flow shunts that develop from meningeal branches of either the ICA or the ECA. Type A is the most frequent of all, appearing mainly in young males with a history of a recent head trauma. In these cases, the main concern is the acute flow of high-pressure arterial blood into a low-pressure venous system, elevating the cavernous sinus pressure and impeding the venous drainage of nearby structures, particularly those of the orbit. This explains the presenting triad of pulsatile exophthalmos, bruit, and conjunctival chemosis. Visual complaints may be due to retinal ischemia and may indicate the need for urgent treatment. Less common presentations like intracerebral or subarachnoid hemorrhage are due to intracranial venous hypertension and also indicate that the fistula must be rapidly treated.

The main objective of CCF treatment is to occlude the fistula while preserving the normal flow of blood through the ICA. There are many treatment options. Conservative management includes manual compression of the ipsilateral ICA. Endovascular treatment includes either transarterial or transvenous embolization, and placement of covered or flow-diverting stents. Surgical intervention may include suturing, clipping, or trapping the fistula, packing the cavernous sinus to occlude the fistula, sealing the fistula with fascia and glue, ligating the ICA, or a combination of these procedures.

Questions for Further Thought

1. What other entities are associated with CCFs?
2. In what group of patients are indirect CCFs often seen?

Reporting Responsibilities

Direct reporting is essential so that urgent treatment might begin. Identify the imaging signs resulting from high pressure in the cavernous sinus, mainly in the orbital structures and in the draining venous structures. Identify enlarged cortical veins that indicate a need for rapid treatment. Describe signs of cerebral edema or infarction that do not follow an arterial territory.

What the Treating Physician Needs to Know

- A high degree of clinical suspicion is needed, especially in the emergency setting
- Absence of compressive lesions such as masses and hematoma responsible for the proptosis or orbital vascular congestion

Answers

1. Fibromuscular dysplasia, Ehlers-Danlos syndrome, and pseudoxanthoma elasticum.
2. Indirect CCFs are generally seen in postmenopausal female patients with subtle clinical symptoms related to them.

CLINICAL HISTORY *3-year-old male presenting with delayed growth and found to have hypopituitarism.*

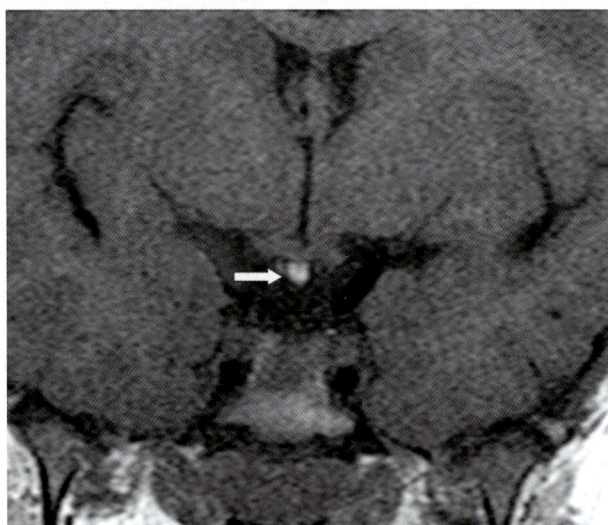

FIGURE 81-1

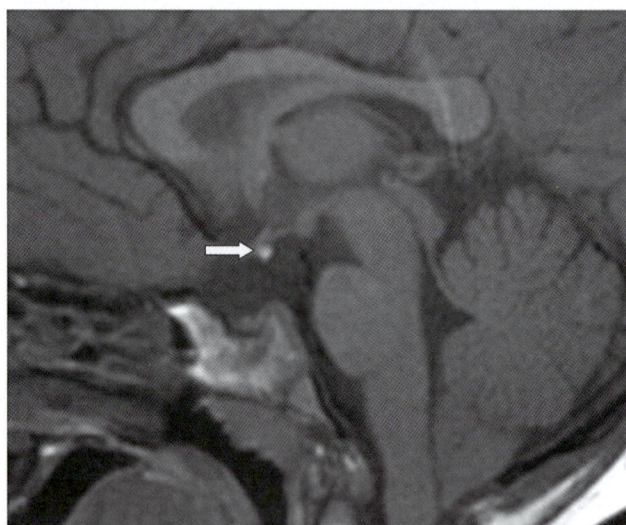

FIGURE 81-2

FINDINGS Figures 81-1 and 81-2. Coronal and sagittal non-contrast T1WI, respectively. There is a hyperintense nodular small mass (neurohypophysis) (arrows) at the expected location of the junction of the infundibulum to the hypothalamus just behind and inferiorly to the chiasm. The infundibulum is absent. The adenohypophysis is barely visible. The normal intrasellar hyperintense posterior pituitary lobe is not seen.

DIFFERENTIAL DIAGNOSIS Suprasellar lipoma, Rathke cleft cyst, basilar artery tip aneurysm (especially if partially or completely thrombosed), small craniopharyngioma, aberrant neurohypophysis (ANH).

DIAGNOSIS Aberrant neurohypophysis (ANH).

DISCUSSION ANH refers to a rare congenital or acquired anomaly of the hypothalamic and pituitary axis whereby the neurohypophysis is located in places other than posteriorly in the sella turcica. ANH include mainly ectopic posterior lobe (EPL) and duplicated pituitary gland (DPG), both found as incidental findings but sometimes found in patients with pituitary deficiency (particularly growth hormone deficiency). EPL can be seen on the undersurface of the median eminence of the hypothalamus or at the inferior end of the truncated pituitary stalk. MRI is the imaging modality of choice. The neurohypophysis is normally hyperintense on T1WI. EPL therefore could be seen as a hyperintense structure on T1WI located at the median eminence in the floor of the third ventricle or along a truncated pituitary stalk since the pituitary stalk is usually absent or thin in this situation. In contrast, DPG usually demonstrates

two stalks and thickening of the tuber cinereum on both T1WI and T2WI. CT shows a small sella turcica in EPL and a wide sella turcica in DPG, as well as other osseous skull base abnormalities. A small lipoma could mimic ANH but the constellation of associated congenital findings should exclude the differentials.

ANH is probably a result of abnormal interaction between the Rathke pouch (ectoderm) and the diencephalic neuroectoderm caused by genetic mutations. The causes of EPL include trauma (particularly at birth) and destruction of the stalk by ischemia. When the stalk is nonfunctioning, hormones produced in the hypothalamus cannot reach the posterior intrasellar lobe reservoir and may accumulate anywhere along the downward path of migration. Because these hormones are lipid rich, the normal positioned and EPLs are hyperintense on T1 sequences. When there is EPL, the adenohypophysis is small due to lack of stimulation by hypothalamic-releasing factors that can no longer use the stalk to migrate inferiorly. Thus, patients tend to present with hormonal abnormalities related to the anterior lobe while posterior lobe hormones continue to be secreted by the EPL into the pituitary portal system. On the other hand, DPG is commonly related to duplication of the stalk and of the sella, and sometimes with hypothalamic dysmorphism such as fusion of mammillary bodies and tuber cinereum. All the cases of DPGs have shown accompanying abnormalities of the face or brain especially midline clefting syndrome or associated with midline brain malformations, pituitary dwarfism, and Kallmann syndrome. Although there is no treatment for these hypothalamic and pituitary anomalies, hormonal supplementary treatment is administered when associated with pituitary dysfunction.

Question for Further Thought

1. What midline anomalies have been associated with EPLs and DPGs?

Reporting Responsibilities

Routine reporting is sufficient. Other associated midline anomalies depending on the type of ANH should be recorded.

What the Treating Physician Needs to Know

- Identifiable hypothalamic–pituitary axis abnormalities that can explain the pituitary dysfunction that occurs in these patients
- Presence of other accompanying midline anomalies

Answer

1. EPLs have been associated with hamartomas of the tuber cinereum, septo-optic dysplasia, Chiari I malformation, lobar holoprosencephaly, olfactory bulb anomalies, agenesis of the corpus callosum, persistent craniopharyngeal canal, and cerebellar vermian dysplasia. DPGs have been associated with hypertelorism, cleft palate, mouth and tongue dysmorphism, persistence of the craniopharyngeal canal, midline clival defects, choanal atresia, and ectopic adenohypophyseal, and hamartomatous pharyngeal masses among other disorders.

CLINICAL HISTORY *34-year-old female with sudden onset of headache and altered mental status.*

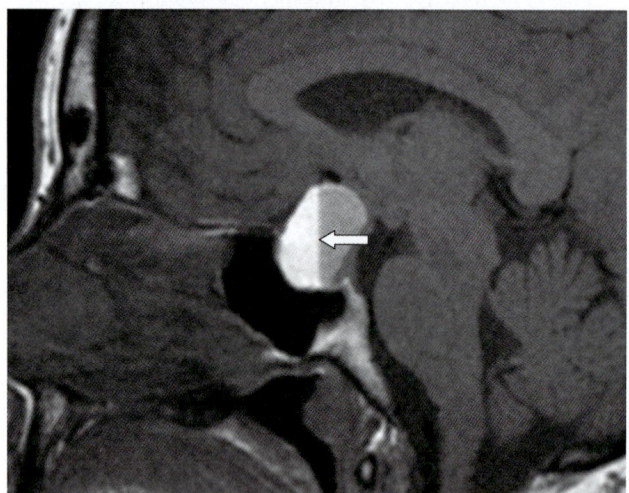

FIGURE 82-1

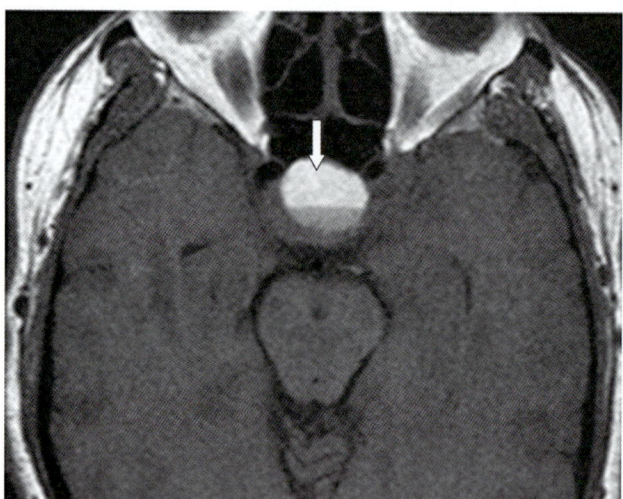

FIGURE 82-2

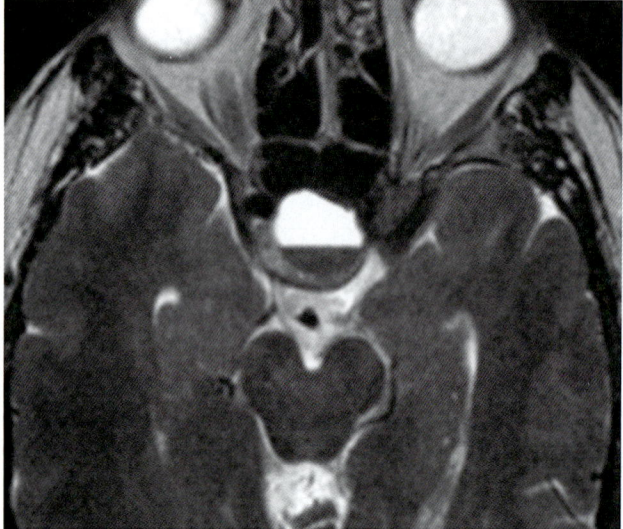

FIGURE 82-3

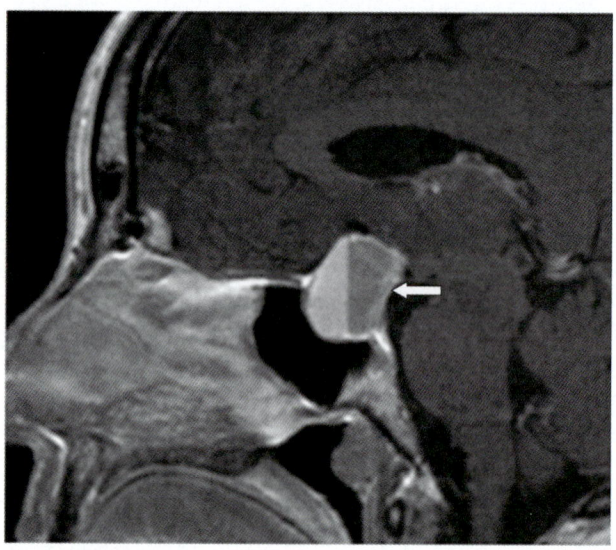

FIGURE 82-4

FINDINGS Figures 82-1 and 82-2. Mid-sagittal and axial non-contrast T1WI, respectively, through the sella turcica. There is a mass in the sella that contains a blood level (arrows). The sella is expanded, implying the presence of a previous mass. Both levels are bright, suggesting methemoglobin. Figure 82-3. Axial T2WI through the sella. The dependent portion of the blood is dark suggesting intracellular methemoglobin, whereas the supernatant remains hyperintense suggesting extracellular methemoglobin. Figure 82-4. Post-contrast sagittal T1WI shows no changes in the contents of the lesion and only posterior enhancement (arrow), where the residual tumor tissue is located.

DIFFERENTIAL DIAGNOSIS Pituitary apoplexy, Rathke cleft cyst, dermoid cyst, craniopharyngioma.

DIAGNOSIS Pituitary hemorrhage.

DISCUSSION Typical MRI findings of pituitary hemorrhage include hyperintensity on T1WI (reflecting acute and subacute blood products such as methemoglobin) with variable contrast enhancement. Restricted diffusion can be seen in solid infarcted components. Hematocrit levels may be present. On CT, the hemorrhagic gland appears hyperdense. Acute hydrocephalus may be present. Large hemorrhage may spill over into the subarachnoid space, resulting in subarachnoid hemorrhage. Fluid level is common in craniopharyngioma and may be present in a dermoid but not in Rathke cleft cyst. The mural nodule is characteristic of Rathke cleft cyst.

Pituitary hemorrhage usually occurs as a result of bleeding into a preexisting adenoma or cyst. If the patient presents with acute decompensation, the diagnosis is referred to as apoplexy, which can result from hemorrhage or infarction of the pituitary gland with mass effect upon surrounding structures. Hemorrhage into pituitary adenomas has been described in several clinical circumstances, including prior radiation treatment, pregnancy (Sheehan syndrome), trauma, anticoagulation therapy, open heart surgery, cerebral angiography, diabetic ketoacidosis, and bromocriptine treatment of a prolactinoma. Symptoms of pituitary apoplexy include acute onset of headache, visual field deficits, ophthalmoplegia, and altered mental status.

Subacute hemorrhage into pituitary adenomas has also been described with a more benign clinical course that can result in hypopituitarism. This is known as subclinical apoplexy. The imaging findings are similar with the differentiating factor being the clinical presentation. The treatment for pituitary apoplexy is urgent surgical decompression with a high mortality rate in patients not receiving surgical treatment if the hematoma is large. Hormonal supplements are also instituted.

Questions for Further Thought

1. What is the incidence of an underlying adenoma in pituitary hemorrhage?
2. What are the different MRI features when evaluating stages of hematoma?

Reporting Responsibilities

Direct reporting is essential as this is an emergency requiring prompt treatment except in the subclinical apoplexy. Describe the abnormalities and their extent.

What the Treating Physician Needs to Know

- Size and extent of the mass effect
- Complications such as compression of the chiasm, subarachnoid hemorrhage, and cavernous sinus compression
- This is an emergency with a high mortality rate in patients not treated promptly

Answers

1. Underlying adenomas are present in up to 90% of cases of pituitary hemorrhage.
2. There are five described stages of degradation of hemorrhage. In the hyperacute stage, intracellular oxyhemoglobin is isointense on both T1WI and T2WI. In the acute stage (1 to 2 days), intracellular deoxyhemoglobin is hypointense on T2WI and isointense on T1WI. In the early subacute stage (2 to 7 days), intracellular methemoglobin is hyperintense on T1WI and hypointense on T2WI. In the late subacute stage (1 to 4 weeks), extracellular methemoglobin is hyperintense on T1WI and T2WI. In the chronic stage (>2 to 4 weeks), hemosiderin is hypointense on T1WI and T2WI.

CLINICAL HISTORY   *Normal variants of cervical arterial anatomy.*

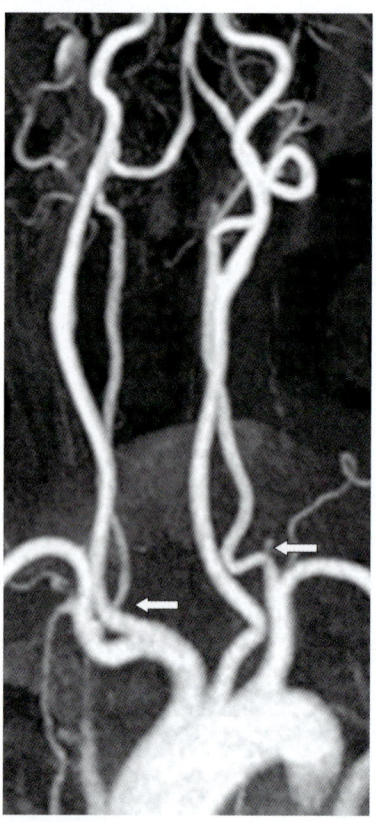

FIGURE 83-1

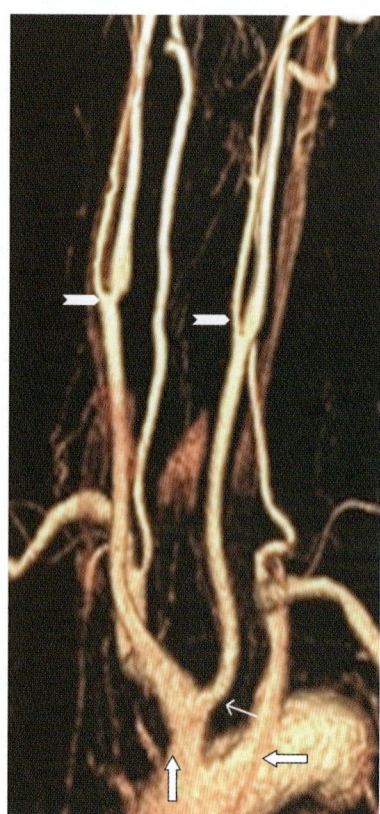

FIGURE 83-2

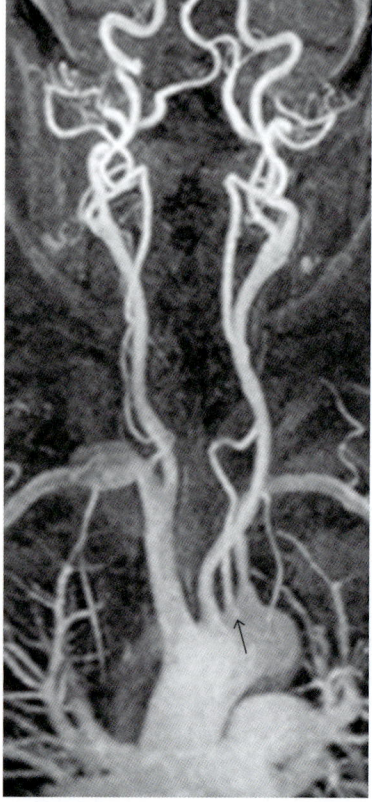

FIGURE 83-3

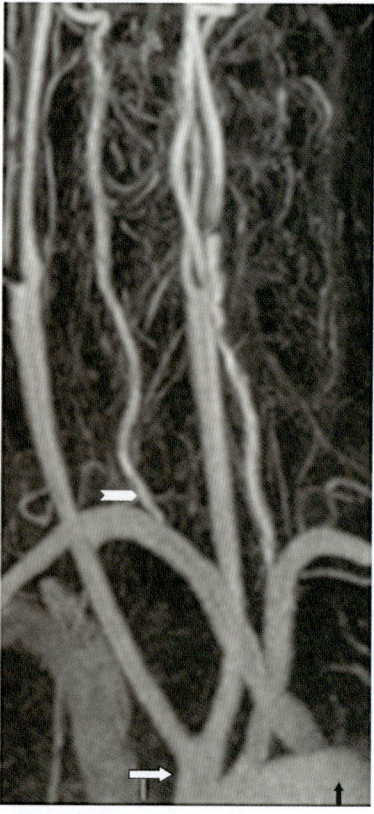

FIGURE 83-4

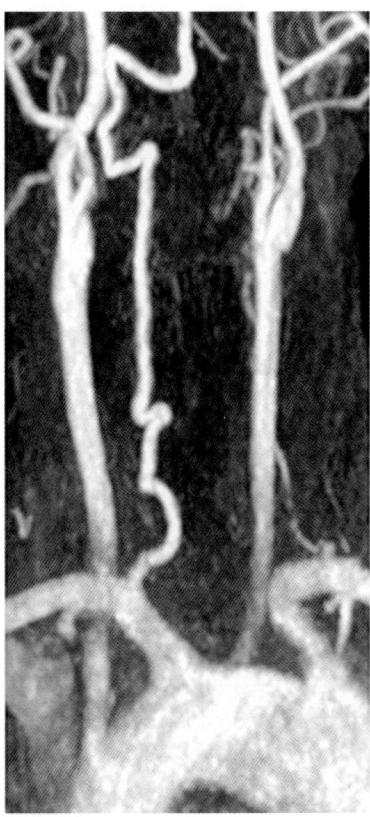

FIGURE 83-5

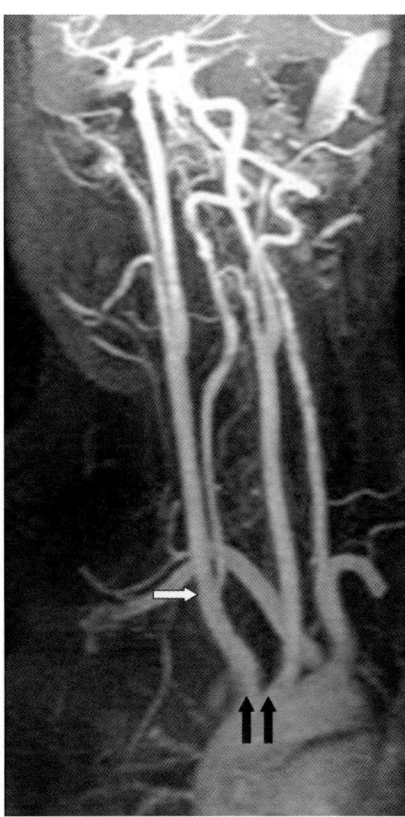

FIGURE 83-6

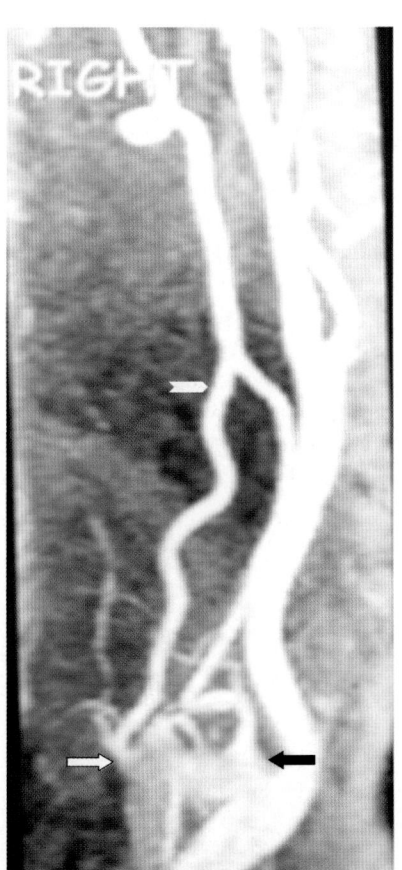

FIGURE 83-7

FINDINGS All figures are contrast-enhanced MIP or volume-rendering neck MRA in different projections to best demonstrate the anatomy. Figure 83-1. Normal three-vessel origins from the aortic arch. From right to left are the brachiocephalic trunk, which divides into the right subclavian artery and the right common carotid artery (RCCA), the left common carotid artery (LCCA), and the left subclavian artery. The vertebral arteries (transverse arrows) originate from the subclavian arteries. The common carotid artery (CCA) divides distally into the internal carotid artery (ICA) and the external carotid artery (ECA) at about C4 level. This is the most common aortic arch configuration encountered. Figure 83-2. There is a common origin of the brachiocephalic trunk and the LCCA—the so-called *bovine* origin (arrow) which is different from the real *bovine* configuration. This is a common anomaly. The true *bovine* configuration has a single trunk from the aortic arch that gives rise to all the neck and head vessels. The LCCA (line arrow) arises as a branch of the brachiocephalic trunk in this case. The left subclavian artery has a separate origin (transverse arrow). The chevrons point to the CCA bifurcations. Figure 83-3. Four-vessel origins from the aortic arch. From right to left are the brachiocephalic trunk, the LCCA, the left vertebral artery (originating directly from the aortic arch) (arrow), and the left subclavian artery. Figure 83-4. There is aberrant origin of the right subclavian artery (vertical black arrow) from the aortic arch distal to the origin of the left subclavian artery. It then courses behind the esophagus to reach the right side. The right vertebral artery originates from the aberrant right subclavian artery (chevron). There is a common origin of the RCCA and LCCA (transverse white arrow). The left subclavian artery originates normally from the aortic arch. Figure 83-5. Each great vessel originates separately from the aortic arch. These are from right to left, RCCA, right subclavian, LCCA, and left subclavian. There is no brachiocephalic trunk. The vertebral arteries emanate from their respective subclavian arteries. Figure 83-6. This is a variant of the aberrant right subclavian artery with the right vertebral artery arising from the RCCA (arrow). There are separate origins of the RCCA and LCCA from the aortic arch (vertical arrows). Figure 83-7. There is duplication of the origin of the right vertebral artery (transverse arrows) from the right subclavian artery and the two duplicated limbs join distally (chevron).

DIFFERENTIAL DIAGNOSIS N/A.

DIAGNOSIS Normal variant vascular anatomy of the origins of the great vessels from the aortic arch.

DISCUSSION The embryology of the aortic arch is complex and will not be described here. More than 20 aortic arch variants have been described. This panel demonstrates some of the normal variant anatomy of the origins of the great vessels from the aortic arch. The commonest encountered pattern of the aortic arch branches is in Figure 83-1, where there are three vessels originating from the aortic arch. This is found in between 75% and 93% of the population depending on the ethnic or racial population studied. The blood supply to the brain is through four major vessels, the bilateral ICA forming the anterior circulation and the bilateral vertebral arteries joining to form the basilar artery and the posterior circulation. In about 10% of the population one vertebral artery terminates in posterior inferior cerebellar artery (PICA) and do not make any significant contribution to the basilar artery. The extracranial circulation and the blood supply to the meninges are provided by the bilateral ECA. The ICA and ECA are the

two branches of the CCA and they both anastomose at the skull base. These anastomoses could be useful compensating for arterial stenosis and occlusions. There are also congenital collateral anastomoses of the carotid and the vertebrobasilar systems; the persistent trigeminal artery, the persistent otic artery, the persistent hypoglossal artery, and the persistent proatlantal artery. The brain is probably the most demanding organ in the body representing about 2% (3 lb) of total body weight yet it receives about 15% (750 mL) of the total cardiac output. Perhaps this is due to the important functions of the brain. This blood supply could be drastically reduced or affected by both congenital and acquired anomalies of the aortic arch and of the individual vessels with significant consequences to the brain and the body in general.

Question for Further Thought

1. What are the common acquired abnormalities of the great neck vessels?

Reporting Responsibilities

Routine reporting of the neck vascular imaging is sufficient. In the case of significant arterial disease due to atherosclerotic stenosis, fibromuscular dysplasia, dissection, pseudoaneurysms, and arterial blowout, additional direct communication with the referring physician becomes essential. However, all anomalies should be carefully categorized and communicated accordingly.

What the Treating Physician Needs to Know

- The pattern of the congenital variants
- Other associated anomalies

Answer

1. The common acquired anomalies of the great vessels of the neck are related to degenerative, inflammatory, and traumatic changes. The predominant degenerative change is atherosclerotic in origin, resulting mostly in luminal narrowing, mural calcifications, artery-to-artery embolism, occlusion, or fusiform aneurysm formation. Inflammatory lesions include vasculitis, vasculopathy, blowout lesions, and mycotic aneurysms. Traumatic lesions include dissections resulting in stenosis, pseudoaneurysms, occlusions, or arteriovenous fistula formation.

CLINICAL HISTORY *57-year-old male with known aneurysm for follow-up MRA.*

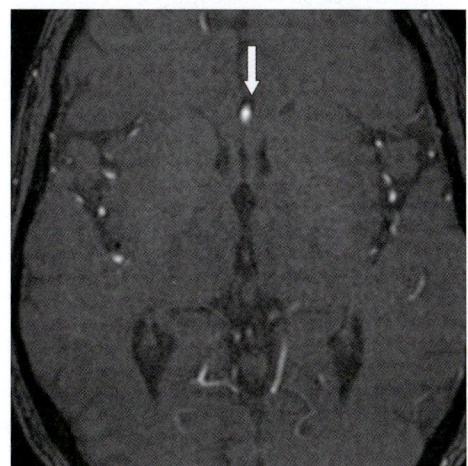

FIGURE 84-1

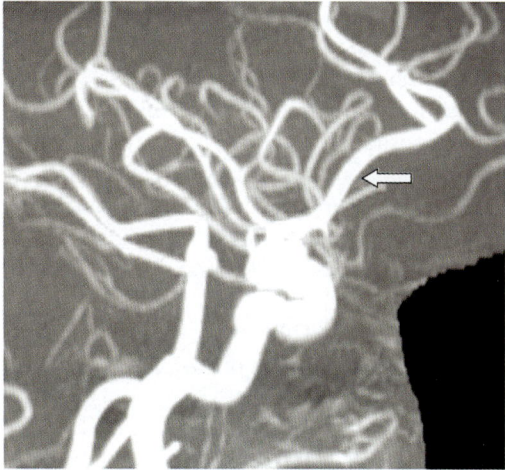

FIGURE 84-2

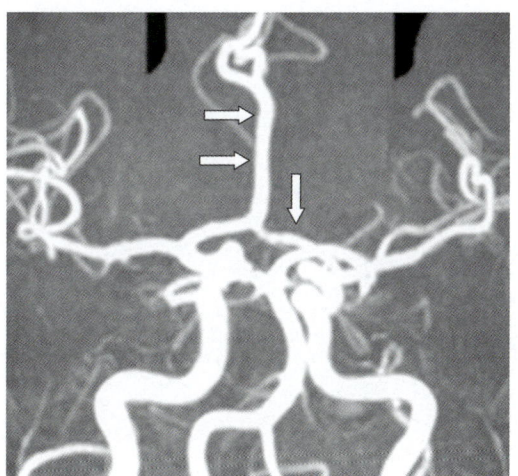

FIGURE 84-3

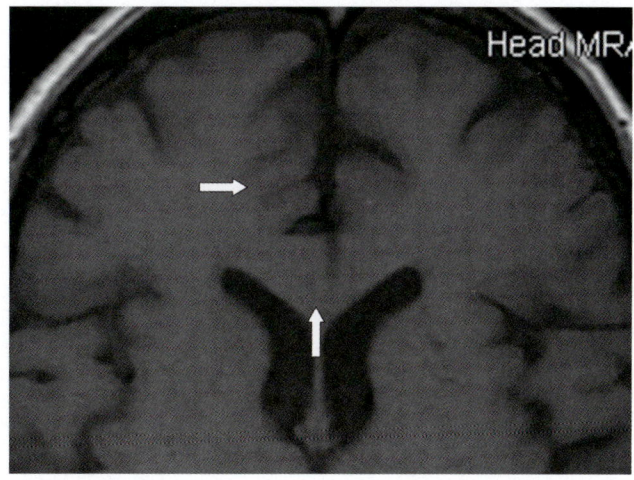

FIGURE 84-4

FINDINGS Figure 84-1. Axial source image from 3D TOF MRA of the head through the third ventricle. There is a single anterior cerebral artery (ACA) within the anterior interhemispheric fissure (arrow). Figure 84-2. Lateral MIP 3D MRA of the brain. There is a single ACA A2 (arrow). Figure 84-3. Submentovertical 3D TOF MRA of the brain. There are two A1s joining together to form a single A2 (transverse arrows). There is no anterior communicating artery. The left A1 is mildly hypoplastic (vertical arrow). Figure 84-4. Axial non-contrast T1WI. Asymmetric frontal medial sulcation abnormality; right parasagittal microgyria (arrow). There is mildly malformed thickening of the genu of corpus callosum (vertical arrow).

DIFFERENTIAL DIAGNOSIS N/A.

DIAGNOSIS Azygos anterior cerebral artery (AACA).

DISCUSSION The single A2 otherwise known as azygos anterior cerebral artery (AACA) is a very rare congenital variant. There is fusion of the two A1. There is no anterior communicating artery (A-com). The single vessel then supplies the bilateral parasagittal frontal lobes. AACA is found in most midline congenital malformations such as agenesis of the corpus callosum, lobar holoprosencephaly, syntelencephaly, and septo-optic dysplasia. There are subtle midline malformations in this case. AACA has also been reported in association with arteriovenous malformation (AVM) and saccular aneurysm. Aneurysm at the bifurcation of the AACA is supposedly common occurring in up to 71% most probably due to hemodynamic stress or due to congenital anomalous histology of the artery. The aneurysm in this patient (not well shown) is on the right supraclinoid ICA. The best imaging technique for demonstrating AACA is either MRA or CTA. DSA demonstration could be very difficult requiring cross-compression of one ICA during contralateral injection. The possibility of bilateral frontal lobe infarction should the AACA be occluded is real. Clipping or embolization of AACA aneurysm could also be challenging.

Question for Further Thought

1. What is the developmental origin of AACA?

Reporting Responsibilities

Routine reporting is sufficient. Presence of aneurysm or vascular malformation, however, demands direct reporting. Presence of other congenital lesions should be documented.

What the Treating Physician Needs to Know

- This could be an incidental finding with very minimal associated lesions elsewhere
- CTA or MRA is equally effective in diagnosing AACA
- Presence of unexplained bifrontal infarcts may suggest presence of occluded AACA

Answer

1. AACA is fairly common in fetuses occurring in 68% of one series of fetal brains examined and 75% of another series of infant brains examined. The incidence in the adult population, however, varies from about 0% to 5%. It does appear that in the developmental process, the single ACA duplicate and the A-com forms. It is not certain at which time this single ACA forms. It has been suggested that this takes place at the 16-mm stage from the medial branch of the olfactory artery or a continuation of the median artery at the 20- to 24-mm stage. AACA is common adult mammals (pigs, squirrels, and rabbits) and lower primates (chimpanzees and monkeys).

CLINICAL HISTORY *22-year-old female with possible stroke. There is a history of connective tissue disease of unknown type.*

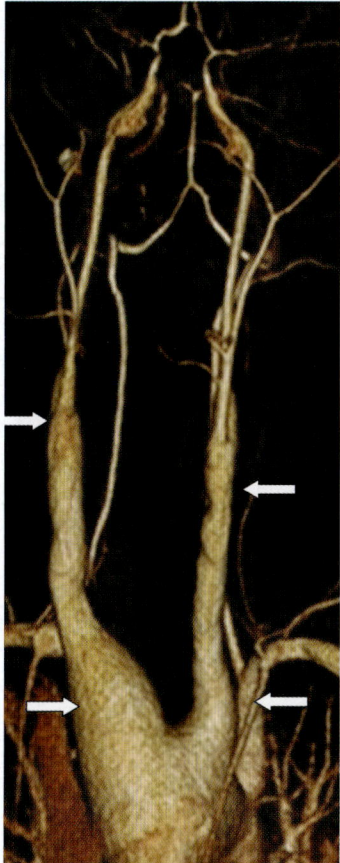

FIGURE 85-1

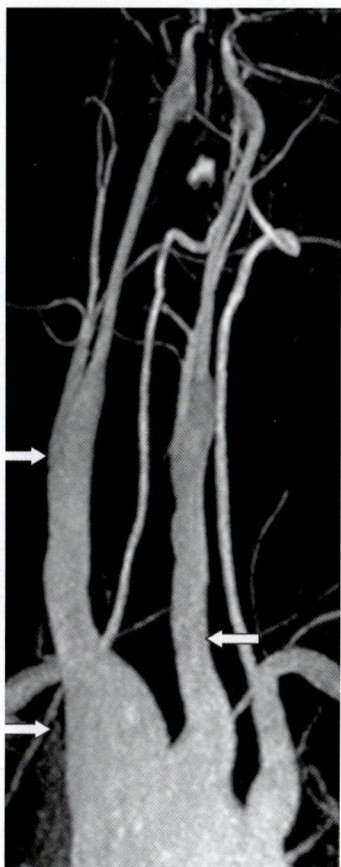

FIGURE 85-2

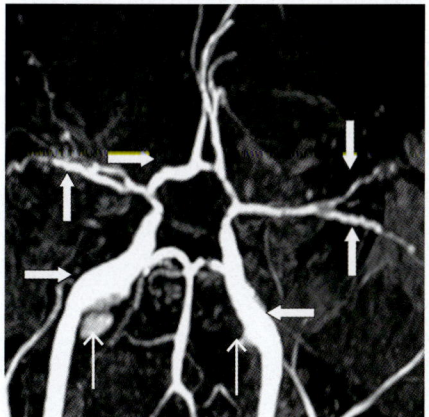

FIGURE 85-3

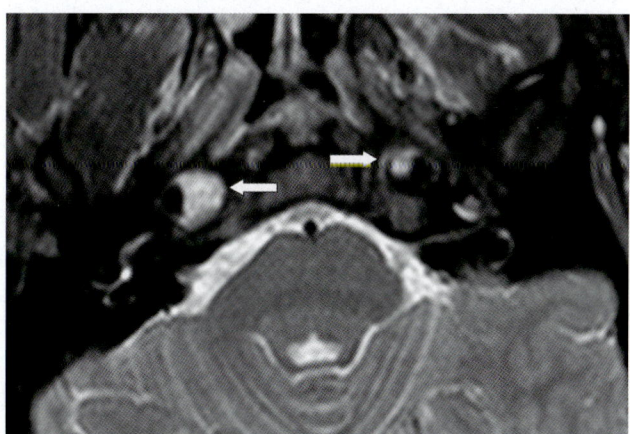

FIGURE 85-4

FINDINGS Figures 85-1 and 85-2. 3D volume rendering with corresponding MIP, respectively at different rotations, of contrast-enhanced MRA of the neck.

There is fusiform dilatation of the aortic arch extending into the origins of all the great vessels, and bilaterally into the common carotid arteries and proximal internal

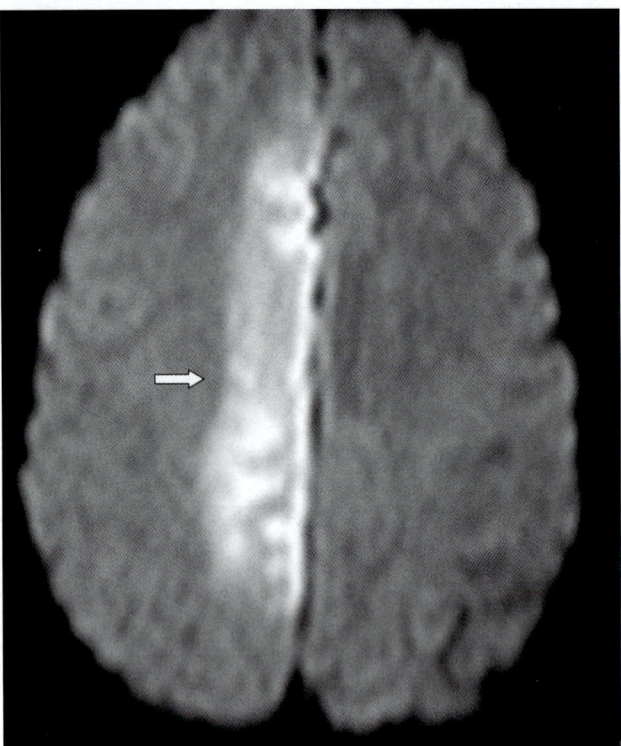

FIGURE 85-5

carotid arteries (ICAs). Figure 85-3. MIP of 3D TOF non-contrast MRA of the head. There is fusiform dilatation of bilateral petrous ICAs and right A1 (transverse arrows) with small out-pouches of the petrous ICAs - pseudo aneurysms (line arrows). There is also "twisted wire" appearance of the branches of the bilateral middle cerebral arteries (MCA) and anterior cerebral arteries (ACA) (vertical arrows). Figure 85-4. Axial T2 proton density (PD) fat sat through the skull base. There is crescentic mural hyperintensity surrounding the flow void in the bilateral ICAs (arrows). Figure 85-5. Axial DWI through the cingulate gyrus. There is right frontal parasagittal restricted diffusion in the right ACA territory consistent with acute infarct (arrow). This was due to distal occlusion of right A2 (not shown).

DIFFERENTIAL DIAGNOSIS Fusiform aneurysm due to vasculopathy, vasculitis, Marfan syndrome, Ehlers-Danlos, neurofibromatosis type 1 (NF1), arterial dissection.

DIAGNOSIS Cylindrical and fusiform aneurysm due to vasculopathy of unknown origin.

DISCUSSION Cylindrical or fusiform aneurysm is a circumferential arterial dilatation resulting from pathologic involvement of the entire artery; if a long segment of the artery is involved it is termed cylindrical, and if a short segment is involved it is termed fusiform. MRI with MRA offers the best method of showing the changes of fusiform or cylindrical aneurysm detailing the pattern of dilatation, presence or absence of mural thrombus, associated brain parenchymal changes, and other related bone or dural changes. There is usually elongation and dilatation of the vessels involved, best demonstrated by MRA or CTA. Axial PD fat sat may show presence of hyperintense mural thrombus or hemorrhage. Associated pseudoaneurysm may present as an outpouch. Distal vascular irregularities such as the twisted wire appearance in this case indicate distal vasculopathic changes. Distal occlusive changes can also be demonstrated. The consequences of the vasculopathy in the form of ischemic changes or infarcts are demonstrated as signal abnormalities on the MRI; in this case, a right distal ACA territory infarct. There were also multifocal white matter (WM) changes consistent with multifocal small infarcts or ischemic changes. CTA and DSA are also useful in demonstrating various aspects of the abnormalities. These changes could be found in the listed differentials. The clinical information will serve as a guide to the correct diagnosis.

Fusiform or cylindrical aneurysms intracranially or extracranially are rare. Intracranially, they are more common in the posterior circulation. The causes may include arterial dissection, atherosclerosis, and disorders of collagen and elastin metabolism, infections, and very rarely neoplastic invasion of the arterial wall. The underlying pathology is usually internal elastic lamina degeneration and fissuring with myxoid changes or altered blood within the wall of the vessel depending on the cause. Serpentine channel forms as disease extends longitudinally, combined with varying degrees of intramural thrombosis. The cervical vessels in this patient did not demonstrate mural thrombosis. Multifocal arterial aneurysms in different parts of the body were present in this patient. The underlying diagnosis was connective tissue disease of unknown type. Known connective tissue or collagen disease responsible for fusiform aneurysms includes lupus, Marfan syndrome, Ehlers-Danlos, and unknown factors. Vascular involvement in NF1 could produce similar findings. Rupture could result in subarachnoid and or parenchymal hemorrhage. Mass effect on critical structures could produce focal neurologic deficit.

Question for Further Thought

1. What are the treatment options?

Reporting Responsibilities

Direct reporting is necessary in view of possible complication of rupture and the presence of acute ischemic changes. The location, extent, and associated parenchymal abnormalities should be tabulated. Presence of underlying pathology if known should also be reported.

What the Treating Physician Needs to Know

- Location, extent, and number of lesions
- Associated intracranial changes (infarcts, parenchymal or subarachnoid hemorrhage, and mass effects if present)
- Underlying cause may not be determinable at imaging

Answer

1. Multifocal extensive changes as in this case could be difficult to manage. Conservative management is recommended with only symptomatic or critical lesions treated. Focal lesions could be wrapped, clipped, coiled, stented, or resected as judged appropriate with or without bypass options.

CLINICAL HISTORY *51-year-old female with a 1-week history of headache. She was brought into the emergency room after developing a new severe headache with loss of consciousness.*

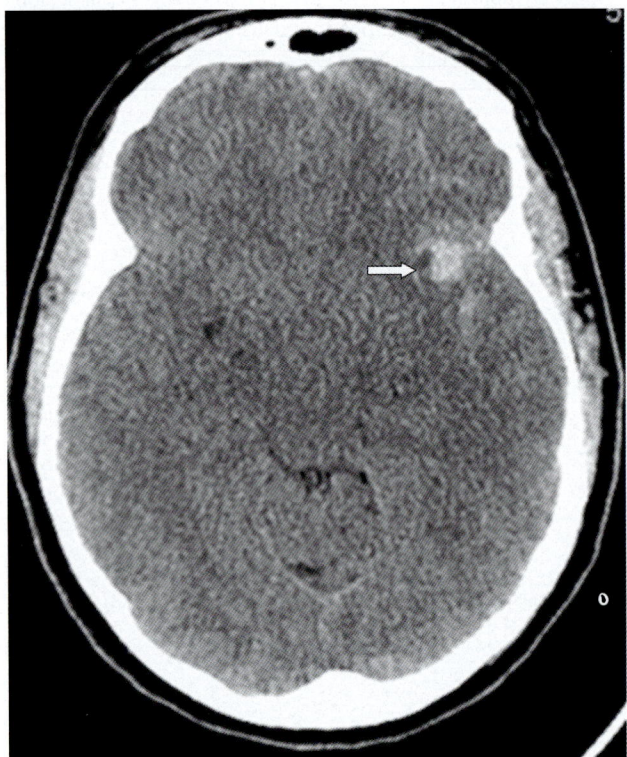

FIGURE 86-1

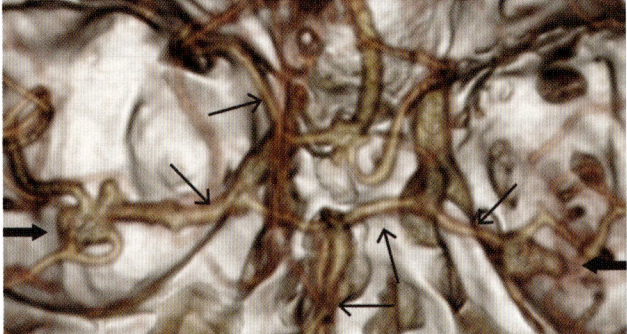

FIGURE 86-2

bilateral irregular, multilobulated middle cerebral artery (MCA) bifurcation aneurysms with nipples (arrows). The right MCA aneurysm has many tits and the neck incorporates the origins of all branches. There is irregularity and multifocal constriction and dilation of the bilateral anterior cerebral artery (ACA), MCA, and posterior cerebral artery (PCA) (line arrows) consistent with vasospasm. Figure 86-3. Axial MIP CTA of the head. The two irregular lobulated MCA aneurysms are again demonstrated (large arrows) with irregularity of the arteries (line arrows) consistent with vasospasm.

DIFFERENTIAL DIAGNOSIS N/A.

DIAGNOSIS MCA aneurysms (bilateral) with subarachnoid hemorrhage and cerebral vasospasm (CVS).

DISCUSSION This patient highlights four important points about aneurysm rupture: how to identify a ruptured aneurysm in the presence of multiple aneurysms, the concept of silent rupture, cerebrovascular spasm, and brain swelling as complications. Multiple aneurysms are present in over 30% of patients with aneurysms. These are more common in women than men in a ratio of 5:1. It is therefore important to scrutinize the entire study for additional aneurysms once one is found. It is always necessary to determine which aneurysm has ruptured once multiple aneurysms are discovered in a patient with subarachnoid hemorrhage (SAH). Since the ruptured aneurysm will be treated first and urgently to prevent further bleeding, it is imperative to identify the one that ruptured. Helpful indicators pointing to a ruptured aneurysm include (a) closeness to the highest concentration of SAH or parenchymal hematoma; (b) larger aneurysm size; (c) aneurysmal wall irregularity such as lobulation, daughter aneurysm, nipples, or tits; (d) local vasospasm; (e) serial change in contour; and (f) obvious contrast extravasation during DSA or CTA. When there are multiple aneurysms, the anterior communicating artery aneurysm is the most likely to

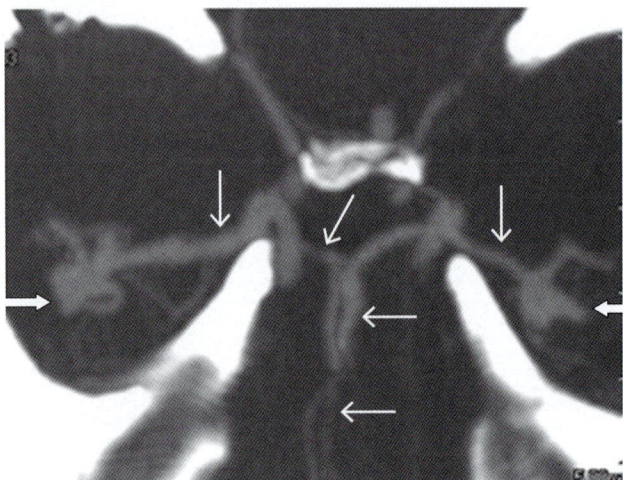

FIGURE 86-3

FINDINGS Figure 86-1. Axial NCCT through the sylvian fissures. There is a rounded hyperdensity with peripheral extensions in the left sylvian fissure (arrow) consistent with hemorrhage. There is effacement of the convexity sulci and basal cisterns, suggesting brain swelling and central herniation. Figure 86-2. Three-dimensional volume rendering CTA head submentovertical (SMV) view. There are

have ruptured with the MCA aneurysm the least likely with all other sites somewhere in between. In this case, the concentration of SAH is in the left sylvian fissure, suggesting the left MCA aneurysm is the recent rupture. Both aneurysms are about the same size and are both irregular in outline, suggesting that both have probably ruptured. The irregularity of the vessels is diffuse consistent with diffuse spasm indicating at least a subacute rupture presumably from the right or both aneurysms since spasm tends to occur 3 to 5 days following SAH. Silent rupture or so-called warning leak may occur in about 50% of patients before the obviously symptomatic one. The headache of the warning leak is not as severe as the usual "worse headache of my life" that patient with SAH presents with. There may have been a warning leak a week before the present presentation in this patient. The effacement of the sulci and basal cisterns is most probably due to brain swelling in the absence of hydrocephalus. This is possibly related to ischemic complications of the CVS.

Question for Further Thought

1. What is the pathogenesis of vasospasm in SAH?

Reporting Responsibilities

This is an acute situation requiring direct reporting. The number of aneurysms, locations of aneurysms and SAH, direction of projection, aneurysm size with measurements, and relationship to vascular branches and surrounding structures should be reported. Complications such as vasospasm, brain swelling, infarction, parenchymal or other extraaxial hematoma, and hydrocephalus should all be carefully tabulated. Other associated lesions coincidental or causative such as AVM and tumors should be reported. A statement should be inserted, suggesting the aneurysm that has ruptured.

What the Treating Physician Needs to Know

- Location and number of aneurysms and SAH
- Which aneurysm has ruptured?
- Complications if any
- What imaging techniques best answer questions regarding evaluation of primary and secondary lesions

Answer

1. CVS is now the leading cause of poor outcome and death affecting about 20% of patients who survive the initial ictus of SAH. The real reason for CVS remains a mystery! It is thought that the primary offending agents are blood products within the subarachnoid space. These products probably set up a cascade of activities driven by several chemicals acting together to cause CVS. These processes may include calcium-dependent and calcium-independent vasoconstriction, effects of chemicals such as superoxide free radicals, endothelins, nitrous oxide, and protein kinase. A disruption of vascular tone autoregulation, endothelial proliferation, and apoptosis along with inflammatory cascades have all been implicated in the development of CVS. Treatment options include nimodipine, hypertensive hypervolemic therapy, and balloon angioplasty along with management of the ischemic complications.

CLINICAL HISTORY *24-year-old female with a 3-day history of right-sided Jacksonian seizures.*

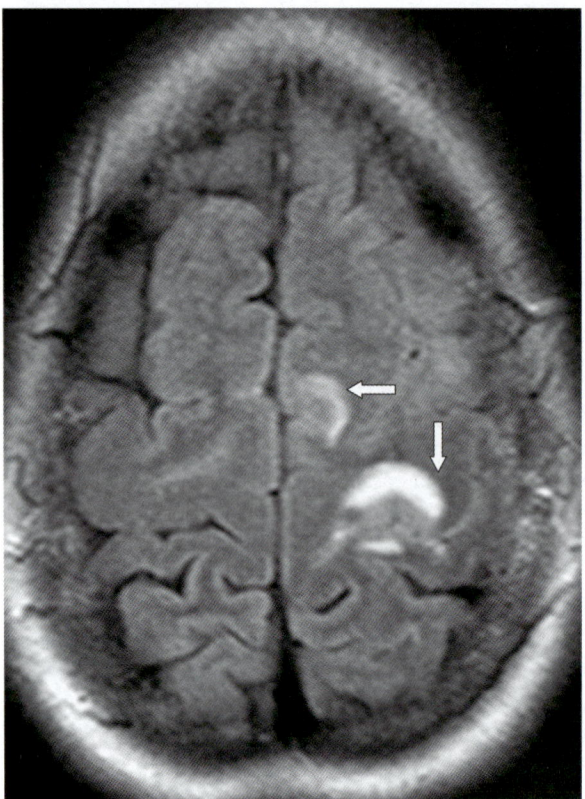

FIGURE 87-1

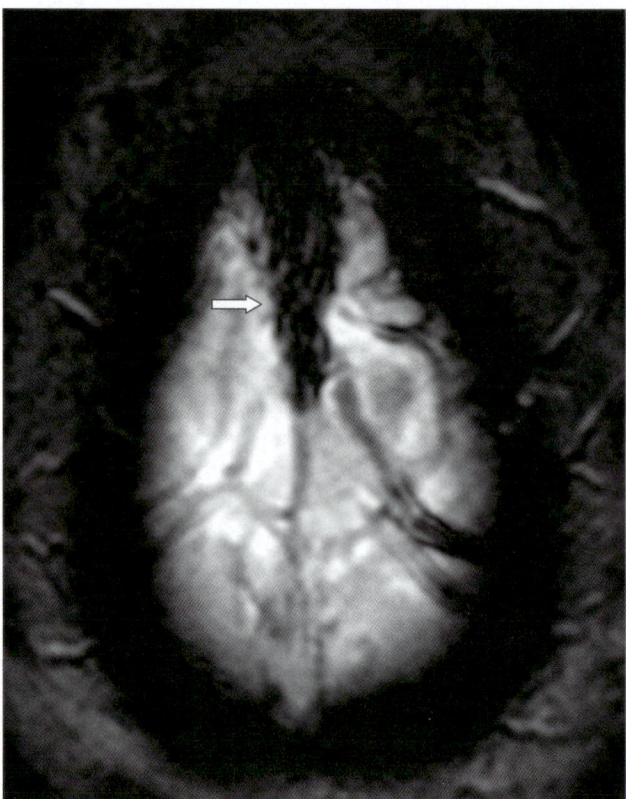

FIGURE 87-2

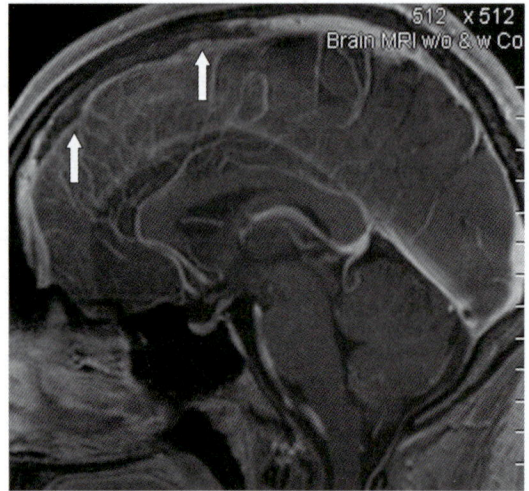

FIGURE 87-3

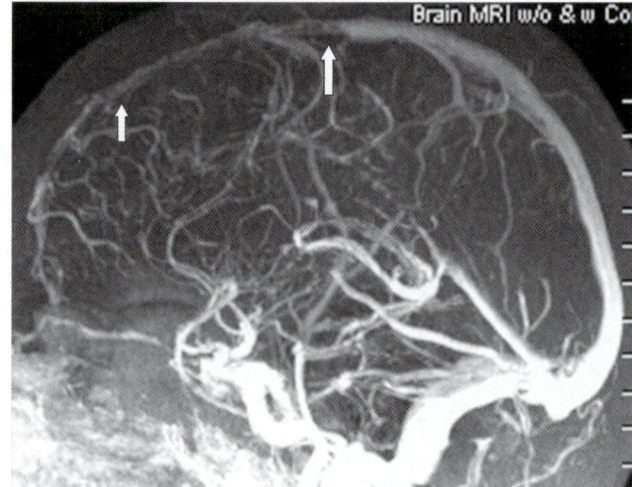

FIGURE 87-4

FINDINGS

Figure 87-1. Axial FLAIR through the vertex. There are thick curvilinear hyperintense foci (arrows) in the posterior left frontal parasagittal convexity with associ-

ated effacement of left frontal sulci. Figure 87-2. Axial GRE through the superior sagittal sinus (SSS). There is enlarged blooming within the anterior SSS (arrow) and within the left vein of Trolard. Figure 87-3. Sagittal post-contrast T1WI. There is iso- to hypointense signal with peripheral enhancement in the anterior SSS (arrows). There is homogeneous opacification of the SSS posteriorly. Figure 87-4. 3D contrast-enhanced MRV. There is irregular severe narrowing of the anterior SSS (arrows) with smooth contrast opacification of the patent posterior SSS. There are multiple irregular collaterals over the frontal lobes.

DIFFERENTIAL DIAGNOSIS Subarachnoid hemorrhage (SAH), cortical infarcts, SSS thrombosis.

DIAGNOSIS SSS thrombosis (acute).

DISCUSSION MRI and contrast-enhanced MRV are the examinations of choice for comprehensive evaluation of SSS or other cerebral venous sinus thrombosis. The MRI demonstrates signal within the sinuses; ordinarily there should be signal void due to flowing blood. Acute thrombosis tends to produce isointensity within the swollen sinuses on T1WI, which may become hyperintense over time. FLAIR and T2WI show iso/hyperintensity within the sinuses. There is blooming within the sinuses and the associated cortical veins on GRE and SWI. Parenchymal changes such as cortical subcortical white matter (WM) hemorrhagic venous infarction are demonstrated on DWI and ADC maps as areas of heterogeneous restricted diffusion with the appropriate blooming on GRE. The hyperintensity of vasogenic edema is well demonstrated on the FLAIR and T2WI. SAH if present could produce sulcal hyperintensity on FLAIR. Post-contrast T1WI shows peripheral enhancement of the clot. Parenchymal enhancement may also be present. MRV demonstrates occlusion, irregularity, or filling defects within the thrombosed sinus along with collaterals, which are generally irregular superficial or transmedullary vessels.

NCCT may demonstrate sinus hyperdensity in about 20% of cases. The so-called empty delta sign refers to filling defect (clot) with peripheral enhancement within the sinus on contrast-enhanced axial CT. Hemorrhagic infarcts and SAH are usually hyperdense. The accuracy of CTA in demonstrating the luminal filling defects and irregularities of the sinuses has been assessed as similar to contrast MRV. DSA is now rarely done for diagnosis and obtained if endovascular treatment is contemplated.

Sinus thrombosis is an uncommon disease of adults. It is more common in women than men. Sinus thrombosis affects the SSS and the transverse sinuses in the majority of patients (70%). Risk factors include pregnancy, oral contraceptive use, prothrombotic state/blood dyscrasias, dehydration, intracranial hypotension, infection, and malignancy. Presenting symptoms and signs could be nonspecific but the common ones are headache in over 95%, seizures, focal neurologic deficit, papilledema, decreased level of consciousness, and coma. The syndrome of benign intracranial hypertension (BIH) (headache, visual disturbances, and papilledema) is common. Treatment is usually anticoagulation and endovascular thrombolysis when deemed appropriate.

Question for Further Thought

1. How do you differentiate congenital hypoplasia of cerebral venous sinus from chronic thrombosis?

Reporting Responsibilities

Direct reporting is required. This is an acute situation. Pattern of occlusion and corresponding parenchymal hemorrhagic infarcts as well as mass effect should be reported. Presence of SAH should be mentioned.

What the Treating Physician Needs to Know

- Extent of thrombosis including all the venous sinuses involved
- Pattern of infarction and complications such as SAH, mass effect, and herniations
- The diagnosis could be made on MRI but MRV confirms the diagnosis
- Progress of recanalization or progression of thrombosis on follow-up
- Patients with suspected benign intracranial hypertension (BIH) should be evaluated for venous sinus thrombosis

Answer

1. It could be difficult differentiating a hypoplastic sinus from chronic thrombosis. Hypoplastic venous sinus is usually small to nonexistent with smooth outline and no filling defects or irregularities. There are usually no irregular collaterals. One of the transverse sinuses is the most likely to be hypoplastic with preferential drainage through the dominant sinus.

CLINICAL HISTORY   *Newborn female with prenatal diagnosis of vein of Galen malformation (VGM) now presents with high-output cardiac failure.*

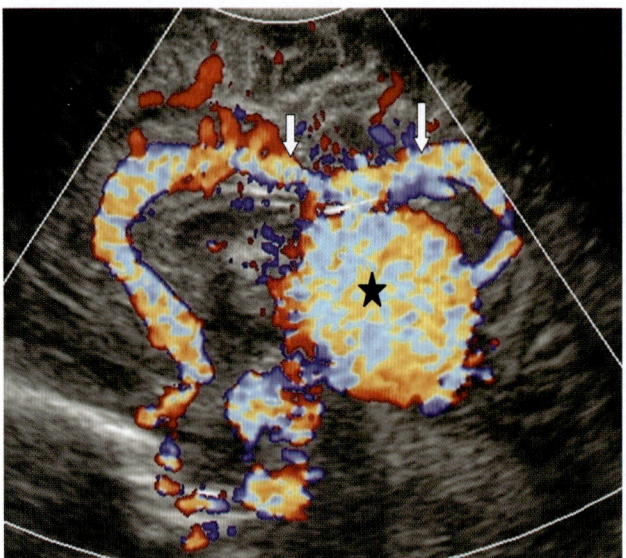

FIGURE 88-1

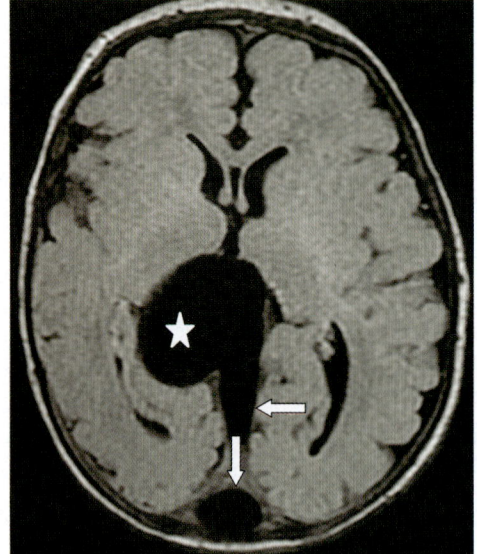

FIGURE 88-2

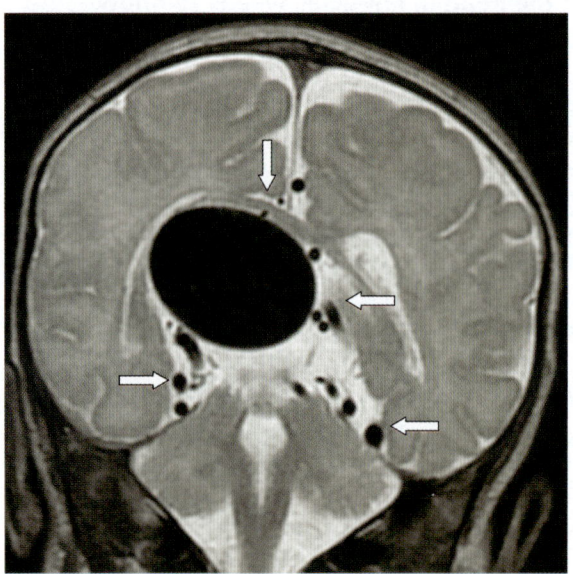

FIGURE 88-3

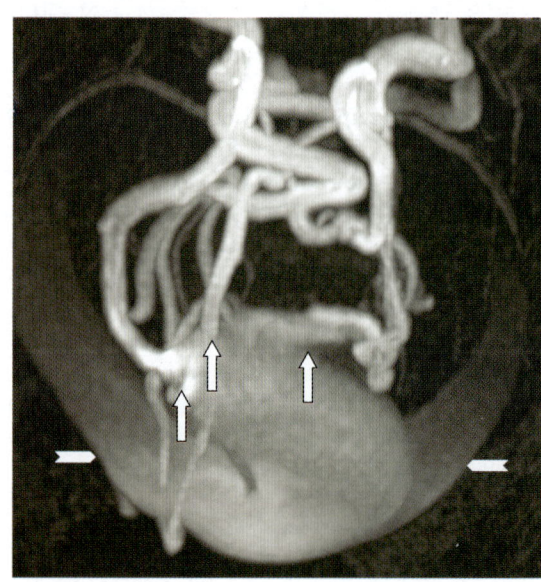

FIGURE 88-4

FINDINGS Figure 88-1. Sagittal Doppler cranial ultrasound. There is a large 3.5-cm vascular structure posteriorly to the third ventricle and splenium of corpus callosum (appropriate position of the vein of Galen) (star) with two large feeding vessels demonstrated: a pericallosal artery and a posterior cerebral artery (arrows). Figure 88-2. Axial FLAIR through the third ventricle. There is a 3.2 cm × 3.1 cm signal void posteriorly to the thalami and third ventricle with mass effect consistent with the vein of Galen aneurysmal malformation (VGAM) (star). Large draining sinus (transverse arrow) and torcula/SSS (vertical arrow) are seen posteriorly to the aneurysm. Figure 88-3. Coronal T2WI through the aneurysm. There is superior displacement of the splenium of the corpus callosum (vertical arrow). Multiple round and tubular signal voids representing large afferent arteries (arrows) are seen surrounding the aneurysm. Figure 88-4. 3D TOF MRA of the head Submentovertical (SMV) view. There is direct connection of all major intracranial vessels (arrows), anterior cerebral artery (ACA), posterior cerebral artery (PCA), and middle cerebral artery

(MCA) to the aneurysmal malformation. Huge bilateral transverse sinuses (chevrons) emanate from the torcula.

DIFFERENTIAL DIAGNOSIS N/A.

DIAGNOSIS VGAM.

DISCUSSION The hallmark of the VGAM is a dilated persistent median prosencephalic vein of Markowski in the usual location of the vein of Galen behind the third ventricle and the splenium of the corpus callosum. There is usually no visible vascular nidus. This is seen on prenatal and postnatal Doppler ultrasound as a vascular pouch with very rich vascular connections. NCCT shows a hyperdense mass with mass effect on surrounding structures, which contrast enhances avidly following contrast administration. MRI particularly FLAIR and T2WI shows a large smooth signal void fed by a collection of tubular signal voids draining into the torcula. It does enhance avidly with significant artifacts due to the turbulent flow. The complications that can be demonstrated on CT and MRI include mass effect, parenchymal and intraventricular hemorrhages, calcifications, volume loss, gliosis, encephalomalacia, and hydrocephalus. CTA and MRA are capable of demonstrating the total geography of the lesion. CTA, however, may be challenging due to the fast flow. The mural type usually shows multiple identifiable feeders to the pouch, while the choroidal type may show poorly defined numerous smaller feeders in a maze configuration anteriorly to the aneurysm. VGAM should be distinguished from aneurysmal dilation of the vein of Galen caused by large arteriovenous malformation (AVM) or dural fistula draining into the true vein of Galen. A definite nidus is present in an AVM unlike VGAM.

VGAM is frequently diagnosed in utero by ultrasound as in this case. It may present in the neonatal period or in infancy usually with high-output cardiac failure or developmental delay. Less severe low-flow VGAM may present later in life. The mural type appears to be less severe compared with the choroidal type. Hence, most of the early presenting VGAMs are the choroidal type, while the late presenting VGAMs are mostly mural type. Up to 80% of the cardiac output may flow through the malformation. Thus, VGAM produces a steal phenomenon, resulting in brain volume loss, encephalomalacia, neurologic deficit, and calcifications. Congested superficial veins develop and these are prone to rupture. Both parenchymal and intraventricular hemorrhages are features of VGAM. Hydrocephalus as a feature of VGAM is fairly common due to obstruction of the aqueduct. Definitive treatment of VGAM is mostly by endovascular route with significant improvement in survival compared with the pre-endovascular therapy time. Radiosurgery has also been utilized.

Question for Further Thought

1. What is the embryologic origin of VGAM?

Reporting Responsibilities

This deserves a direct reporting if the find is unsuspected. A confirmation of a suspected VGAM also deserves direct reporting. Size of the malformation, afferent arteries, efferent veins, and complications should be enumerated. DSA is usually necessary to complete the evaluation of VGAM.

What the Treating Physician Needs to Know

- Size of malformation, afferent arteries, and the efferent veins/sinuses
- Associated parenchymal or extraaxial changes
- Follow up changes. Some of these malformations have been known to thrombose spontaneously
- Complications following treatment

Answer

1. It is generally believed that VGAM forms between the 6 and 11 weeks of gestation following the development of the Circle of Willis (COW). It is an arteriovenous fistula of the median prosencephalic vein (the precursor of the vein of Galen) and the primitive choroidal arteries. This prevents the regression of this precursor vein and therefore formation of the proper vein of Galen and straight sinus. It also retards proper brain development. Efferent flow is usually through a falcine sinus or other anomalous veins or sinuses into the SSS.

CLINICAL HISTORY *22-year-old male with history of cystic fibrosis and seizure disorder presents with the worst headache of his life. Imaging was obtained to rule out subarachnoid hemorrhage or aneurysm.*

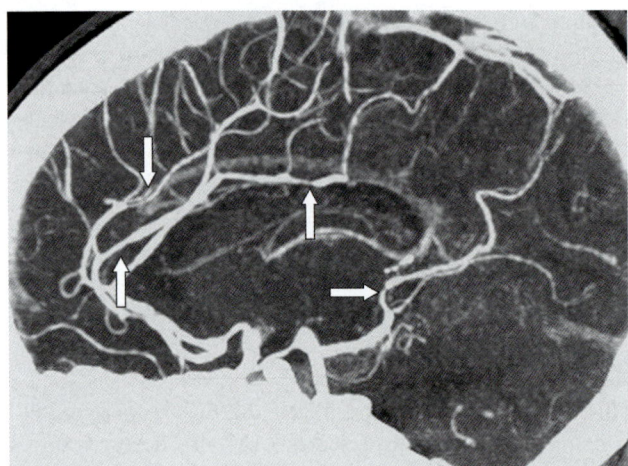

FIGURE 89-1

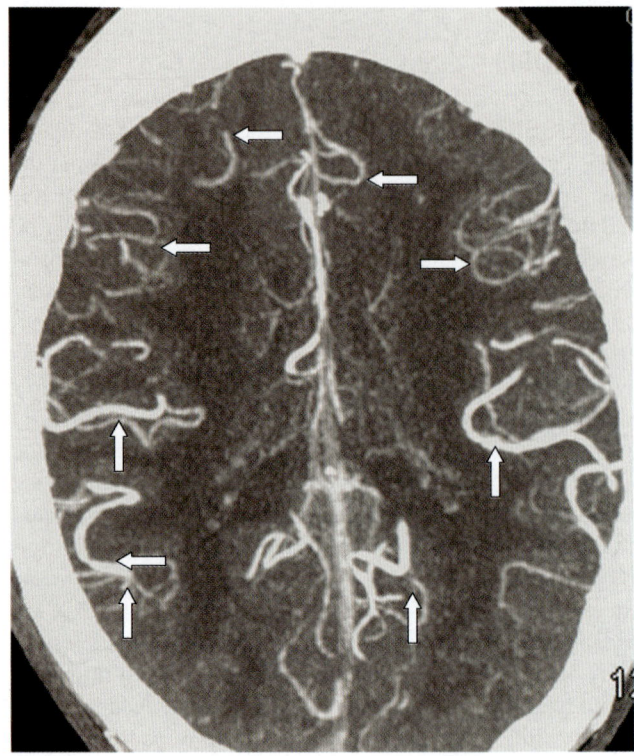

FIGURE 89-2

FINDINGS The initial NCCT was normal. Figure 89-1. Sagittal CTA MIP. There are multiple segmental vascular irregularities involving multiple territories (arrows). Figure 89-2. Axial MIP through the centrum semiovale. There is extensive vascular irregularity—significant bifrontal arterial attenuation and beading (transverse arrows) with some dilated vessels posteriorly (vertical arrows).

DIFFERENTIAL DIAGNOSIS Vasculitis, vasculopathy, vasospasm.

DIAGNOSIS Reversible cerebral vasoconstriction syndrome (RCVS).

DISCUSSION The imaging findings in RCVS are usually nonspecific. Initial imaging could be normal in up to 55% of the patients and becoming subsequently abnormal. MRI or CT could be abnormal in 12% to 81% with abnormalities consisting of focal mainly convexity subarachnoid hemorrhages, parenchymal hemorrhage, ischemic infarcts mainly in watershed locations, posterior reversible encephalopathy syndrome, and brain edema. MRA and/or CTA tend to demonstrate changes that suggest vasculitis—vascular irregularities, string of beads pattern, alternating constriction, and vasodilation of vessels. The initial angiogram could be normal and repeat angiogram may show resolution of lesions. Based on the angiographic findings, the differential should include vasculitis, vasculopathy, and vasospasm. Occasional aneurysm and vascular dissections have been reported.

RCVS is increasingly recognized. It is more common in women than men. Generally, it is presumed that there is a trigger. It is common in the postpartum period, during stressful periods, physical and emotional exertion, and has

been reported in all ages but appears to peak in the fifth decade. The syndrome is characterized by severe thunderclap headaches with features suggestive of subarachnoid hemorrhage, with or without other symptoms such as focal neurologic deficits. Laboratory investigations including erythrocyte sedimentation rate (ESR) and lumbar puncture (LP) are usually normal or minimally abnormal with minimally raised cell count or elevated protein in the cerebrospinal fluid (CSF) without any evidence to support vasculitis. RCVS is presumably due to a transient disturbance in the control of cerebrovascular tone presumably due to vasoactive substances. The disease is self-limited and the symptoms tend to resolve spontaneously if there are no complications. The vascular imaging changes tend to resolve within 3 months. Persistent headache may require a more aggressive treatment with nimodipine or corticosteroids. Death has been reported in a few cases.

Question for Further Thought

1. How do you differentiate vasculitis from RCVS?

Reporting Responsibilities

Direct reporting is necessary. The clinical concern is usually for subarachnoid hemorrhage. Findings such as convexity subarachnoid hemorrhage, ischemic infarcts, parenchymal hemorrhage, and brain swelling should be reported if present.

What the Treating Physician Needs to Know

- Location of lesions and associated parenchymal changes or complications
- Imaging may not be able to differentiate vasculitis from vasculopathy or RCVS; the findings are similar
- Changes of RCVS may not be present on initial imaging and may take up to 2 weeks to appear. It is therefore necessary to repeat the imaging if symptoms persist. Maximum vasoconstriction could take up to 16 days to occur after the ictus. Reversal of angiographic findings takes up to 12 weeks

Answer

1. It could be difficult to distinguish between the two entities. Helpful hints to the diagnosis of RCVS include thunderclap headache, various patterns of cerebrovascular events, normal or near-normal CSF, and ESR. There is usually reversal of the vascular irregularities on angiography without treatment. Vasculitis or angiitis, on the other hand, has an insidious onset of the headache; cerebrovascular changes are usually of ischemic infarcts, CSF changes of inflammatory reaction, and an elevated ESR.

CLINICAL HISTORY *13-year-old female with dystonia and contractions of the right hand.*

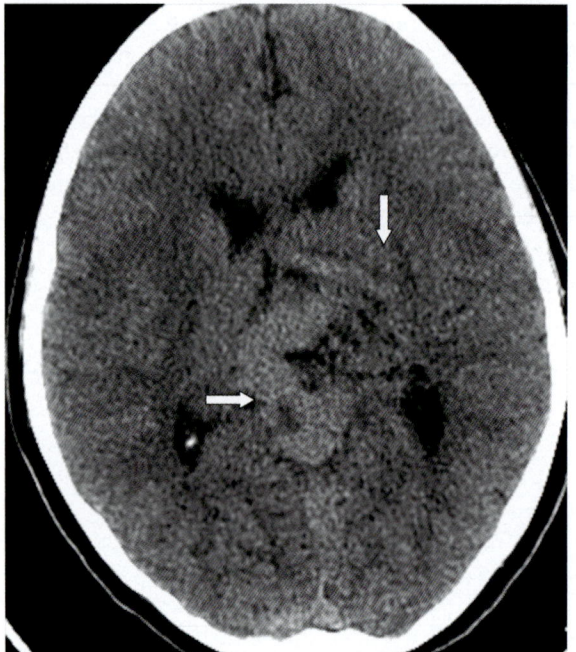

FIGURE 90-1

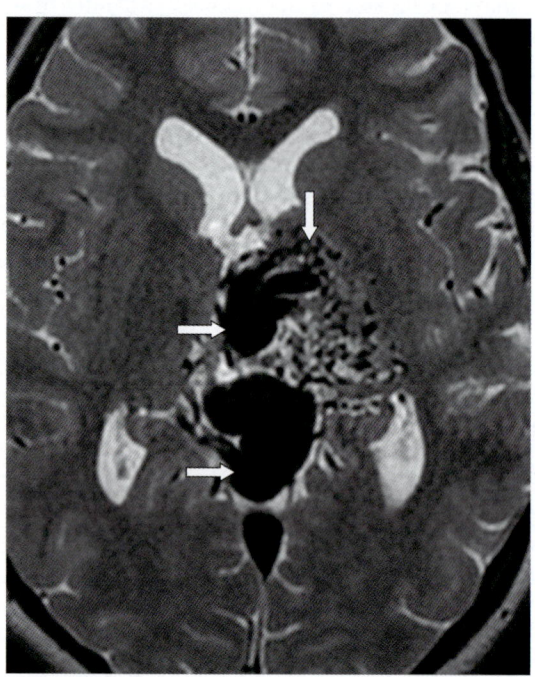

FIGURE 90-2

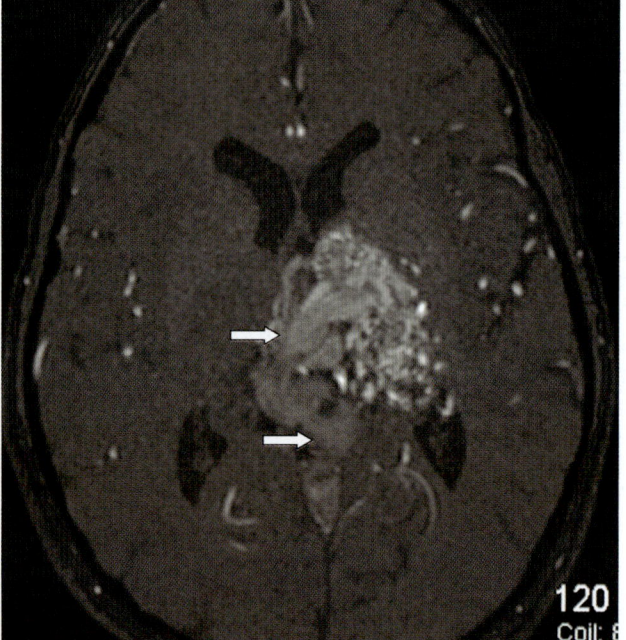
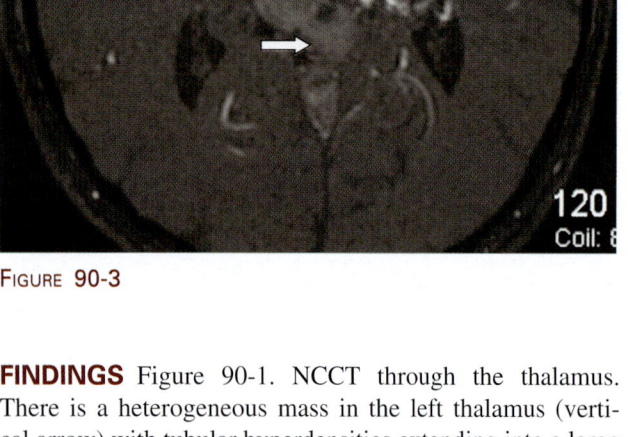

FIGURE 90-3

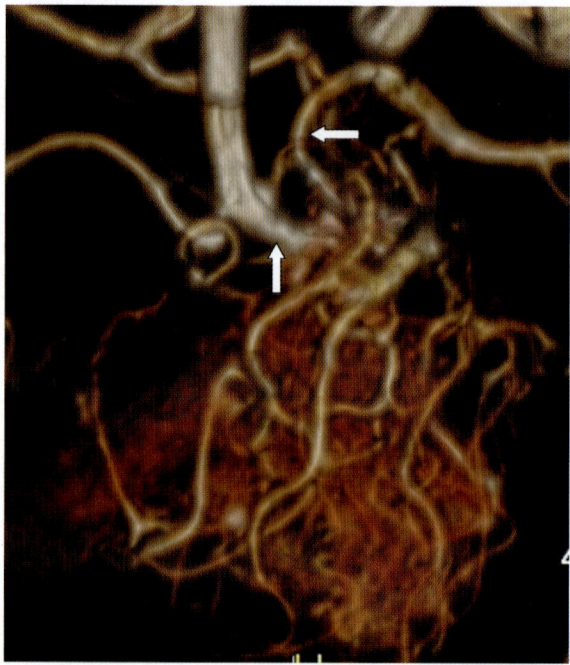

FIGURE 90-4

FINDINGS Figure 90-1. NCCT through the thalamus. There is a heterogeneous mass in the left thalamus (vertical arrow) with tubular hyperdensities extending into a large tortuous midline hyperdense tubular structure—enlarged internal cerebral vein (transverse arrow). There is local mass effect. Figure 90-2. Axial T2WI through the thalamus. There is a collection of tubular signal voids in the left thalamus (vertical arrow) extending into a large tortuous signal void in the midline consistent with a large internal cerebral vein and great vein of Galen (transverse arrows). Areas of hyperintensity are seen surrounding the tubular signal voids in the left thalamus. These areas possibly represent gliosis. Figure 90-3. Axial 3D TOF MRA source image through the thalamus. There is a collection of serpentine tubular structures in the left thalamus. Large tortuous internal cerebral vein and vein of Galen are visualized (arrows). Figure 90-4. Volume-rendered 3D TOF MRA best projection. There is a left thalamic tangle of vessels (the nidus) with many large feeding arteries from the enlarged left P-Com artery and the left posterior cerebral artery (PCA) (arrows).

DIFFERENTIAL DIAGNOSIS Arteriovenous malformation (AVM), vein of Galen aneurysmal malformation (VGAM).

DIAGNOSIS Left thalamic AVM.

DISCUSSION Both MRI and CT are complementary in the evaluation of AVM. MRI, however, presents comprehensive topographical and parenchymal details unmatched by CT. CT, however, is better at distinguishing between calcifications and hemorrhage. CTA and MRA are equally effective in evaluating the afferent, nidus, and efferent vascular patterns of the AVM. The classic AVM has afferent vessels or arteries that are usually larger than other arteries in the vicinity. There is a nidus that contains a tangle of small vessels that are hyperdense on CT and show signal voids on T2WI, some of which could dilate into aneurysmal proportion. T2 hyperintense areas present within the nidus probably represent gliosis. Calcifications and old and new hemorrhages could be present. Calcification and acute hemorrhage are usually hyperdense on CT but could be differentiated by measuring the Hounsfield unit. Both may be hypointense on T2WI and GRE. Surrounding volume loss due to steal phenomenon or edema due to recent bleed could be visible. The draining or efferent veins are also usually larger than other veins in the vicinity. The afferent and efferent vessels could be single or multiple. Accelerated atherosclerotic changes on the afferent vessels could result in irregularities, stenosis, or aneurysmal formation that could alter the flow dynamics of the AVM. The details of the vasculature are well demonstrated by CTA or MRA. DSA now plays a role in endovascular treatment of AVM, with the primary diagnosis being made by CT/CTA and MRI/MRA.

The DSA confirmed in this case that most of the afferent supply was from the left thalamoperforators. Strategically placed AVM could produce mass effect and hydrocephalus. The presence of a parenchymal nidus indicates an AVM draining into the vein of Galen rather than VGAM.

AVMs are rare and considered congenital but de novo AVMs are reported. They have been described in all age groups. Common presentations include headache, numbness, neurologic deficit, intracranial hemorrhages (subarachnoid hemorrhage [SAH], intracranial hemorrhage [ICH], and intraventricular hemorrhage [IVH]), mental status changes, and coma. The risk of hemorrhage depends on the hemodynamic of the AVM, its location, and the presence of prior hemorrhage. This risk is estimated at 1% to 4% per year. In rare situations, AVMs could thrombose spontaneously. Multimodal treatment is usually advocated. This includes endovascular treatment, radiosurgery, and surgical intervention.

Question for Further Thought

1. What are the complications of AVM?

Reporting Responsibilities

Direct reporting is necessary in this circumstance as it is unpredictable when AVM will rupture. Location, number if more than one, origin and number of feeders, number and termination of efferent veins, associated parenchymal changes including new or old hemorrhage, gliosis, volume loss, mass effect, calcifications, and hydrocephalus should be reported.

What the Treating Physician Needs to Know

- Location, size, and number if more than one
- Pattern of afferent and efferent vessels regarding origins, number, stenosis, and aneurysms
- Evidence of prior hemorrhage or new hemorrhage
- Presence of steal phenomenon, gliosis, atrophy, calcification, mass effect, hydrocephalus, etc

Answer

1. Complications of AVM include accelerated atherosclerosis on afferent arteries, hemorrhage, mass effect, volume loss, hydrocephalus, dementia, and high cardiac output failure.

CLINICAL HISTORY *65-year-old female with history of breast cancer.*

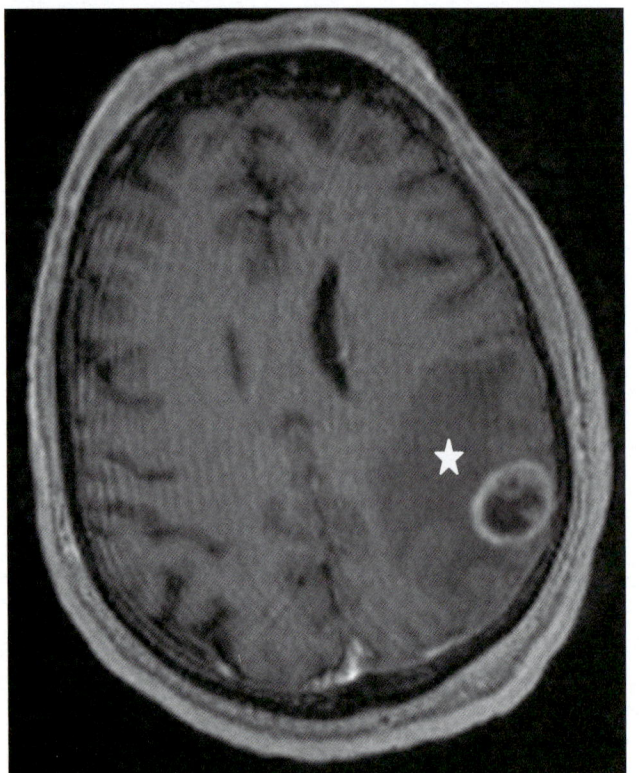

FIGURE 91-1

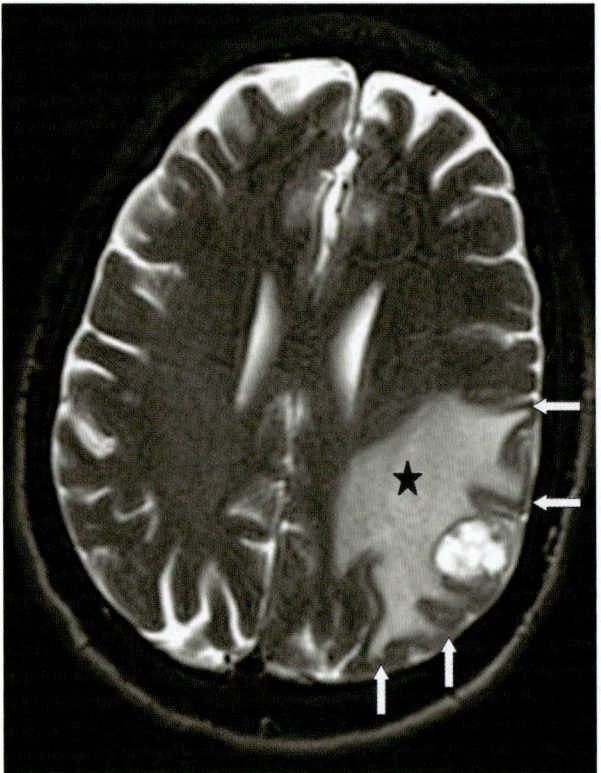

FIGURE 91-2

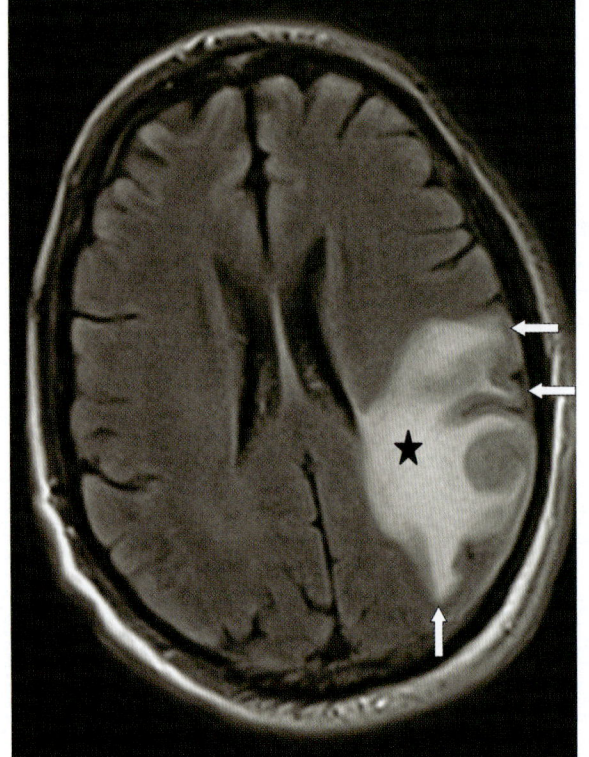

FIGURE 91-3

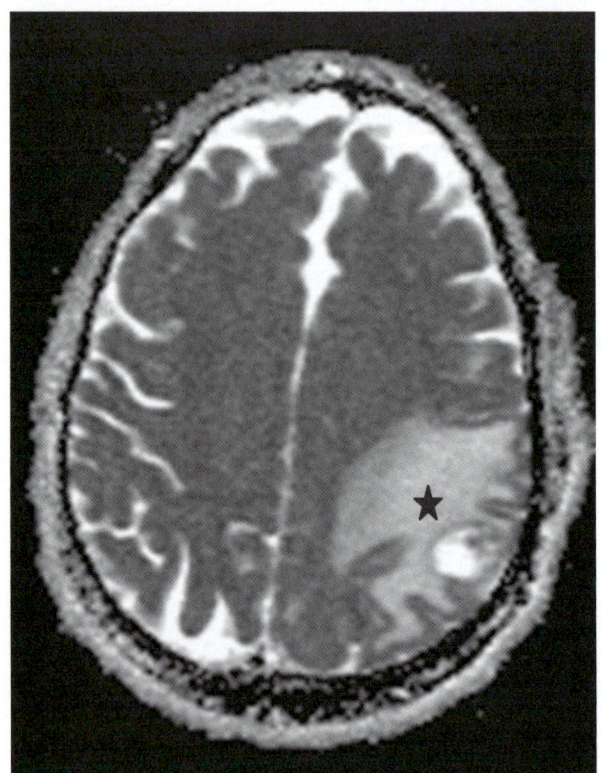

FIGURE 91-4

FINDINGS Figure 91-1. Axial post-contrast T1WI through the corona radiata/centrum semiovale. There is a ring-enhancing mass in the left frontoparietal junction with surrounding white matter (WM) hypointensity (star). Figures 91-2 and 91-3. Axial T2WI and FLAIR through the mass. The mass is surrounded by confluent WM hyperintensity (star) extending into the corona radiata/centrum semiovale and the subcortical WM in a finger-like fashion into the gyri sparing the cortical gray matter (GM) (arrows). The intervening sulci are effaced by mass effect. Figure 91-4. Axial ADC map through the lesion. There is confluent hyperintensity (star) of the WM around the mass (star) indicative of increased diffusivity and lack of restricted diffusion.

DIFFERENTIAL DIAGNOSIS Vasogenic edema, cytotoxic edema, encephalitis, primary malignancy, metastasis, toxoplasmosis, and abscess.

DIAGNOSIS Vasogenic edema secondary to brain metastasis.

DISCUSSION Both CT and MRI are capable of demonstrating the features of vasogenic edema. Typically on CT, vasogenic edema manifests as area of confluent hypodensity relative to normal brain parenchyma. It predominantly involves the WM and spares the GM even when it involves the deep structures. It insinuates into the subcortical WM and produces mass effect with effacement of the sulci. Within the deep structures, it involves the internal, external, and extreme capsules without involvement of the basal ganglia or the thalami. Mass effect on these structures may be present. On MRI, vasogenic edema manifests as areas of confluent hypointensity on T1WI with corresponding confluent hyperintensity on FLAIR and T2WI (although not to the degree of normal cerebrospinal fluid [CSF] hyperintensity). The typical finger-like insinuations into the subcortical WM are better demonstrated on the FLAIR with suppression of the CSF hyperintensity. Additionally, vasogenic edema is either iso- or hypointense on DWI with corresponding hyperintensity on ADC maps (in contrast to cytotoxic edema that is hyperintense on DWI but hypointense on ADC map—restricted diffusion). It does not restrict diffusion. Invariably, there is diffuse mass effect depending on the size of the edema. The underlying cause of the edema may be visible as in this case here—metastatic breast cancer. Causes of vasogenic edema include metastases, primary malignant or high-grade brain tumors such as glioblastoma (GB), sarcomas, and oligodendroglioma (ODG), and inflammatory lesions or infections such as tumefactive demyelination and abscesses. In some forms of encephalitis, the vasogenic edema may be the manifestation of the disease. It could be present around subacute contusions and hematomas.

Vasogenic edema results from a breakdown of the normal blood-brain barrier (BBB) and tight junctions in the arterial walls. Proteins and fluid that are normally intravascular penetrate into the cerebral parenchyma and extracellular space through the disrupted BBB. The extravascular fluid primarily affects WM and spreads along WM fiber tracts; only rarely does it affect GM. The most common causes of vasogenic edema are tumor, infection, trauma, and inflammation. Vasogenic edema generally takes time to develop, in contrast to cytotoxic edema that develops rapidly and typically involves both WM and GM. Management consists of treatment of the underlying pathology. Primary management of the edema may include osmotherapy with the use of diuretics, hypertonic saline, glycerol, and mannitol to reduce fluid load by osmotic diuresis, corticosteroids that suppress the expression of the edema-producing factor vascular endothelial growth factor (VEGF) and somehow tighten the BBB and in the extreme, surgical decompression to relieve the compression of the underlying brain.

Questions for Further Thought

1. Why do brain gliomas result in vasogenic edema?
2. Can vasogenic edema and cytotoxic edema coexist?

Reporting Responsibilities

Direct reporting is essential. Vasogenic edema is usually an indication of an acute or subacute condition requiring immediate resolution. Describe the location of abnormality and any associated important findings such cause of the edema if present, mass effect, herniation, and hydrocephalus. Present reasonable differential diagnosis and recommend further workup or follow-up studies, if deemed necessary.

What the Treating Physician Needs to Know

- Relevant differential diagnosis and the most likely cause of the vasogenic edema
- What further workup is needed to evaluate the abnormality?
- Degree of mass effect produced by the edema

Answers

1. It is believed that gliomas produce VEGF that is involved in angiogenesis. Newly formed arteries are not normal and lack tight junctions between their endothelial cells leading to escape of fluids into the extracellular space. Additionally, other factors such as the hypoxia-inducible factor and the vascular permeability factor also increase this process.
2. Yes. Vasogenic and cytotoxic edema can coexist in several situations, such as PRES, venous thrombosis, trauma, hypoxic ischemic encephalopathy, and large infarction.

CLINICAL HISTORY *7-year-old male who had been developing normally started 12 months before with hearing loss which progressed to visual and coordination problems followed by an overall decline of intellectual and motor milestones.*

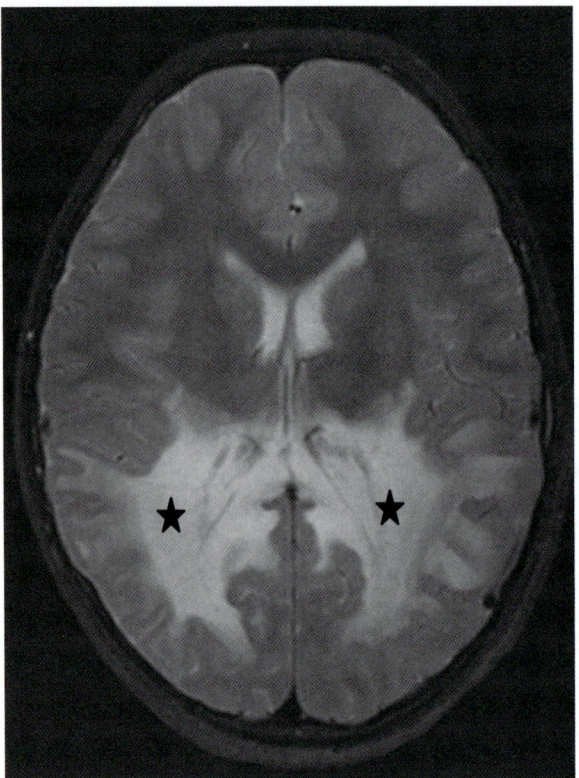

FIGURE 92-1

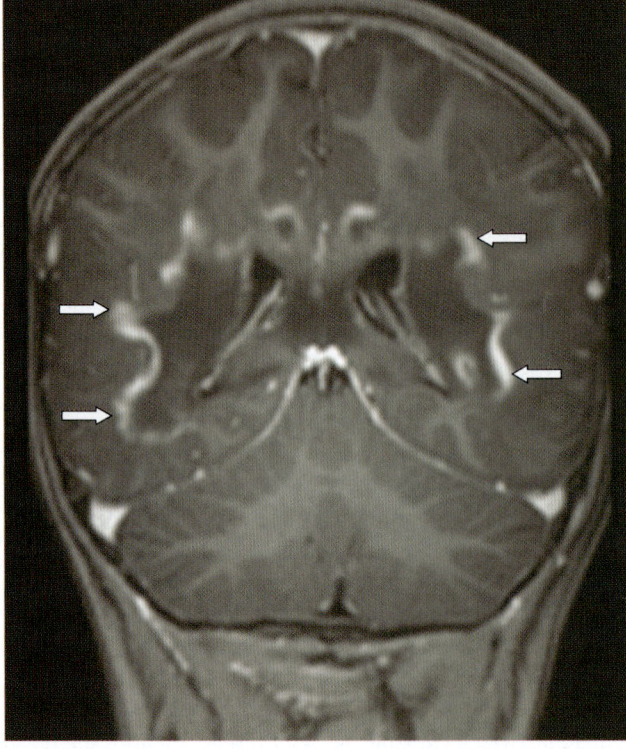

FIGURE 92-2

FINDINGS Figure 92-1. Axial T2WI through the trigones. There is bilateral symmetrical peritrigonal confluent white matter (WM) hyperintensity extending from the ventricular walls to the subcortical U fibers (stars) crossing the midline through the splenium of corpus callosum. Figure 92-2. Coronal post-contrast T1WI through the trigones. There is bilateral symmetrical centrally affected WM hypointense with peripheral wavy contrast enhancement following the pattern of the subcortical U fibers (arrows).

DIFFERENTIAL DIAGNOSIS Krabbe disease, metachromatic leukodystrophy (MLD), Alexander disease, Adrenoleukodystrophy (ALD), Canavan disease.

DIAGNOSIS Adrenoleukodystrophy (ALD).

DISCUSSION ALD describes several closely related inherited disorders that affect the metabolism of certain lipids resulting in the accumulation of very long chain fatty acids (VLCFAs) in the affected tissues, including the myelin of the nervous system, the Leydig cells of the testes, and the adrenal cortex. There is, however, no clear genotype–phenotype correlation. Imaging of ALD is best achieved by

contrast-enhanced MRI. However, on CT, the affected WM is hypodense and generally located in the posterior aspects of the brain surrounding the trigones. MRI especially T2WI and FLAIR show confluent symmetrical hyperintensity of the peritrigonal WM linking up across the splenium. The affected cerebral WM typically has three different zones. The central or inner zone appears moderately hypointense on T1WI and markedly hyperintense on T2WI. This zone corresponds to irreversible gliosis and scarring. The intermediate zone represents active inflammation and breakdown in the blood–brain barrier. This zone may appear isointense or slightly hypointense on T2WI and readily enhances in a wavy pattern after contrast administration. The peripheral or outer zone represents the leading edge of active demyelination. It appears moderately hyperintense on T2WI and demonstrates no enhancement. MR spectroscopy obtained from the enhancing region shows elevated choline reflecting active inflammation, low N-acetyl aspartate (NAA), and lipids. When performed in the nonenhancing region, most metabolites are low, and lipids and lactate are abundant. The abnormalities initially affect the periventricular WM with eventual spread to the subcortical regions. Symmetric abnormal areas of T2 hyperintensity along the descending pyramidal tract may be present. Atypical cases with unilateral or predominantly frontal lobe involvement may occur. The brain retains its volume until late in the disease. The abnormalities may extend inferiorly to involve the midbrain. During the latter stages of the disease, the affected WM may show calcifications. Krabbe and MLD are global affection of the centrum semiovale and corona radiata, while ALD is confined posteriorly. Canavan tends to affect posterior corona radiata and centrum predominantly, while Alexander favors the frontal WM.

ALD is a genetic metabolic disorder inherited in an X-linked pattern. Therefore, the majority of affected individuals are male as they are homozygous for the affected gene. Women carriers can have milder forms of the disease. It has an incidence of 1:20,000 people with no ethnic predilection. Three subtypes of the disease are recognized: the childhood cerebral form which appears in mid-childhood ages 4 to 8 years, adrenomyelopathy occurs in men in their twenties or later, and impaired adrenal function, called Addison disease or Addison-like phenotype in adult. The typical clinical presentation of the childhood cerebral form is that of a hither to healthy young boy, 4 to 8 years old, with new-onset emotional instability and disruptive behavior at school. Other symptoms may include adrenal insufficiency, decreased fine motor control (deterioration of handwriting), decreased muscle tone, aphasia, hearing loss, strabismus, visual disturbances, difficulty swallowing, and possible seizures. This is a progressive disease that leads to a persistent vegetative state anywhere from 2 to 10 years after onset of neurologic symptoms.

The adrenomyelopathy form presents with difficulty controlling urination, muscle weakness or leg stiffness, and decreased mentation and visual memory. These patients are also at risk for adrenal insufficiency. Lastly, the adrenal gland failure or Addison type shows signs of adrenal insufficiency such as increased skin pigmentation, decreased appetite, vomiting, weight loss, loss of muscle mass, muscle weakness, and possible coma.

Question for Further Thought

1. In a male child with WM changes on MR and the clinical suspicion of ALD what are some appropriate tests for further workup and diagnosis?

Reporting Responsibilities

Direct reporting is important because dietary intervention may halt progression of the disease. The Loes score is a severity rating of the abnormalities in the brain found on MRI. It ranges from 0 to 34 based on a point system derived from the location and extent of disease and the presence of atrophy in the brain, either localized to specific points or generally throughout the brain. A Loes score of 0.5 or less is classified as normal, while a Loes score of 14 or greater is considered as severe.

What the Treating Physician Needs to Know

- Genetic counseling is recommended for prospective parents with a family history of ALD
- Prenatal diagnosis from chorionic villus sampling is available

Answer

1. Blood tests can detect VLCFA or these may also be found in skin biopsies.

CLINICAL HISTORY *2-year-old female with progressive difficulty walking, deterioration of coordination, and speech disturbances.*

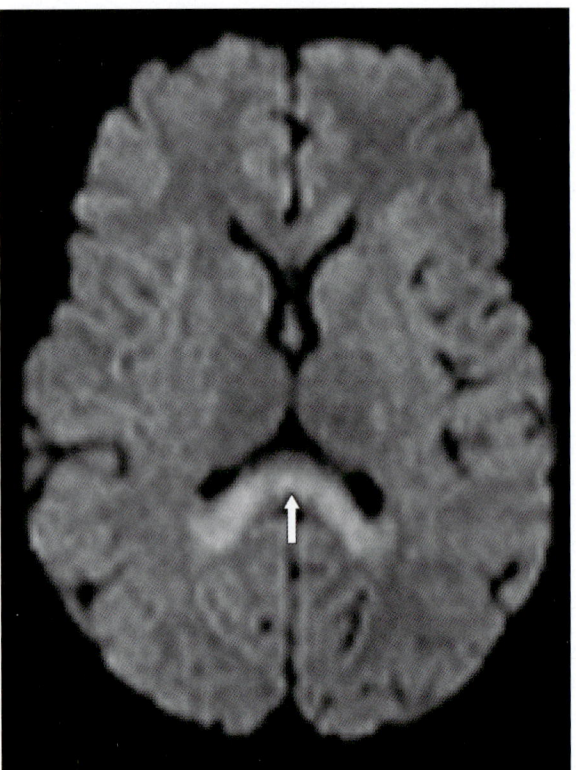

FIGURE 93-1

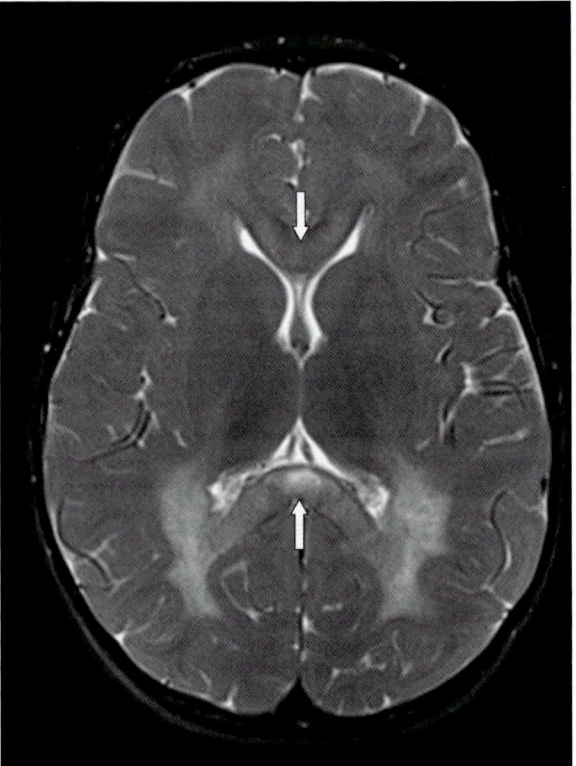

FIGURE 93-2

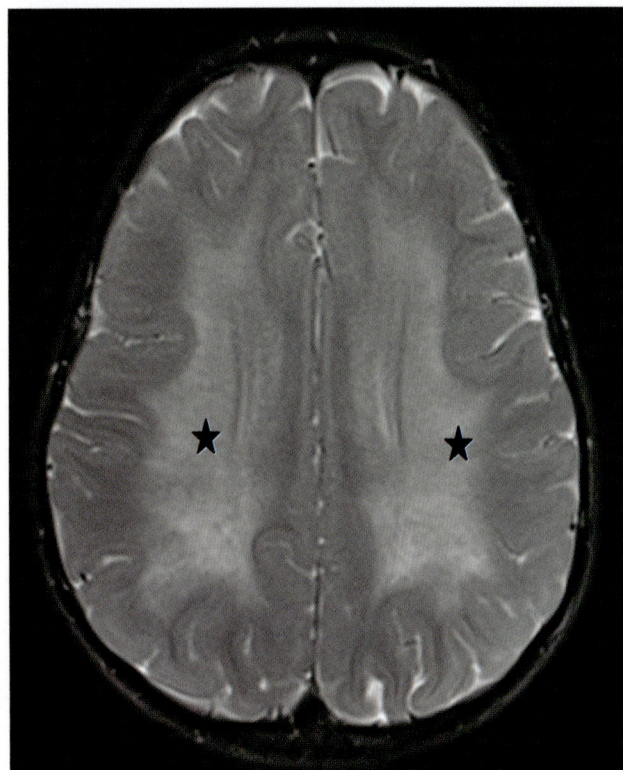

FIGURE 93-3

FINDINGS Figure 93-1. Axial DWI through the splenium of corpus callosum. There is hyperintensity of the splenium (arrow). The ADC map (not shown) is consistent with restricted diffusion. Figures 93-2 and 93-3. Axial T2WI through the splenium and centrum semiovale, respectively. There is symmetric confluent white matter (WM) (sometimes called "butterfly") hyperintensity (stars) extending from the ventricular walls to the subcortical WM. The splenium and genu of the corpus callosum (arrows) are involved. Linear tubular and punctate hypointensities are present within the confluent WM changes consistent with the so-called tigroid pattern.

DIFFERENTIAL DIAGNOSIS Pelizaeus-Merzbacher, TORCH, periventricular leukomalacia, metachromatic leukodystrophy (MLD), Krabbe disease.

DIAGNOSIS Metachromatic leukodystrophy (MLD).

DISCUSSION MLD is a devastating demyelinating disease due to lysosomal storage disorder resulting in the accumulation of galactosylceramide sulfatide, a lipid component of myelin with a characteristic metachromatic histologic staining. The most common form of MLD (50% to 80%) is the late infantile form. Typical MRI findings in this form of the disease include symmetric confluent T2 hyperintensity in the corona radiata and the centrum semiovale. There is posterior predominance and sparing of the subcortical U fibers. There is occasional cerebellar WM involvement in late stages of the disease. Various portions of the corpus callosum, the internal capsules, and the claustrum may be involved. Multiple linear and punctate radiating hypointensities, so-called tigroid pattern, are usually present within the confluent WM hyperintensities. There is usually no contrast enhancement. An MRI severity scoring system has been proposed to provide a measure of brain involvement in this disease.

MLD is a rare disease directly caused by a deficiency of the enzyme arylsulfatase A (ASA) and is characterized by enzyme activity that is less than 10% of human controls leading to buildup of sulfatides in many tissues of the body and in the brain eventually destroying the myelin sheath. The ARSA gene responsible for ASA is located on the long arm of chromosome 22. It has autosomal recessive inheritance. More than 110 mutations have been identified in the ARSA gene resulting in MLD.

Three forms of the disease are recognized: late infantile MLD with symptoms usually beginning by ages 1 to 2 years, juvenile MLD with symptoms usually beginning between ages 4 and 12 years, adult (and late-stage juvenile MLD) with symptoms occurring between age 14 and adulthood (over age 16), but may begin as late as the 40s or 50s. Symptoms include muscle wasting and weakness, muscle rigidity, developmental delays, progressive loss of vision leading to blindness, convulsions, impaired swallowing, paralysis, and dementia and eventually coma. Untreated, most children with this form of MLD die by the age of 5 or sooner. The adult form usually manifests as a psychiatric disorder or progressive dementia after the age of 16 years. There is no cure for MLD. Care is mostly supportive.

Question for Further Thought

1. What is the appropriate workup for patients with suspected MLD?

Reporting Responsibility

Although there is no cure for this disease and it is not an acute situation, a direct report may be appreciated so that appropriate genetic testing to confirm the diagnosis may begin.

What the Treating Physician Needs to Know

- This is a heritable disorder. The families of patients with suspected MLD should be referred for genetic counseling
- Progression of disease on follow-up

Answer

1. Urine and blood samples are required for a formal diagnosis of MLD (an MRI is not definitive in diagnosing the disease because the appearance may overlap with many other conditions). The blood ASA enzyme levels are measured first, followed by urine sulfatide levels. An increased amount of sulfatide in the urine indicates that the ASA enzyme is not breaking down sulfatides, which usually suggests MLD. A low level of ASA enzyme in the blood is not a definitive test for MLD because these same low levels of ASA are also found in a condition called ASA pseudo-deficiency prevalent in up to 5% of people with European ancestry.

CLINICAL HISTORY *2-year-old child with progressive psychomotor retardation and loss of developmental milestones, megalencephaly and frontal bossing, seizures, hyperreflexia and pyramidal signs, and ataxia.*

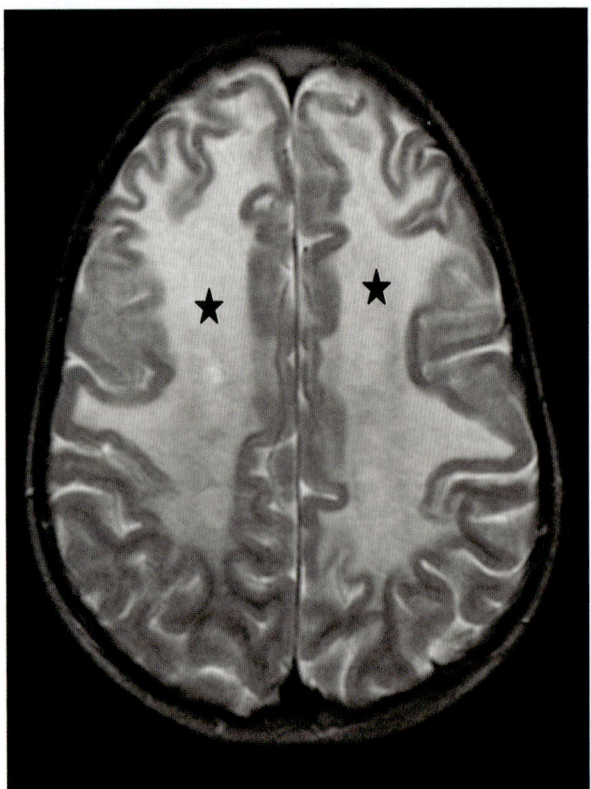

FIGURE 94-1

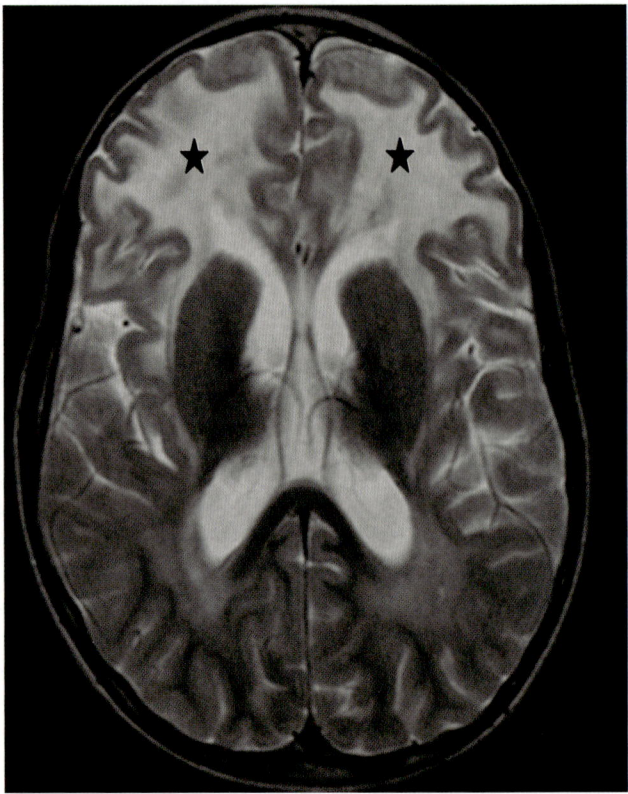

FIGURE 94-2

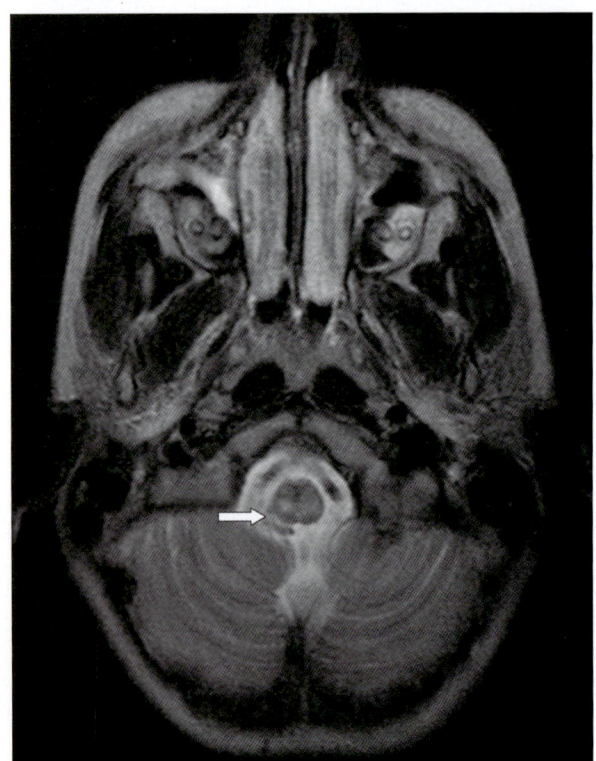

FIGURE 94-3

FINDINGS Figure 94-1. Axial T2WI through the centrum semiovale. There is extensive confluent frontal and parietal white matter (WM) hyperintensity involving deep and subcortical regions (stars). Figure 94-2. Axial T2WI at the level of the lateral ventricles. There is predominant bilateral frontal lobe WM confluent hyperintensity (stars). Figure 94-3. Axial T2WI through the medulla. Areas of hyperintensity (arrow) are seen in the upper medulla too. (Case courtesy of Dr. Karuna Shekdar, University of Pennsylvania, Philadelphia.)

DIFFERENTIAL DIAGNOSIS Canavan disease, megalencephalic leukoencephalopathy with subcortical cysts (MLC), mucopolysaccharidoses (MPS), Alexander disease.

DIAGNOSIS Alexander disease.

DISCUSSION The hallmark of the imaging findings in Alexander disease is extensive cerebral WM T2 hyperintensity with frontal predominance. There is a periventricular rim of T1 hyperintensity which is hypointense on T2WI and often contrast enhances. The enhancement may also involve the frontal WM, basal ganglia, thalami, parts of the midbrain, fornix, brainstem, optic chiasm, and dentate nucleus of the cerebellum. These areas may also demonstrate T2 hyperintensities. Volume loss is a prominent feature late in the disease, not only affecting the WM but also the deep gray matter with cystic degeneration. Hydrocephalus is often a feature of Alexander disease.

First described in 1949 by William Stuart Alexander, a pathologist in New Zealand, Alexander disease is a rare, sporadic, progressive, and fatal leukodystrophy or WM disease. The classic presentation is of an infant with macrocephaly, seizures, and rapid neurologic deterioration. There are less common juvenile/adult variants. Alexander disease is caused by a sporadic mutation of the glial fibrillary acid protein (GFAP) gene that maps to chromosome 17. Histologically, it is characterized by marked cytoplasmic accumulations containing GFAP and heat shock proteins, known as Rosenthal fibers. More specifically, Rosenthal fibers are abnormal intracytoplasmic proteinaceous inclusions in fibrous astrocytes; therefore, the disease can be thought of a disease not of WM but of astrocytes proper. These are present in great quantities throughout the brain in patients with Alexander disease but may also be found in more limited distribution in other conditions, including multiple sclerosis (MS), pilocytic astrocytoma, and the lining of syrinx cavities. Interestingly, the noncommunicating hydrocephalus observed in Alexander disease is caused by swelling of the astrocytes that line the cerebral aqueduct. The accumulation of Rosenthal fibers eventually produces narrowing or occlusion of the aqueduct. There is no cure for Alexander disease. Treatment is supportive.

Questions for Further Thought

1. What other variants of Alexander disease are known?
2. Is there an inherited pattern of Alexander disease?

Reporting Responsibilities

Routine reporting is sufficient unless there are some acute changes such as hydrocephalus. However, in most of these infant or juvenile diseases with rapid deterioration, direct reporting may be appreciated so that prompt genetic testing may begin.

What the Treating Physician Needs to Know

- There is no known treatment, care is supportive and palliative
- There may be a familial association in many cases of Alexander disease; therefore, genetic counseling may be indicated

Answers

1. There are four described variants: neonatal, infantile, juvenile, and adult forms of the disease. The neonatal form is very rare and rapidly fulminant with death occurring within 2 years. The infantile form is the most common affecting 63% of patients presenting with those classical presentations described above. Affected children survive weeks to several years. The juvenile form, 24% of cases, usually presents between ages 4 and 10 years, occasionally in the mid-teens. Findings include bulbar/pseudobulbar signs, ataxia, gradual loss of intellectual function, seizures, megalencephaly, and breathing problems. Survival ranges from the early teens to the twenties to thirties. The adult form is the most variable both in severity and in progression. Bulbar and pseudobulbar symptoms as well as spasticity are seen, and the disease may resemble MS.

2. Although adult-onset Alexander disease seems to be sporadic in most cases, familial segregation, suggesting an autosomal dominant mode of transmission, has been reported. In these families, a new mutation in the GFAP gene (17q21) has been identified. Affected adults may transmit the mutation to their offspring in an autosomal dominant fashion.

CLINICAL HISTORY *48-year-old male with traumatic brain injury.*

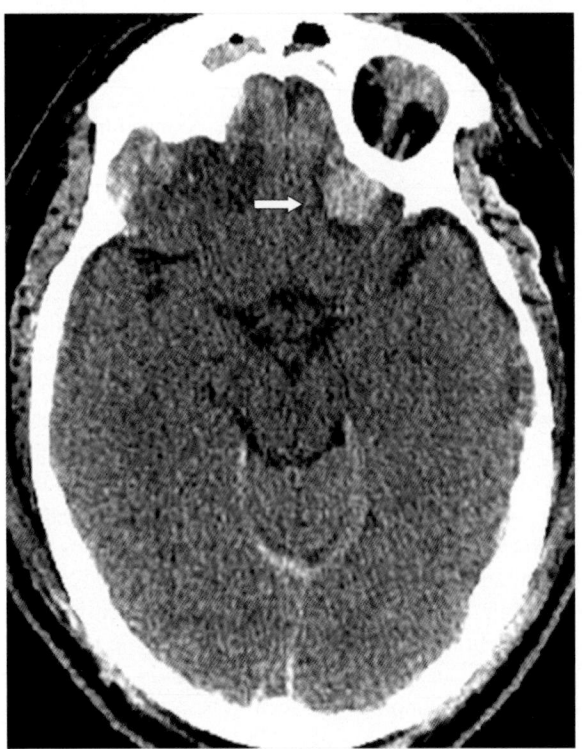

FIGURE 95-1

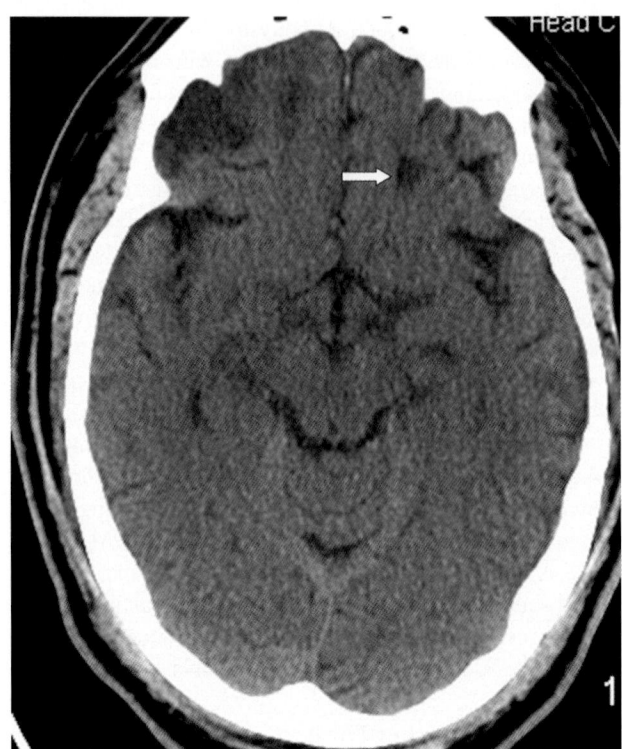

FIGURE 95-2

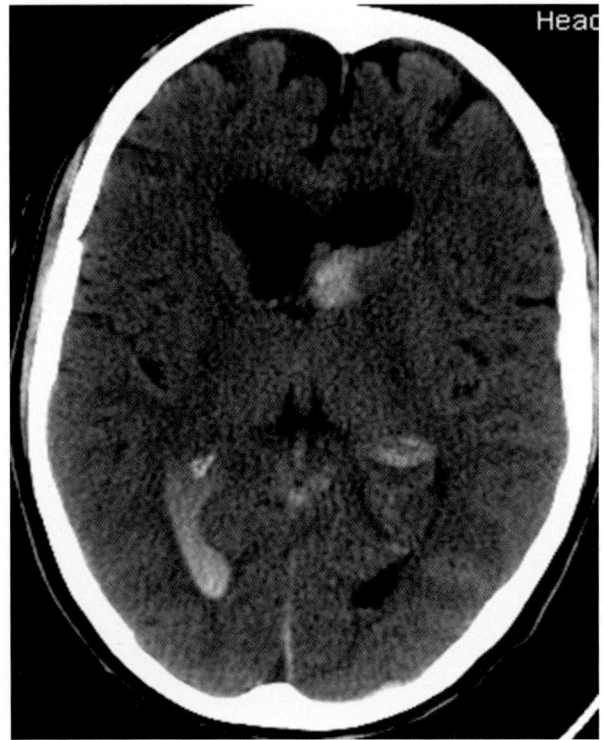

FIGURE 95-3

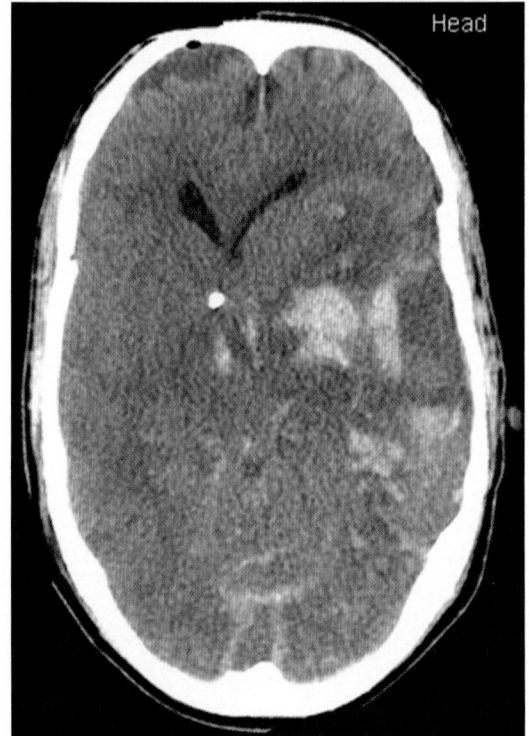

FIGURE 95-4

FINDINGS Figure 95-1. Axial NCCT through inferior frontal lobes. There is a 1.5-cm round hyperdensity surrounded by a hypodense halo in the left frontal lobe just posterior and superior to the left orbital roof (arrow) consistent with hematoma. There are contusions in the right frontal and left temporal lobes. Figure 95-2. Axial NCCT through the frontal lobes 6 months after Figure 95-1. The area of hematoma is now represented by a well-defined hypodensity (encephalomalacia) significantly smaller than the original lesion (arrow). Figures 95-3 and 95-4. Axial NCCT 24 hours apart in another patient. There are new and expanding hematomas (arrows in Figure 95-4) on follow-up. There is significant brain swelling, mass effect, and herniation.

DIFFERENTIAL DIAGNOSIS N/A.

DIAGNOSIS Traumatic intracerebral hematoma (TICH).

DISCUSSION TICH is a hyperdense mass on CT. TICH is usually superficial and more common in the frontal and temporal lobes than elsewhere. They are rarely deep seated. A hypodense halo of edema is usually present. The hematoma and surrounding edema frequently increase in size over the following few days. New foci or so-called delayed hematoma may develop up to 15 days after the initial injury. Presence of mass effect depends on the size of the hematoma and its surrounding edema. While CT is usually the method of choice for evaluation of acute TICH, MRI is more sensitive in the subacute and chronic stages of the hematomas and could show many more smaller hematomas using various sequences. The MRI presentation depends on the age of the hematomas.

TICH is due to shearing or rapid deceleration injury, resulting in rupture of superficial/subcortical blood vessels with extravasation of blood into the brain parenchyma. A large hematoma can cause secondary brain damage by compression and displacement or herniation of surrounding structures. TICH is invariably associated with other primary intracranial injuries. Follow-up imaging is usually necessary for assessment of the status of the hematoma particularly when the patient is not doing well. The natural history is that of a gradual resorption and transformation from hyperdensity to hypodensity. The end result is a much smaller focal encephalomalacia and volume loss while smaller hematomas may completely disappear. The clinical presentation depends on size, number, and other associated injuries. It could include headaches, focal neurologic deficit,

and seizures. Surgical intervention may be indicated if there is significant mass effect or herniations depending on other variables. Patient outcome depends very much on the age of the patient and admission Glasgow Coma Scale (GCS) score; the higher the GCS score, the better the outcome.

Question for Further Thought

1. What is responsible for the delayed and expanding TICH in traumatic brain injury?

Reporting Responsibilities

TICH is an emergency requiring direct reporting. Location and number if more than one should be categorized. Associated complications such as swelling, compartmental shifts or herniations, and other associated primary injuries should be enumerated. Significant changes on follow-up should also be communicated directly.

What the Treating Physician Needs to Know

- Location and number if more than one
- Other primary injuries such as contusions, extraaxial hemorrhages, and intraventricular hemorrhages
- Complications and secondary injuries such as brain swelling, infarcts, herniations, hydrocephalus, expansion, and new hematomas on follow-up

Answer

1. The incidence of delayed traumatic intracerebral hematoma (DTICH) is less than 10% in most series. DTICH can be superficial or deep and may occur up to 15 days following the initial insult. It may or may not be heralded by new symptoms or deterioration of clinical status. It has been observed to occur in patients with or without decompressive surgery. Several theories for the formation of new and expanded hematoma include presence of existing injury such as necrosis and vascular injury with subsequent coagulopathy, presence of infarction with secondary hemorrhagic conversion, loss of local autoregulation resulting in coalescing small hemorrhages, and venous congestions resulting in blood exudation among others. Secondary hypoxic insult is more common in this subset of patients. DTICH is therefore regarded as an epiphenomenon likely to represent hemorrhage into an existing traumatized area and could be ascribed to local hypoxia and hypercapnia following the vascular damage.

CLINICAL HISTORY *26-year-old female was involved in a motor vehicle collision. She lost consciousness at the site of collision. She is not waking up.*

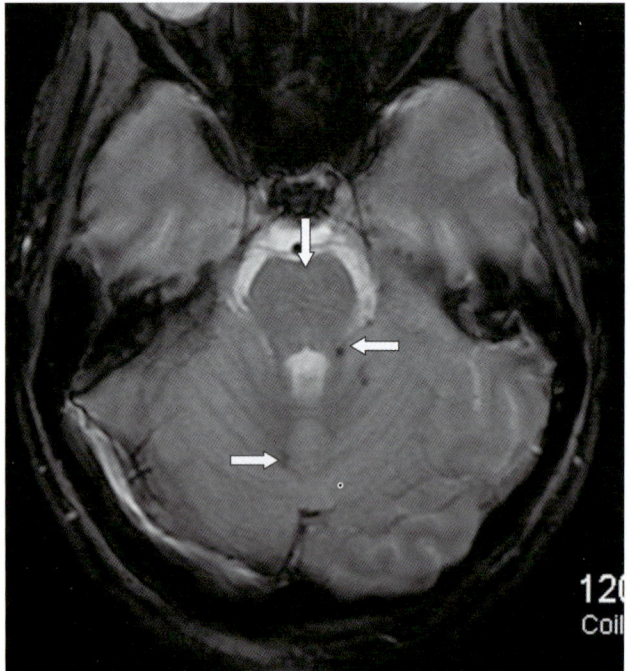

FIGURE 96-1

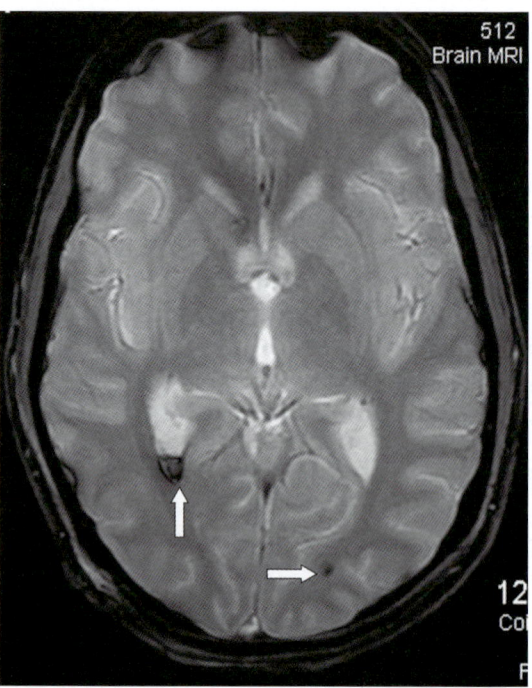

FIGURE 96-2

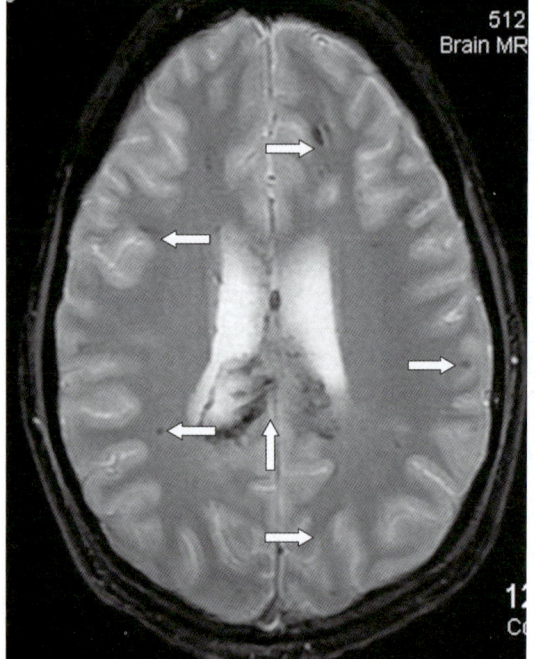

FIGURE 96-3

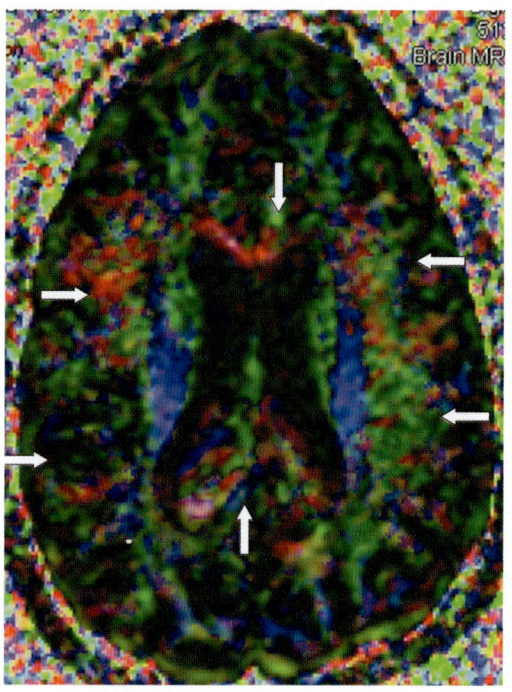

FIGURE 96-4

FINDINGS Figure 96-1. Axial MRI GRE through the fourth ventricle. There are multifocal bilateral cerebellar, pons, and left superior cerebellar peduncle punctate hypointensities (arrows show some of them) consistent with hemorrhagic products. Figure 96-2. Axial GRE through the trigones. There is hypointense sedimentation with fluid-fluid level in the right trigone consistent with intraventricular hemorrhage (vertical arrow). There is visible subcortical punctate hypointensity in the left occipital lobe (transverse arrow). Figure 96-3. Axial GRE through the corpus callosum (CC). There is heterogeneous enlargement of the posterior body and splenium of the CC (vertical arrow). There are numerous bilateral frontal and parietal subcortical hypointensities (transverse arrows identify some of them). Figure 96-4. Color directional MRI DTI map through the CC. There is disorganization and asymmetry of fiber tracts (transverse arrows). There is disruption, enlargement, and heterogeneity of the usual red transverse fiber tracts of the CC (vertical arrows).

DIFFERENTIAL DIAGNOSIS N/A.

DIAGNOSIS Traumatic brain injury with diffuse axonal injury (TBI/DAI).

DISCUSSION This is a grade III DAI involving the subcortical white–gray matter regions of the brain, the cerebellum, the CC, and the brainstem. Grade I DAI usually involves the subcortical white matter of the brain mainly frontotemporal lobes but elsewhere and the cerebellum. Grade II involves the CC mostly splenium and posterior body in addition to areas involved in grade I. Grade III encompasses grades I and II along with brainstem injury involving mostly fiber tracts, rostral brainstem, and superior cerebellar peduncles. Diagnosis of DAI could be difficult to make on CT since up to 80% of nonhemorrhagic DAI may have normal CT. Hemorrhagic lesions could be visible on CT depending on their size. A few hemorrhagic lesions in the appropriate locations are usually enough to suspect that there are widespread lesions. Presence of intraventricular hemorrhage may lead to elevated intracranial pressure that is associated with significant mortality.

DAI lesions are better categorized by MRI. MRI is the modality of choice in suspected DAI. Unfortunately, it may not be feasible to obtain MRI in the acute phase. Specifically, DWI, FLAIR, GRE, and SWI show both nonhemorrhagic and hemorrhagic DAI lesions. They restrict diffusion on DWI and are hyperintense on FLAIR and T2WI, while the hemorrhagic lesions are hypointense on GRE and SWI. The age of the hemorrhagic lesions determines their intensity on FLAIR, T1WI, and T2WI. Associated brain swelling could be diffuse or regional. DAI lesions are usually widespread varying from small to large. DTI usually shows decreased fractional anisotropy, with the color directional maps showing disruption and disorganization of fiber tracts. Brain perfusion studies may show patchy areas of hypoperfusion. Perfusion abnormalities tend to correlate with poor outcome in TBI.

Most patients with DAI are usually unconscious at the site of injury. They are more likely to suffer posttraumatic coma, fail to recover neurologically, and remain in vegetative state. Mild forms do exist. Young men are overrepresented. Unfortunately, there is no known treatment.

Question for Further Thought
1. What is the pathogenesis of DAI?

Reporting Responsibilities
This is an emergency requiring direct reporting. General location, size, and number of lesions should be noted. Other associated primary injuries such as fractures, soft tissue injuries, contusions, major hematomas, extraaxial hemorrhages, and hygromas should be reported. Presence of secondary injuries or complications such as brain swelling, herniations, intraventricular hemorrhage, infarcts, and hydrocephalus are categorized. Significant changes on follow-up should also be directly communicated.

What the Treating Physician Needs to Know
- NCCT may be normal. Clinical suspicion should encourage the use of MRI
- Locations and number of visible lesions
- Other primary and secondary injuries
- Other imaging modalities that could help resolve inconclusive findings
- Significant changes on follow-up particularly new and secondary injuries

Answer
1. DAI is a common primary injury in patients with severe TBI. It is generally regarded as due to widespread shearing injury during acceleration and rotation of the brain at impact. DAI lesions depend on the magnitude and direction of the shearing forces during impact and the relative rigidity and density of contiguous tissues. Lesions are more commonly found in subcortical white matter particularly of the centrum semiovale, the basal ganglia, CC, cerebellum, and brainstem. Lesions are usually multifocal, hemorrhagic or nonhemorrhagic, and vary in size from punctate to over 1.5 cm. Initial CT imaging may not detect these lesions but as surrounding edema develops over the next few days they become visible and their impact results in deterioration of clinical symptoms. Hemorrhagic lesions may expand substantially. The natural history is that of brain atrophy. The clinical outcome is generally very poor.

CASE 97

CLINICAL HISTORY *91-year-old male fell 2 days earlier and now has a change in mental status.*

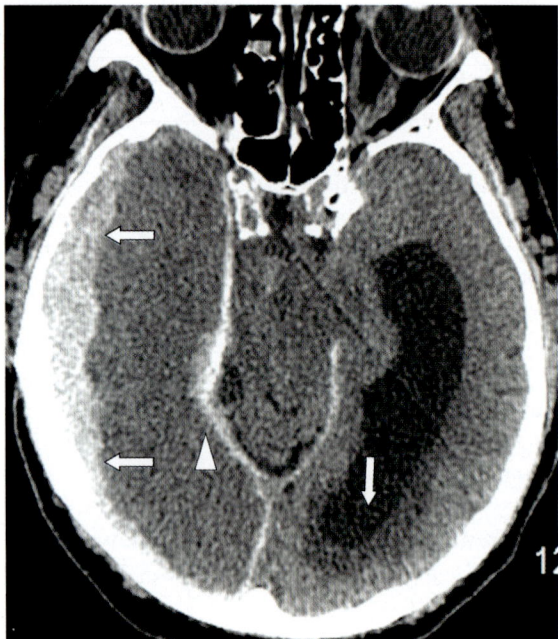

FIGURE 97-1

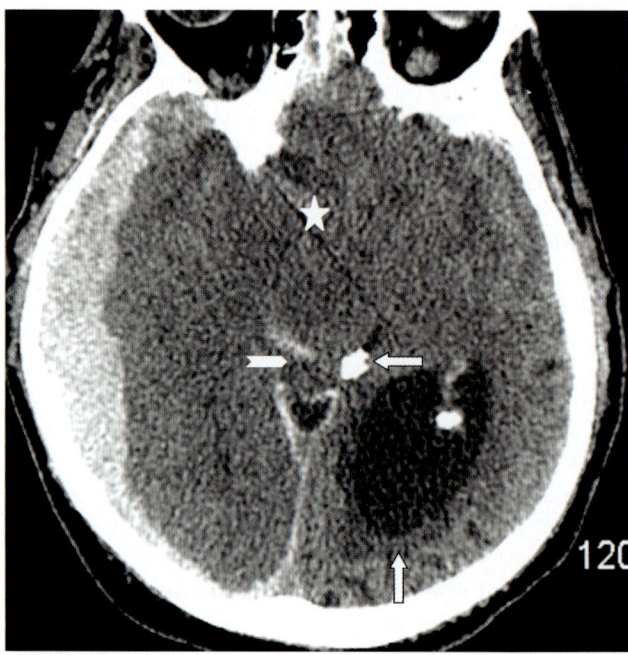

FIGURE 97-2

FINDINGS Figure 97-1. Axial NCCT through the tentorial incisura. There is a 1.5-cm thick crescentic hyperdense right temporal–occipital extraaxial collection displacing the right temporal and occipital lobes from the inner skull table consistent with acute subdural hematoma (ASDH) (transverse arrows). There is hyperdense subdural hematoma (SDH) around the right tentorium (triangle). There is crowding of the incisura with effacement of the cerebrospinal fluid (CSF) spaces. The right temporal horn is obliterated. The left temporal horn is severely dilated with periventricular hypodensity (vertical arrow) consistent with transependymal CSF permeation due to the acute hydrocephalus. Figure 97-2. Axial NCCT through the suprasellar cistern. There is obliteration of the suprasellar (star), interpeduncular, perimesencephalic, and quadrigeminal cisterns by a right uncal and transtentorial herniation. The left trigone is massively dilated (vertical arrow). There is acute hemorrhage (hyperdensity) in the right quadrigeminal cistern/midbrain (chevron). The calcified pineal gland is displaced inferiorly and to the left—midline shift (transverse arrow).

DIFFERENTIAL DIAGNOSIS N/A.

DIAGNOSIS Acute subdural hematoma (ASDH) with complications.

DISCUSSION The hallmark of ASDH on CT is the crescentic hyperdense extraaxial collection. The collection can freely distribute around the cerebral hemisphere,

layering on the tentorium and along the falx. The cerebral hemisphere is displaced away from the inner table of the skull or falx with compression and effacement of the sulci. Medium- and large-sized ASDH tend to displace midline structures, resulting in subfalcine, uncal, and transtentorial herniations. Massive transtentorial herniation could produce Duret hemorrhages of the brainstem. The ipsilateral lateral ventricle is usually compressed and obliterated along with the basal cisterns. Compression of the third ventricle and the foramen of Monro tend to create obstruction to CSF flow from the contralateral lateral ventricle resulting in acute hydrocephalus. Acute periventricular edema may surround the dilated ventricle. The contralateral convexity sulci may be effaced by the increased pressure in the lateral ventricle. Compression of ipsilateral cortical veins may result in venous congestion and edema of the cerebral white matter particularly in the subcortical regions. The other complications of the herniations may include infarctions in the vascular territories of the posterior cerebral artery (PCA), superior cerebellar artery (SCA), anterior choroidal artery, and anterior cerebral artery (ACA) due to compression of these arteries.

There is occasional hypodense or isodense ASDH, which has been explained on the basis of severe anemia or dilution of the ASDH by CSF that has entered the subdural space through an arachnoid tear. This is actually a rare phenomenon. Active bleeding into the ASDH may result in a mixed density hematoma. This is present about 40%

of the time. ASDH is more common supratentorially than infratentorially. SDH is generally believed to be due to rupture of cortical veins as they cross the potential subdural space caused by minor or severe abnormal brain rotations or skull fractures. It has also been postulated that arterial bleed could cause ASDH. Such bleed tends to be large and rapidly progressive. SDH may be associated with other brain parenchymal injuries or traumatic subarachnoid hemorrhage. Other causes of SDH include coagulopathies, surgical trauma, ventriculoperitoneal shunts, and neoplastic lesions of the dura or arachnoid. It has no gender predilection and occurs in all ages. Presentation may include headache, focal neurologic deficit, seizures, changes in mental status, and coma.

The management of ASDH depends on several factors that include the Glasgow Coma Scale (GCS) score, neurologic state of the patient, the size and acuity of the SDH along with degree of midline shift, associated primary injuries and herniations on CT, clinical condition of the patient at presentation and over time, as well as the age of the patient. Small ASDH in a clinically stable patient could be conservatively managed. Symptomatic lesions are generally surgically treated. Outcome generally depends on the GCS score at presentation; the lower the score, the higher the mortality. ASDH thicker than 1 cm, producing more than 5 mm of midline shift, the presence of transtentorial herniation, and elevated intracranial pressure (ICP) are all associated with significant morbidity and mortality.

Questions for Further Thought

1. Is MRI essential in the management of ASDH?
2. Are there other imaging modalities that could be useful in the management of SDH?

Reporting Responsibilities

This is an emergency and should be directly reported. Size, location, complications such as herniations, infarcts, hydrocephalus and presence of active bleed should be reported. Significant changes on follow-up should also be directly reported. Presence of other primary and secondary brain injuries should be mentioned.

What the Treating Physician Needs to Know

- Location, size, complications, other primary and secondary injuries
- Usefulness of other imaging modalities in defining clinical outcome
- Significant changes on follow-up

Answers

1. MRI is not essential in making the diagnosis of ASDH. The patient's clinical condition usually does not permit MRI evaluation in the acute phase. In the long term, however, MRI could be useful in evaluation of inappropriate response to management such as stagnant or deteriorating clinical state. MRI could better define the extent of contusions, infarctions, or DAI that may have been missed or not visualized on CT. These could help in defining prognosis in such cases. MRI could also be useful in evaluation of SDH due to underlying meningeal pathologies such as neoplasm or vascular malformations.
2. The role of MRI has been described above. CTA or DSA could be useful in defining bleeding vessels and such bleeding points could be treated via the endovascular route. Perfusion studies may be able to define abnormal blood flow in the brain. Such perfusion abnormalities have been associated with poor outcome in SDH.

CLINICAL HISTORY *41-year-old male fell from a height. He was stuporous on arrival.*

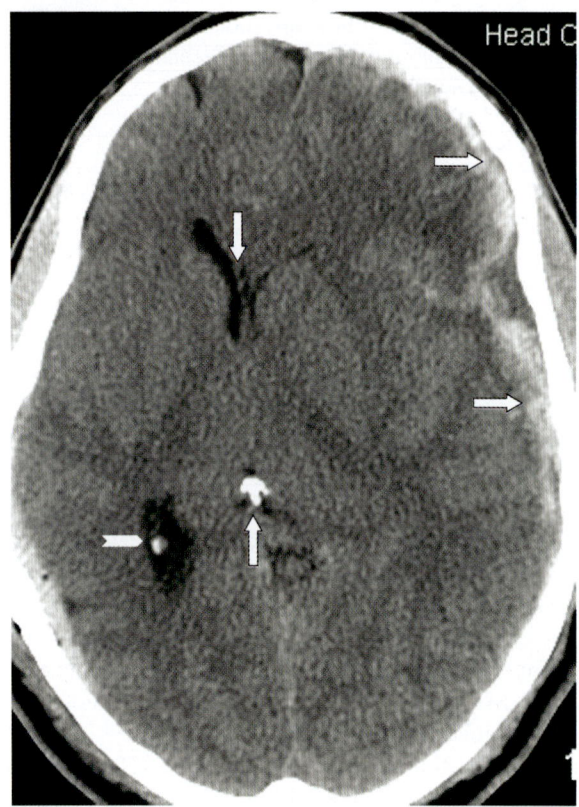

FIGURE 98-1

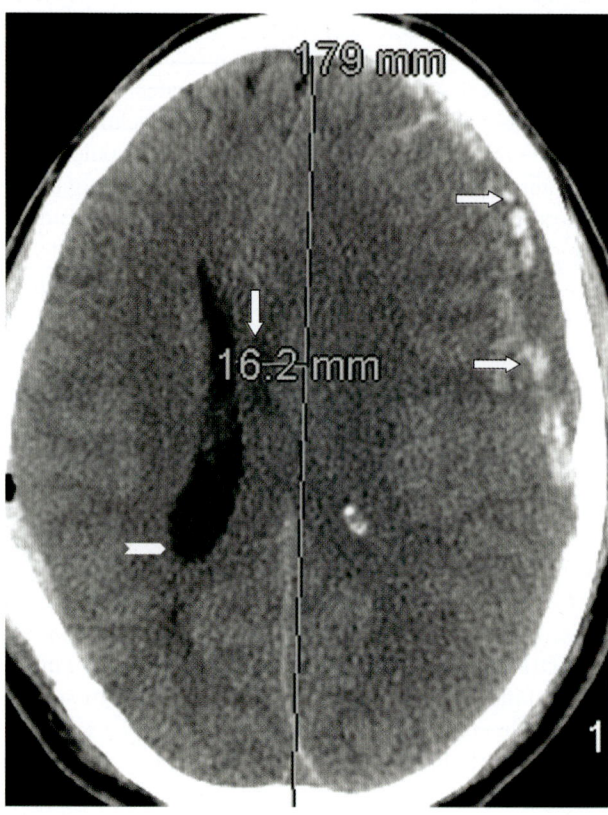

FIGURE 98-2

FINDINGS Figure 98-1. Axial NCCT through the basal ganglia. There is a left hemispheric mixed density (hyperacute) subdural hematoma (SDH) (transverse arrows). There is also some subarachnoid hemorrhage (SAH) beneath the SDH. The midline structures such as the septum pellucidum, third ventricle, and the calcified pineal gland (vertical arrows) have moved to the right of midline. The third and left lateral ventricles are compressed. Convexity sulci are effaced. There is mild dilation of the right lateral ventricle (chevron). Figure 98-2. Axial NCCT through the corona radiata. This demonstrates how to measure the shift; the septum pellucidum (vertical arrow) represents the midline structure measured against a line connecting the anterior and posterior attachment of the falx. The falx itself may bend away from the side of the mass or collection (transverse arrows point to the SDH). There is dilation of the right lateral ventricle (chevron).

DIFFERENTIAL DIAGNOSIS N/A.

DIAGNOSIS Subfalcine herniation (SFH) due to acute subdural hematoma.

DISCUSSION SFH is the most common brain herniation. The cause of SFH in this patient is the large left hemispheric hyperacute SDH. SFH is easily and readily imaged by CT. There is usually a unilateral hemispheric mass, extraaxial mass, or collection of bilateral hemispheric masses or collection with a dominant side. This pushes the midline structures of the septum pellucidum, third ventricle, pineal gland, internal cerebral veins (ICVs), to the contralateral side away from the dominant mass. A high convexity mass/collection may also push down on the ipsilateral cingulate gyrus, which subsequently slides medially under the falx to the contralateral side. These structures could therefore be found on the contralateral side of the midline. There is usually compression or effacement of the ipsilateral convexity sulci, lateral ventricle, and the third ventricle. A few complications can occur. Obstruction at the level of the third ventricle and the foramina of Monro prevents cerebrospinal fluid (CSF) from exiting the contralateral lateral ventricle resulting in trapping or hydrocephalus of that ventricle. This could be associated with periventricular edema. Compression or wedging of the ACA branches against the inferior edge of the falx by the herniating brain could produce stenosis or occlusion of the pericallosal or callosomarginal arteries resulting in ischemic infarction in the ipsilateral ACA territory. If these vessels rupture, SAH could occur. Compression of the ICV, vein of Galen, or the straight sinus could result in deep venous system obstruction with venous congestion, further raised intracranial pressure, and venous infarction. Although MRI is not necessary to demonstrate SFH, it has a capacity to show early complications of SFH.

Massive SFH may also be associated with transtentorial and ipsilateral uncal herniations. Patients usually show deterioration in clinical status. If the brainstem is compressed, Duret hemorrhages may occur and cardiac and respiratory functions may be affected. Significant shift that alters patient's clinical status may be an indication for decompressive surgery.

Question for Further Thought

1. What is paradoxical brain herniation?

Reporting Responsibilities

SFH is an emergency requiring direct reporting. The size is usually measured in relation to displacement of midline structures away from the midline. It is important that comparison measurement should be done at about the same level. Whatever is causing the herniation should be documented. Other primary intracranial injuries should be categorized. Complications such as infarcts, trapping of the contralateral lateral ventricle, and significant changes on follow-up should be reported directly as well. There may be other associated herniations in massive midline shifts such as uncal/transtentorial herniations that are all reportable.

What the Treating Physician Needs to Know

- Size of shift measured in millimeters or centimeters
- Offending mass or collection; location and size
- Other primary injuries such as fractures, epidural hematoma (EDH), SDH, hygromas, contusions, hematoma, and diffuse axonal injury (DAI)
- Complications and other associated herniations

Answer

1. Paradoxical herniation is the phenomenon of SFH following brain decompressive surgery without evidence of raised intracranial pressure or any extraaxial lesion that could account for the herniation. Paradoxical herniation can occur following a lumbar puncture, upright position, CSF leak, or dehydration in the presence of a large craniectomy. The explanation is that gravity on the decompressed brain creates a negative pressure gradient between atmospheric and intracranial pressure under these circumstances and this allows the brain to be sucked into the low-pressure infratentorial compartment and through the foramen magnum. The clinical condition tends to deteriorate suddenly. Focal neurologic deficit and mental status changes occur. The patient may become unarousable and comatose. It could be fatal. These changes could also be delayed a few days after a lumbar puncture (LP). The CT scan usually demonstrates a midline shift or SFH with a sunken brain or a concavity of the brain at the site of craniectomy. Recommended treatment has included the Trendelenburg position, hydration, blood patch, and early cranioplasty with varying degrees of success. It is recommended that an LP be withheld in a patient who has a large craniectomy. If, however, an LP becomes necessary, then it is done with the patient in the Trendelenburg position.

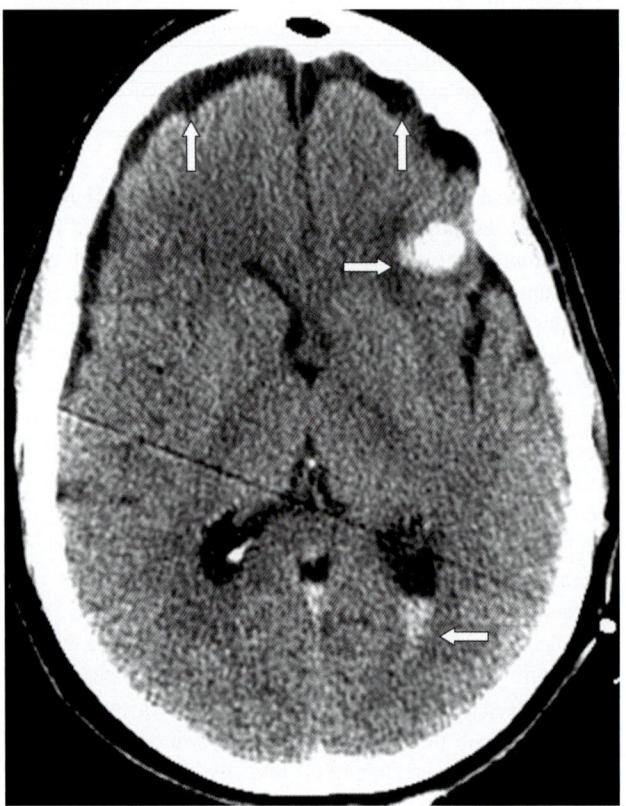

FIGURE 99-1

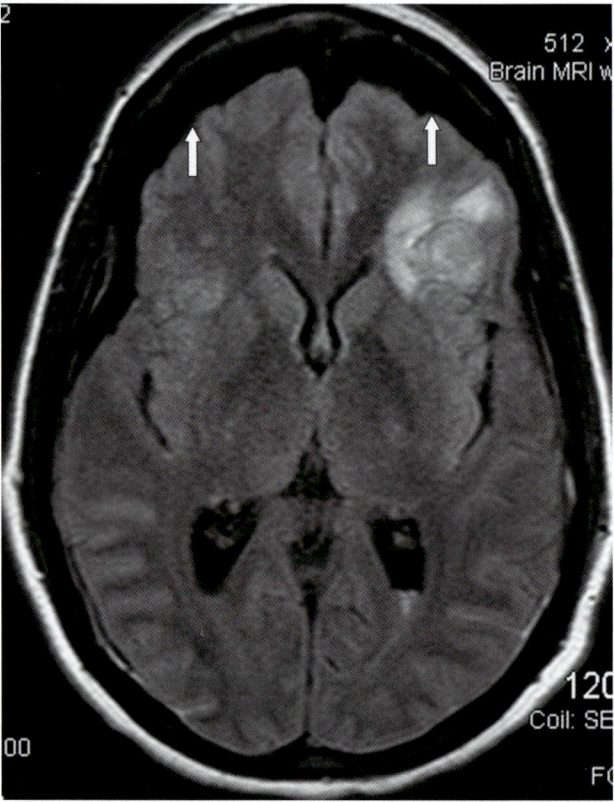

FIGURE 99-2

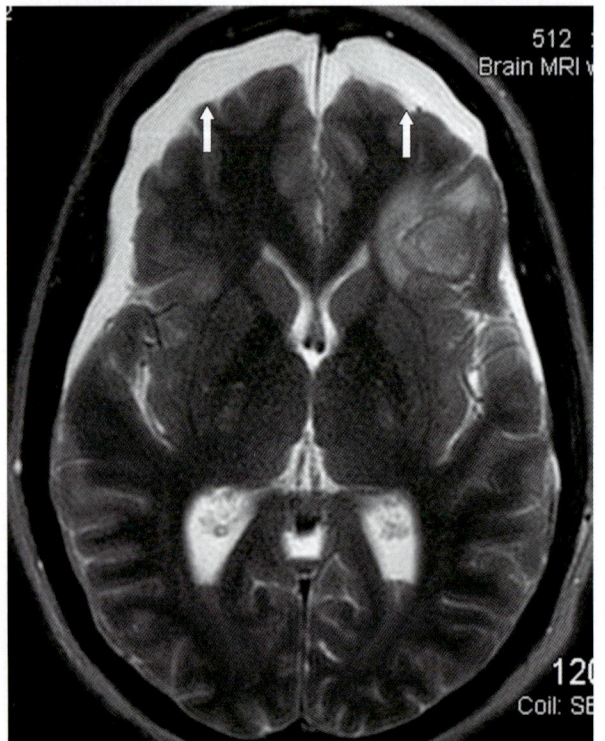

FIGURE 99-3

FINDINGS Figure 99-1. NCCT through the inferior frontal lobes. There is extraaxial crescentic large cerebrospinal fluid (CSF) density space measuring about 1 cm thick over both frontal lobes with effacement of underlying sulci (vertical arrows). There is associated left frontal opercula hematoma (transverse arrow) and IVH in left trigone (posterior left arrow). Figures 99-2 and 99-3. Axial FLAIR and T2WI through the frontal lobes respectively. The bifrontal extraaxial collections have CSF intensity on all sequences (arrows). The left frontal opercula hematoma and IVH are again visualized.

DIFFERENTIAL DIAGNOSIS Atrophy or volume loss, subdural hygroma (SDG), chronic subdural hematoma (CSDH).

DIAGNOSIS Traumatic subdural hygroma (TSDG).

DISCUSSION TSDG is defined as crescentic collection of CSF, xanthochromic, or slightly hemorrhagic fluid in the subdural space at least 3 mm thick following trauma. This may be preceded by what has been described as a subdural effusion (SDE) usually same fluid less than 3 mm thick in 50% of SDG population. Some literature treats SDG and SDE as the same entity. It has also been known as subdural hydroma or subdural fluid collection. The fluid is usually hypodense or CSF density on CT with CSF intensity pattern on MRI. There is effacement of the underlying sulci and depending on its size and lateralization could be associated with midline shift. It is unilateral in 65% and bilateral but asymmetric in 35% of one particular series. SDG could be detected immediately following minor or severe head trauma or delayed. Association with ventriculomegaly occurs in about a third of the patients. It is most commonly supratentorial and frontal but posterior fossa occurrence has been reported. SDG is considered benign but could progress significantly over time resulting in significant mass effect. TSDG is found in about 6% of traumatic head injuries. Brain contusions, diffuse axonal injury, subdural hematoma, fractures, and subarachnoid hemorrhage or other forms of intracranial injuries occur in about 45.8% as in this patient. Differentiating this entity from atrophy in the elderly could be difficult but the presence of sulcal effacement is key to the differentiation. A small proportion of SDG evolve into CSDH. This evolution has not been fully explained. The enhancing membrane of CSDH differentiates it from SDG.

SDG is more common in men and occurs in all age groups. Apart from trauma, SDG could be found as a complication of meningitis, craniotomy, shunt, subarachnoid hemorrhage, or arachnoid cyst. Presentation depends on other associated traumatic findings. A stand-alone SDG could present with headache, seizures, and altered mental status. It is usually considered benign, and treatment is conservative but operative treatment may include craniotomy or CSF diversion if associated with significant growth or ventriculomegaly.

Question for Further Thought

1. What is the pathogenesis of TSDG?

Reporting Responsibilities

Presence of any extraaxial collections including SDG following trauma requires direct reporting. Other associated traumatic findings should be enumerated. Presence of mass effect or ventricular dilatation should be reported. Follow-up imaging changes in size, associated CSDH, or associated ventriculomegaly are reportable.

What the Treating Physician Needs to Know

- Size and location
- Growth on follow-up imaging
- Presence of mass effect, ventriculomegaly, or CSDH

Answer

1. The basic explanation for TSDG is the presence of an arachnoid tear, allowing CSF to accumulate in the subdural space. Presence of a flap valve provides a one-way mechanism that allows continuing accumulation of CSF. A second explanation is that the fluid is an effusion due to increased permeability of the traumatized vessels rather than CSF. Yet another explanation particularly in those associated with ventriculomegaly is that of impaired CSF absorption resulting in some form of external hydrocephalus. These are usually the patients that may require CSF diversion.

CASE 100

CLINICAL HISTORY   *52-year-old female with prior multiple craniotomies and ventriculoperitoneal shunts on follow-up for seizure disorder.*

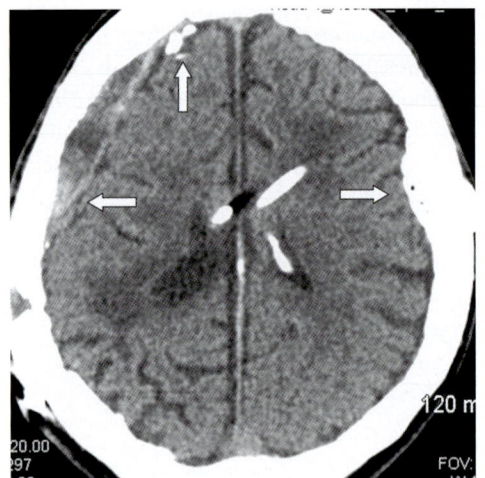

FIGURE 100-1

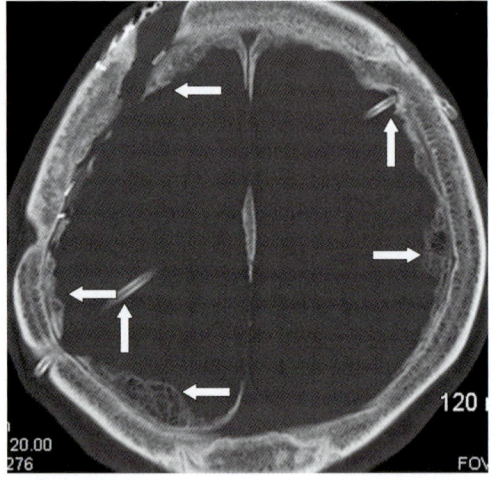

FIGURE 100-2

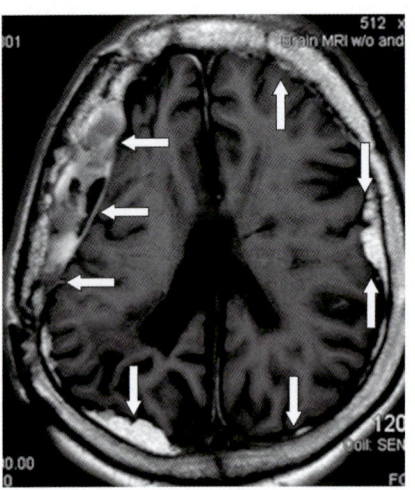

FIGURE 100-3

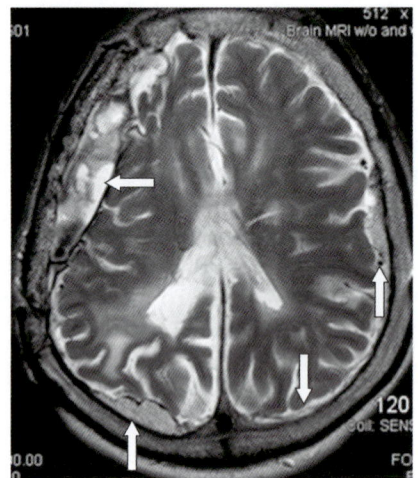

FIGURE 100-4

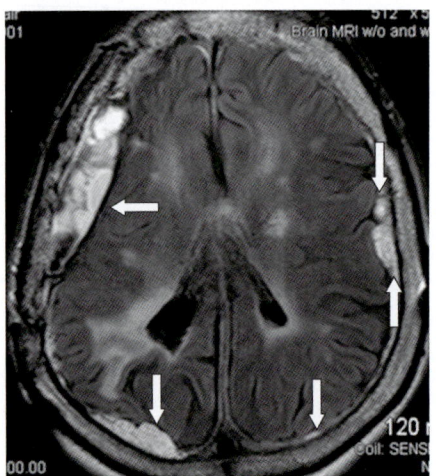

FIGURE 100-5

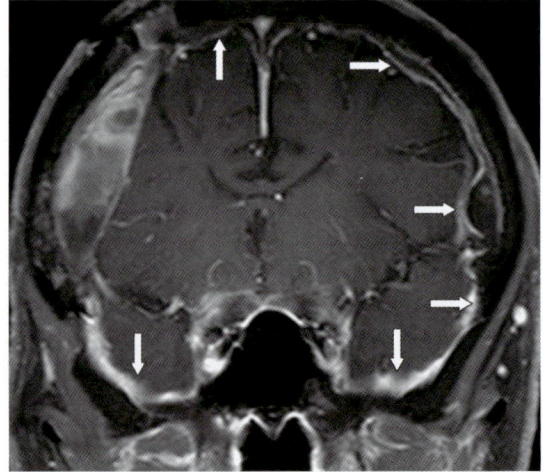

FIGURE 100-6

FINDINGS Figure 100-1. Axial NCCT through the centrum semiovale. There is a mixed density right frontal extraaxial collection (right transverse arrow). There is an area of focal hyperdensity (calcification/ossification) at the anterior end of the collection (vertical arrow). Left-sided dural bony excrescences are present (transverse left arrow). Figure 100-2. Axial NCCT bone window setting through the lateral ventricles. There is a left anterior transfrontal and a right posterior transparietal ventriculoperitoneal (VP) shunts (vertical arrows). Ossified excrescences are present along the inner table bilaterally with ossification of the falx (transverse arrows). Figures 100-3 to 100-5. Axial T1WI, T2WI, and FLAIR, respectively, through the inferior lateral ventricles. There is a large biconvex heterogeneous right frontal convexity extraaxial mass compressing the brain under the right frontoparietal craniotomy consistent with a large organized chronic subdural hematoma (CSDH) (transverse arrows). There are multiple hyperintense bony excrescences on all sequences along the inner table bilaterally (vertical arrows). Figure 100-6. Coronal post-contrast fat sat T1WI through the level of the cavernous sinuses. There is thickened pachymeningeal contrast enhancement (vertical arrows) around the brain and surrounding the convexity calcified extraaxial masses. A double layer is present along the left inner table surrounding the fat-suppressed extraaxial calcified SDH (transverse arrows). These changes have remained stable for 8 years of follow-up.

DIFFERENTIAL DIAGNOSIS Calvarial mass, chronic calcified/ossified subdural hematoma (CCSDH), hyperostosis frontalis interna.

DIAGNOSIS Chronic calcified/ossified subdural hematoma (CCSDH).

DISCUSSION The CCSDH may present as a thin hyperdense (calcified) shell surrounding the crescentic or biconvex CSDH or as irregular sheaths of extraaxial hyperdensities of varying sizes and shapes which could be continuous or fragmentary on CT. There may be varying degrees of brain compression depending on the size and location. Woven bone configuration is not uncommon as shown in Figure 100-2. The MRI changes parallel the CT changes with extraaxial masses presenting as heterogeneous, hypointense, or hyperintense structures depending on whether the content is organized blood, calcification, or woven bone on all sequences. The calcification could be hypointense, while the fatty woven bone is usually hyperintense on MRI. There is invariably avid contrast enhancement of the dura and the membrane. The pattern could be mistaken for calvarial masses. If the woven bone pattern is confined to the frontal lobes, it may be mistaken for hyperostosis frontalis interna in the appropriate age group.

CCSDH is a very rare condition that is more common in children than in adults. Because of its rarity, the incidence is not definitely known but said to occur in up to 10% of CSDH. It has been reported in association with chronic ventriculoperitoneal shunts, postmeningitic subdural effusions, and late complications of head injuries in atrophic brains. The pathogenesis is not known and calcification may take 3 to 12 months to develop, while ossification takes much longer. The membrane could calcify in an eggshell fashion or the entire collection could ossify. Presentation is much varied from asymptomatic to symptoms and signs of raised intracranial pressure, seizures, neurologic deficit, decreased level of consciousness, calvarial masses, and cortical hemorrhage. Asymptomatic cases do not require treatment unless there is significant compression of the brain. Symptomatic cases have been surgically resected.

Question for Further Thought

1. What is armored brain?

Reporting Responsibilities

Unless there are complications such as cortical hemorrhage, brain edema, or herniations, routine reporting is sufficient. Complications should be communicated urgently and directly. Circumferential calcification tightly adherent to the brain should be reported as this could pose a potential problem if surgical excision is envisaged.

What the Treating Physician Needs to Know

- Location and size and effect on the underlying brain
- Presence of armored brain may be a contraindication if surgery is contemplated

Answer

1. An armored brain is a form of CCSDH where there is circumferential calcification of the subdural membrane encasing the brain with tight adhesion to the arachnoid membrane and the brain. Attempt to remove such a CCSDH surgically may result in damage to the underlying brain.

TREATMENT-RELATED CHANGES
CASE 1
- Constine LS, Konski A, Ekholm S, McDonald S, Rubin P. Adverse effects of brain irradiation correlated with MR and CT imaging. *Int J Radiat Oncol Biol Phys.* 1988;15:319–330.
- Lai R, Abrey LE, Rosenblum MK, DeAngelis LM. Treatment-induced leukoencephalopathy in primary CNS lymphoma. *Neurology* 2004;62:451–456.

BRAINSTEM ENCEPHALITIS
CASE 2
- Odaka M, Yuki N, Yamada M. Bickerstaff's brainstem encephalitis: clinical features of 62 cases and a subgroup associated with Guillain–Barré syndrome. *Brain* 2003;126:2279–2290.
- Roos RP, Soliven B, Goldenberg F, Badruddin A, Baron JM. An elderly patient with Bickerstaff brainstem encephalitis and transient episodes of brainstem dysfunction. *Arch Neurol.* 2008;65:821–824.

CEREBELLOPONTINE ANGLE MENINGIOMA
CASE 3
- Bonneville F, Sarrazin JL, Marsot-Dupusch K, et al. Unusual lesions of the cerebellopontine angle: a segmental approach. *Radiographics* 2001;21:419–438.
- Voss NF, Vrionis FD, Hellman CB, Robertson JH. Meningiomas of the cerebellopontine angle. *Surg Neurol.* 2000;53:439–446.

FIBROUS DYSPLASIA
CASE 4
- Lustig LR, Holliday MJ, McCarthy EF, Nager GT. Fibrous dysplasia involving the skull base and temporal bone. *Arch Otolaryngol Head Neck Surg.* 2001;127:1239–1247.
- Osborn AG. *Osborn's Brain: Imaging, Pathology, and Anatomy.* Salt Lake City/Philadelphia, PA: Amirsys/LWW Publishers; 2013:727–731.

INTRALABYRINTHINE (COCHLEA) SCHWANNOMA
CASE 5
- Salzman KL, Childs AM, Davidson HC, Kennedy RJ, Shelton C, Harnsberger HR. Intralabyrinthine schwannomas: imaging diagnosis and classification. *AJNR Am J Neuroradiol.* 2012;33:104–109.
- Tsang Juliano AF, Maya MM, Lo WWM, Kovanlikaya I. Temporal bone tumors and cerebellopontine angle lesions. In: Som PM, Curtin, HD, eds. *Head and Neck Imaging.* 5th ed. Philadelphia, PA: Elsevier Health Sciences; 2011:1263–1407.

ENLARGED ENDOLYMPHATIC SAC SYNDROME
CASE 6
- Okamoto K, Ito J, Furusawa T, et al. MRI of enlarged endolymphatic sacs in the large vestibular aqueduct syndrome. *Neuroradiology* 1998;40:167–172.
- Vijayasekaran S, Halsted MJ, Boston M, et al. When is the vestibular aqueduct enlarged? A statistical analysis of the normative distribution of vestibular aqueduct size. *AJNR Am J Neuroradiol.* 2007;28:1133–1138.

PAGET DISEASE
CASE 7
- Resnick D. *Diagnosis of Bone and Joint Disorders.* 3rd ed. Philadelphia, PA: Saunders; 1995.
- Smith SE, Murphey MD, Motamedi K, Mulligan ME, Resnik CS, Gannon FH. From the archives of the AFIP. Radiologic spectrum of Paget disease of bone and its complications with pathologic correlation. *Radiographics* 2002;22:1191–1216.

HEMANGIOMA OF CRANIAL VAULT
CASE 8
- Lloret I, Server A, Taksdal I. Calvarial lesions: a radiological approach to diagnosis. *Acta Radiol.* 2009;50(5):531–542.
- Naama O, Gazzaz M, Akhaddar A, et al. Cavernous hemangioma of the skull: 3 case reports. *Surg Neurol.* 2008;70(6):654–659.

CAROTID CAVERNOUS FISTULA (I)
CASE 9
- Gemmete JJ, Chaudhary N, Pandey A, Ansari S. Treatment of carotid cavernous fistulas. *Curr Treat Options Neurol.* 2010;12:43–53.
- Théaudin M, Saint-Maurice JP, Chapot R, et al. Diagnosis and treatment of dural carotid-cavernous fistulas: a consecutive series of 27 patients. *J Neurol Neurosurg Psychiatry* 2007;78:174–179.

ORBITAL AND NASOFRONTAL CEPHALOCELE
CASE 10
- Huisman TA, Schneider JF, Kellenberger CJ, Martin-Fiori E, Willi UV, Holzmann D. Developmental nasal midline masses in children: neuroradiological evaluation. *Eur Radiol.* 2004;14:243–249.
- Wani BN, Jajoo SN, Bhole AM. Transilluminant naso-orbital dermoid cyst masquerading as meningocele. *J Craniofac Surg.* 2010;21:930–932.

SINUS PERICRANII
CASE 11
- Akram H, Prezerakos G, Haliasos N, O'Donovan D, Low H. Sinus pericranii: an overview and literature review of a rare cranial venous anomaly (a review of the existing literature with case examples). *Neurosurg Rev.* 2012;35:15–26; discussion 26.
- Gandolfo C, Krings T, Alvarez H, et al. Sinus pericranii: diagnostic and therapeutic considerations in 15 patients. *Neuroradiology* 2007;49:505–514.

HEMANGIOBLASTOMA
CASE 12
- Conway JE, Chou D, Clatterbuck RE, Brem H, Long DM, Rigamonti D. Hemangioblastomas of the central nervous system in von Hippel-Lindau syndrome and sporadic disease. *Neurosurgery* 2001;48:55–62.
- Jagannathan J, Lonser RR, Smith R, et al. Surgical management of cerebellar hemangioblastomas in patients with von Hippel-Lindau disease. *J Neurosurg.* 2008;108:210.

POSTERIOR FOSSA EPENDYMOMA
CASE 13
- McLendon RE, Wiestler OD, Kros JM, Korshunov A, Ng H-K. Ependymoma and anaplastic ependymoma. In: Louis DN, Ohgaki H, Wiestler OD, Cavenee WK. eds. *WHO Classification of Tumours of the Central Nervous System.* Lyon, France: IARC; 2007: 74–80.
- Yuh EL, Barkovich AJ, Gupta N. Imaging of ependymomas: MRI and CT. *Childs Nerv Syst.* 2009;25:1203–1213.

HYPERTROPHIC OLIVARY DEGENERATION
CASE 14
- Kitajima M, Korogi Y, Shimomura O, et al. Hypertrophic olivary degeneration: MR imaging and pathologic findings. *Radiology* 1994;192:539–543.
- Sanverdi SE, Oguz KK, Haliloglu G. Hypertrophic olivary degeneration in children: four new cases and a review of the literature with an emphasis on the MRI findings. *Br J Radiol.* 2012;85:511–516.

CROSSED CEREBELLAR DIASCHISIS AND ATROPHY
CASE 15
- O'Gorman RL, Siddiqui A, Alsop DC, Jarosz JM. Perfusion MRI demonstrates crossed-cerebellar diaschisis in sickle cell disease. *Pediatr Neurol.* 2010;42:437–440.
- Poretti A, Boltshauser E. Crossed cerebro-cerebellar diaschisis. *Neuropediatrics* 2012;43:53–54.

POSTERIOR FOSSA ATYPICAL TERATOID RHABDOID TUMOR
CASE 16
- Bing F, Nugues F, Grand S, Bessou P, Salon C. Primary intracranial extra-axial and supratentorial atypical rhabdoid tumor. *Pediatr Neurol.* 2009;41:453–456.
- Meyers SP, Khademian ZP, Biegel JA, Chuang SH, Korones DN, Zimmerman RA. Primary intracranial atypical teratoid/rhabdoid tumors of infancy and childhood: MRI features and patient outcomes. *AJNR Am J Neuroradiol.* 2006;27:962–971.

JOUBERT SYNDROME
CASE 17
- Brancatil F, Dallapiccola B, Valente EM. Joubert syndrome and related disorders. *Orphanet J Rare Dis.* 2010;5:20–29.
- Poretti A, Bolshauser E, Loenneker T, et al. Diffusion tensor imaging in Joubert syndrome. *AJNR Am J Neuroradiol.* 2007; 28:1929–1933.

CHIARI II MALFORMATION (CIIM) MR
CASE 18
- El Gammal T, Mark EK, Brooks BS. MR imaging of Chiari II malformation. *AJR Am J Roentgenol.* 1988;150:163–170.
- Geerdink N, der Vliet TV, Rotteveel JJ, Feuth T, Roeleveld N, Mullaartal RA. Essential features of Chiari II malformation in MR imaging: an interobserver reliability study-part I. *Childs Nerv Syst.* 2012;28:977–985.

RHOMBENCEPHALOSYNAPSIS
CASE 19
- Ishak GE, Dempsey JC, Shaw DWW, et al. Rhombencephalosynapsis: a hindbrain malformation associated with incomplete separation of midbrain and forebrain, hydrocephalus and a broad spectrum of severity. *Brain* 2012;135:1370–1386.
- Patel S, Barkovich AJ. Analysis and classification of cerebellar malformations. *AJNR Am J Neuroradiol.* 2002;23:1074–1087.

CREUTZFELD-JAKOB DISEASE
CASE 20
- Zerr I, Kallenberg K, Summers DM, et al. Updated clinical diagnostic criteria for sporadic Creutzfeldt-Jakob disease. *Brain* 2009;132:2659–2668.

ALZHEIMER DISEASE
CASE 21
- Petrella JR, Coleman RE, Doraiswamy PM. Neuroimaging and early diagnosis of Alzheimer's disease: a look to the future. *Radiology* 2003;226:315–336. doi:10.1148/radiol.2262011600.

NORMAL PRESSURE HYDROCEPHALUS
CASE 22
- Hashimoto M, Ishikawa M, Mori E, Kuwana N. Diagnosis of idiopathic normal pressure hydrocephalus is supported by MRI-based scheme: a prospective study. *Cerebrospinal Fluid Res.* 2010;7:18. Published online Oct 31, 2010. doi:10.1186/1743-8454-7-18.

DURAL METASTASIS BREAST
CASE 23
- Kremer S, Grand S, Rémy C, et al. Contribution of dynamic contrast MR imaging to the differentiation between dural metastasis and meningioma. *Neuroradiology* 2004;46:642–648.
- Lee EK, Lee EJ, Kim MS, et al. Intracranial metastases: spectrum of MR imaging findings. *Acta Radiol.* 2012;53(10):1173–1185.

IDIOPATHIC HYPERTROPHIC PACHYMENINGITIS
CASE 24
- Poon CS, Chang J, Swarnkar A, Johnson MH, Wasenko J. Radiologic diagnosis of cerebral venous thrombosis: pictorial review. *AJR Am J Roentgenol.* 2007;189:S64–S75.
- Sze, G. Diseases of the intracranial meninges: MR imaging features. *AJR Am J Roentgenol.* 1993;160:727–733.

NEUROSARCOIDOSIS
CASE 25
- Christoforidis GA, Spickler EM, Recio MV, Mehta BM. MR of CNS sarcoidosis: correlation of imaging features to clinical symptoms and response to treatment. *AJNR Am J Neuroradiol.* 1999;20:655–669.
- Shah R, Roberson GH, Cure JK. Correlation of MR imaging findings and clinical manifestations in neurosarcoidosis. *AJNR Am J Neuroradiol.* 2009;30:953–961.

POSTTRAUMATIC CSF COLLECTION
CASE 26
- Muhonen MG, Piper JD, Menezes AH. Pathogenesis and treatment of growing skull fractures. *Surg Neurol.* 1995; 43:367–373.
- Sherif C, Di Ieva A, Gibson D, et al. Management algorithm for cerebrospinal fluid leak associated with anterior skull base fractures: detailed clinical and radiological follow-up. *Neurosurg Rev.* 2012;35:227–238.

BACTERIAL MENINGITIS

CASE 27

- Castillo M. Imaging of meningitis. *Semin Roentgenol.* 2004;39:458–464.
- Hughes DC, Raghavan A, Mordekar SR, Griffiths PD, Connolly DJA. Role of imaging in the diagnosis of acute bacterial meningitis and its complications. *Postgrad Med J.* 2010;86:478–485.

EPIDERMOID CYST

CASE 28

- Aribandi M, Wilson NJ. CT and MR imaging features of intracerebral epidermoid—a rare lesion. *Br J Radiol.* 2008;81:e97–e99.
- Nagasawa D, Yew A, Safaee M, et al. Clinical characteristics and diagnostic imaging of epidermoid tumors. *J Clin Neurosci.* 2011; 18:1158–1162. Epub Jul 13, 2011. doi:10.1016/j.jocn.2011.02.008.

SUBARACHNOID HEMORRHAGE (NONANEURYSMAL)

CASE 29

- Whiting J, Reavey-Cantwell J, Velat G, et al. Clinical course of nontraumatic, nonaneurysmal subarachnoid hemorrhage: a single-institution experience. *Neurosurg Focus* 2009;26:E21. doi:10.3171/2009.2.FOCUS092.
- Wohaibi MA, Russell NA, Ferayan AA, Awada A, Jumah MA, Omojola M. Pituitary apoplexy presenting as massive subarachnoid haemorrhage. *J Neurol Neurosurg Psychiatry* 2000;69:692–709.

ARACHNOID CYST

CASE 30

- Huang D, Abe T, Kojima K, et al. Intracystic hemorrhage of the middle fossa arachnoid cyst and subdural hematoma caused by ruptured middle cerebral artery aneurysm. *AJNR Am J Neuroradiol.* 1999;20:1284–1286.
- Yildiz H, Erdogan C, Yalcin R, et al. Evaluation of communication between intracranial arachnoid cysts and cisterns with phase-contrast cine MR imaging. *AJNR Am J Neuroradiol.* 2005;26:145–151.

PILOCYTIC ASTROCYTOMA

CASE 31

- Horger M, Vogel MN, Beschorner R, et al. T2 and DWI in pilocytic and pilomyxoid astrocytoma with pathologic correlation. *Can J Neurol Sci.* 2012;39:491–498.
- Lee IH, Kim JH, Suh YL, et al. Imaging characteristics of pilomyxoid astrocytomas in comparison with pilocytic astrocytomas. *Eur J Radiol.* 2011;79:311–316.

GRANULAR CELL ASTROCYTOMA

CASE 32

- Brat DJ, Scheithauer BW, Medina-Flores R, Rosenblum MK, Burger PC. Infiltrative astrocytomas with granular cell features (granular cell astrocytomas): a study of histopathologic features, grading, and outcome. *Am J Surg Pathol.* 2002; 26:750–757.
- Schittenhelm J, Psaras T. Glioblastoma with granular cell astrocytoma features: a case report and literature review. *Clin Neuropathol.* 2010;29:323–329.

PLEOMORPHIC XANTHOASTROCYTOMA

CASE 33

- Goncalves VT, Reis F, Queiroz Lde S, Franca M Jr. Pleomorphic xanthoastrocytoma: magnetic resonance imaging findings in a series of cases with histopathological confirmation. *Arq Neuropsiquiatr.* 2013;71:35–39.
- Yu S, He L, Zhuang X, Luo B. Pleomorphic xanthoastrocytoma: MR imaging findings in 19 patients. *Acta Radiol.* 2011;52:223–228.

DYSEMBRYOPLASTIC NEUROEPITHELIAL TUMOR

CASE 34

- Bulakbasi N, Kocaoglu M, Sanal TH, Tayfun C. Dysembryoplastic neuroepithelial tumors: proton MR spectroscopy, diffusion and perfusion characteristics. *Neuroradiology* 2007;49:805–812.
- Campos AR, Clusmann H, von Lehe M, et al. Simple and complex dysembryoplastic neuroepithelial tumors (DNT) variants: clinical profile, MRI, and histopathology. *Neuroradiology* 2009;51:433–443.

LYMPHOMA

CASE 35

- Harting I, Hartmann M, Jost G, et al. Differentiating primary central nervous system lymphoma from glioma in humans using localised proton magnetic resonance spectroscopy. *Neurosci Lett.* 2003;342:163–166.
- Jensen-Kondering U, Henker C, Dorner L, Hugo HH, Jansen O. Differentiation of primary central nervous system lymphomas from high grade astrocytomas by qualitative analysis of the signal intensity curves derived from dynamic susceptibility-contrast magnetic resonance imaging. *Neurol Res.* 2012;34:984–988.

CORTICAL EPENDYMOMA

CASE 36

- Van Gompel JJ, Koeller KK, Meyer FB, et al. Cortical ependymoma: an unusual epileptogenic lesion. *J Neurosurg.* 2011;114:1187–1194.
- Vitanovics D, Balint K, Hanzely Z, Banczerowski P, Afra D. Ependymoma in adults: surgery, reoperation and radiotherapy for survival. *Pathol Oncol Res.* 2010;16:93–99.

BILATERAL THALAMIC GLIOMA

CASE 37

- Hegde AN, Mohan S, Lath N, et al. Differential diagnosis for bilateral abnormalities of the basal ganglia and thalamus. *Radiographics* 2011;31:5–30.
- Khanna PC, Iyer RS, Chaturvedi A, et al. Imaging bithalamic pathology in the pediatric brain: demystifying a diagnostic conundrum. *AJR Am J Roentgenol.* 2011;197:1449–1459.

ARTERY OF PERCHERON INFARCTS

CASE 38

- Hegde AN, Mohan S, Lath N, Tchoyoson Lim CC. Differential diagnosis for bilateral abnormalities of the basal ganglia and thalamus. *Radiographics* 2011;31:15–30.
- Lazzaro NA, Wright B, Castillo M, et al. Artery of Percheron infarction: imaging patterns and clinical spectrum. *AJNR Am J Neuroradiol.* 2010;31:1283–1289.

HYPOXIC-ISCHEMIC ENCEPHALOPATHY IN TERM INFANT

CASE 39

• Badve CA, Khanna PC, Ishak GE. Neonatal ischemic brain injury: what every radiologist needs to know. *Pediatr Radiol.* 2012;42:606–619.

• Chao CP, Zaleski CG, Patton AC. Neonatal hypoxic-ischemic encephalopathy: multimodality imaging findings. *Radiographics* 2006;26(Suppl 1):S159–S172.

HUNTINGTON DISEASE

CASE 40

• Ho VB. Juvenile Huntington disease: CT and MR features. *AJNR Am J Neuroradiol.* 1995;16:1405–1412.

• Sturrok A. Magnetic resonance spectroscopy biomarkers in premanifest and early Huntington disease. *Neurology* 2010;75:1702–1710.

POSTTRANSPLANT LYMPHOPROLIFERATIVE DISEASE

CASE 41

• Cavaliere R, Petroni G, Lopes MB, Schiff D; International Primary Central Nervous System Lymphoma Collaborative Group. Primary central nervous system post-transplantation lymphoproliferative disorder: an International Primary Central Nervous System Lymphoma Collaborative Group Report. *Cancer* 2010;116:863–870.

• Lieberman F, Yazbeck V, Raptis A, Felgar R, Boyiadzis M. Primary central nervous system post-transplant lymphoproliferative disorders following allogeneic hematopoietic stem cell transplantation. *J Neurooncol.* 2012;107:225–232.

MITOCHONDRIAL ENCEPHALOPATHY WITH LACTIC ACIDOSIS AND STROKES (MELAS)

CASE 42

• Chinnery PF. Mitochondrial disorders review. 2010. http://www.ncbi.nlm.nih.gov/books/NBK1224. Accessed on May 25, 2013.

• Debrosse S, Parikh S. Neurologic disorders due to mitochondrial DNA mutations. *Semin Pediatr Neurol.* 2012;19:181–193.

FAHR DISEASE (BILATERAL STRIOPALLIDODENTATE CALCINOSIS)

CASE 43

• Ashtari F, Fatehi F. Fahr's disease: variable presentations in a family. *Neurol Sci.* 2010;31:665–667.

• Hedge A, Mohan S, Lath N, Lim CCT. Differential diagnosis for bilateral abnormalities of the basal ganglia and thalamus. *Radiographics* 2011;31:5–30.

INTRAVENTRICULAR SIMPLE CYST

CASE 44

• Park SW, Yoon SH, Cho KH, et al. A large arachnoid cyst of the lateral ventricle extending from the supracerebellar cistern—case report. *Surg Neurol.* 2006;65:611–614.

• Xi-an Z, Songtao Q, Yuping P. Endoscopic treatment of intraventricular cerebrospinal fluid cysts: 10 consecutive cases. *Minim Invasive Neurosurg.* 2009;52:158–162.

CHOROID PLEXUS PAPILLOMA WHO I

CASE 45

• Naeini RM, Yoo JH, Hunter JV. Spectrum of choroid plexus lesions in children. *AJR Am J Roentgenol.* 2009;192:32–40.

• Paulus W, Brandner S. Choroid plexus tumours. In: Louis DN, Ohgaki H, Wiestler OD, Cavenee WK, eds. *WHO Classification of Tumours of the Central Nervous System.* Lyon, France: IARC; 2007:82–85.

INTRAVENTRICULAR MENINGIOMA

CASE 46

• Nakamura M, Roser F, Bundschuh O, Vorkapic P, Samii M. Intraventricular menigiomas: a review of 16 cases with reference to the literature. *Surg Neurol.* 2003;59:491–504.

• Stemmer-Rachamimov AO, Wiestler OD, Louis DN. Neurofibromatosis type 2. In: Louis DN, Ohgaki H, Wiestler OD, Cavenee WK, eds. *WHO Classification of Tumours of the Central Nervous System.* Lyon, France: IARC; 2007:210–214.

CHOROID PLEXUS METASTASIS

CASE 47

• Leach JCD, Garrott H, King JAJ, Kaye AH. Solitary metastasis to the choroid plexus of the third ventricle mimicking a colloid cyst: report of two cases. *J Clin Neurosci.* 2004;11:521–523.

• Raila FA, Bottoms WT, Fratkin JD. Solitary choroid plexus metastasis from renal cell carcinoma. *South Med J.* 1998;91:1159–1162.

CENTRAL NEUROCYTOMA

CASE 48

• Kocaoglu M, Ors F, Bulakbasi N, Onguru O, Ulutin C, Secer HI. Central neurocytoma: proton MR spectroscopy and diffusion weighted MR imaging findings. *Magn Reson Imaging* 2009;27:434–440.

• Schmidt MH, Gottfried ON, von Koch CS, Chang SM, McDermott MW. Central Neurocytoma: a review. *J Neurooncol.* 2004;66:377–384.

CORPUS CALLOSUM OLIGODENDROGLIOMA WHO II

CASE 49

• Ho ML, Moonis G, Ginat DT, Eisenberg RL. Lesions of the corpus callosum. *AJR Am J Roentgenol.* 2013;200:W1–W16.

• Monaco EA 3rd, Armah HB, Nikiforova MN, Hamilton RL, Engh JA. Grade II oligodendroglioma localized to the corpus callosum. *Brain Tumor Pathol.* 2011;28:305–309. Epub Jul 22, 2011. doi:10.1007/s10014-011-0054-0.

AGENESIS OF CORPUS CALLOSUM

CASE 50

• Griffiths PD, Batty R, Reeves MJ, Connolly DJ. Imaging the corpus callosum, septum pellucidum and fornix in children: normal anatomy and variations of normality. *Neuroradiology* 2009;51:337–345.

• Santo S, D'Antonio F, Homfray T, et al. Counseling in fetal medicine: agenesis of the corpus callosum. *Ultrasound Obstet Gynecol.* 2012;40:513–521.

CORPUS CALLOSUM LIPOMA

CASE 51

• Jabot G, Stoquart-Elsankari S, Saliou G, Toussaint P, Deramond H, Lehmann P. Intracranial lipomas: clinical appearances on neuroimaging and clinical significance. *J Neurol.* 2009; 256:851–855.

• Tart RP, Quisling RG. Curvilinear and tubulonodular varieties of lipoma of the corpus callosum: an MR and CT study. *J Comput Assist Tomogr.* 1991;15:805–810.

CORPUS CALLOSUM TUMEFACTIVE DEMYELINATION
CASE 52
- Given CA, Stevens BS, Lee C. The MRI appearance of tumefactive demyelinating lesions: a diagnostic challenge. *AJR Am J Roentgenol*. 2004;182:195–199.
- Kim DS, Na DG, Kim KH, et al. Distinguishing tumefactive demyelinating lesions from glioma or central nervous system lymphoma: added value of unenhanced CT compared with conventional contrast enhanced MR imaging. *Radiology* 2009;251:467–475.

BILATERAL MIDDLE CEREBRAL ARTERY TERRITORY INFARCTION
CASE 53
- Heinsius T, Bogousslavsky J, Van Melle G. Large infarcts in the middle cerebral artery territory. Etiology and outcome patterns. *Neurology* 1998;50:341–350.
- Kim KK, Kim DG, Ku YH, et al. Bilateral cerebral hemispheric infarction associated with sildenafil citrate (Viagra) use. *Eur J Neurol*. 2008;15:306–308.

CEREBRAL ARTERIAL GAS EMBOLISM
CASE 54
- Donepudi S, Chavalitdhamrong D, Pu L, Draganov PV. Air embolism complicating gastrointestinal endoscopy: a systematic review. *World J Gastrointest Endosc*. 2013;5:359–365.
- Rangappa P, Uhde B, Byard RW, Wurm A, Thomas PD. Fatal cerebral arterial gas embolism after endoscopic retrograde cholangiopancreatography. *Indian J Crit Care Med*. 2009;13:108–112.

POSTERIOR REVERSIBLE ENCEPHALOPATHY SYNDROME
CASE 55
- Hugonnet E, Da Ines D, Boby H, et al. Posterior reversible encephalopathy syndrome (PRES): features on CT and MR imaging. *Diagn Interv Imaging* 2013;94(1):45–52.
- Roth C, Ferbert A. The posterior reversible encephalopathy syndrome: what's certain, what's new? *Pract Neurol*. 2011;11(3):136–144.

ACUTE HYPERTENSIVE BASAL GANGLIA HEMATOMA
CASE 56
- Awada A, Russell N, al Rajeh S, Omojola M. Non-traumatic cerebral hemorrhage in Saudi Arabs: a hospital-based study of 243 cases. *J Neurol Sci*. 1996;144:198–203.
- Parizel PM, Makkat S, Van Miert E, Van Goethem JW, van den Hauwe L, De Schepper AM. Intracranial hemorrhage: principles of CT and MRI interpretation. *Eur Radiol*. 2001;11:1770–1783.

MOYAMOYA DISEASE
CASE 57
- Jang DK, Lee KS, Rha HK, et al. Clinical and angiographic features and stroke types in adult moyamoya disease. *AJNR Am J Neuroradiol*. 2014;35:1124–1131 Originally published online on Jan 2, 2014. doi:10.3174/ajnr.A3819.
- Scott RM, Smith ER. Moyamoya disease and moyamoya syndrome. *N Engl J Med*. 2009;360:1226–1237.

THALAMIC HEMATOMA WITH SPOT SIGN
CASE 58
- Gazzola S, Aviv RI, Gladstone DJ. Vascular and nonvascular mimics of the CT angiography "spot sign" in patients with secondary intracerebral hemorrhage. *Stroke* 2008; 39:1177–1183.
- Wada R, Aviv RI, Fox AJ, et al. CT angiography "spot sign" predicts hematoma expansion in acute intracerebral hemorrhage. *Stroke* 2007;38:1257–1262. Epub Feb 22, 2007.

SPONTANEOUS THROMBOSIS OF ARTERIOVENOUS MALFORMATION
CASE 59
- DeCesare B, Omojola MF, Fogarty EF, Brown JC, Taylon C. Spontaneous thrombosis of congenital cerebral arteriovenous malformation complicated by subdural collection: in utero detection with disappearance in infancy. *Br J Radiol*. 2006;79:e140–e144.
- Omojola MF, Fox AJ, Vinuela FV, et al. Spontaneous regression of intracranial arteriovenous malformations. Report of three cases. *J Neurosurg*. 1982;57:818–22.

BRAIN PYOGENIC ABSCESS WITH VENTRICULITIS
CASE 60
- Luthra G, Parihar A, Nath K, et al. Comparative evaluation of fungal, tubercular, and pyogenic brain abscesses with conventional and diffusion MR imaging and proton MR spectroscopy. *AJNR Am J Neuroradiol*. 2007;28:1332–1338.
- Rana S, Albayram S, Lin DDM, Yousem DM. Diffusion-weighted imaging and apparent diffusion coefficient maps in a case of intracerebral abscess with ventricular extension. *AJNR Am J Neuroradiol*. 2002;23:109–112.

BRAIN TUBERCULOMATA AND TUBERCULOUS ABSCESS
CASE 61
- Trivedi R, Saksena S, Gupta RK. Magnetic resonance imaging in central nervous system tuberculosis. *Indian J Radiol Imaging* 2009;19:256–265.
- Whiteman M, Espinosa L, Donovan Post MJ, Bell MD, Falcone S. Central nervous system tuberculosis in HIV-infected patients: clinical and radiographic findings. *AJNR Am J Neuroradiol*. 1995;16:1319–1327.

NEUROCYSTICERCOSIS VESICULAR/COLLOIDAL
CASE 62
- Coyle CM, Tanowitz HB. Diagnosis and treatment of neurocysticercosis. *Interdiscip Perspect Infect Dis*. 2009;2009:ID 180742, 9 pages. doi:10.1155/2009/180742.
- Kimura-Hayama ET, Higuera JA, Corona-Cedillo R, et al. Neurocysticercosis: radiologic-pathologic correlation. *Radiographics* 2010;30:1705–1719.

MYCOTIC ANEURYSM LEFT INTERNAL CAROTID ARTERY
CASE 63
- Allen LM, Fowler AM, Walker C, et al. Retrospective review of cerebral mycotic aneurysms in 26 patients: focus on treatment in strongly immunocompromised patients with a brief literature review. *AJNR Am J Neuroradiol*. 2013;34:823–827.

- Kannoth S, Thomas SV. Intracranial microbial aneurysm (infectious aneurysm): current options for diagnosis and management. *Neurocrit Care* 2009;11:120–129.

VARICELLA-ZOSTER VIRUS ENCEPHALITIS
CASE 64
- Amlie-Lefond C, Kleinschmidt-DeMasters BK, Mahalingam R, Davis LE, Gilden DH. The vasculopathy of varicella-zoster virus encephalitis. *Ann Neurol*. 1995;37:784–790.
- Kleinschmidt-DeMasters BK, Amlie-Lefond C, Gilden DH. The patterns of varicella zoster virus encephalitis. *Hum Pathol*. 1996;27:927–938.

HIV ENCEPHALOPATHY
CASE 65
- Balakrishnan J, Becker PS, Kumar Ashok, Zinreich SJ, McArthur JC, Bryan RN. Acquired immunodeficiency syndrome: correlation of radiologic and pathologic findings in the brain. *Radiographics* 1990;10:201–215.
- Smith AB, Smirniotopoulos JG, Rushing EJ. Central nervous system infections associated with human immunodeficiency virus infection: radiologic-pathologic correlation. *Radiographics* 2008;28:2033–2058.

MULTIPLE SCLEROSIS
CASE 66
- Noseworthy JH, Lucchinetti C, Rodriguez M, Weinshenker BG. Multiple sclerosis. *N Engl J Med*. 2000;343:938–952.
- Polman CH, Reingold SC, Banwell B, et al. Diagnostic criteria for multiple sclerosis: 2010 revisions to the McDonald criteria. *Ann Neurol*. 2011;69:292–302.

TUMEFACTIVE MULTIPLE SCLEROSIS
CASE 67
- Fallah A, Banglawala S, Ebrahim S, Paulseth JE, Jha NK. Tumefactive demyelinating lesions: a diagnostic challenge. *Can J Surg*. 2010;53:69–70.
- Kepes J. Large focal tumor-like demyelinating lesions of the brain: intermediate entity between multiple sclerosis and acute disseminated encephalomyelitis? *Ann Neurol*. 1993;33:18–27.

SUSAC SYNDROME
CASE 68
- Susac JO. Susac's syndrome. Editorial. *AJNR Am J Neuroradiol*. 2004;25:351–352.
- White ML, Zhang Y, Smoker WR. Evolution of lesions in Susac syndrome at serial MR imaging with diffusion-weighted imaging and apparent diffusion coefficient values. *AJNR Am J Neuroradiol*. 2004;25:706–713.

DELAYED POSTHYPOXIC LEUKOENCEPHALOPATHY
CASE 69
- Chalela JA, Wolf RL, Maldjian JA, et al. MRI identification of early white matter injury in anoxic-ischaemic encephalopathy. *Neurology* 2001;56:481–485.
- Molloy S, Soh C, Williams TL. Reversible delayed posthypoxic leukoencephalopathy. *AJNR Am J Neuroradiol*. 2006;27:1763–1765.

PARANEOPLASTIC LIMBIC ENCEPHALITIS
CASE 70
- Schott JM. Limbic encephalitis: a clinician's guide. *Pract Neurol*. 2006;6:143–153.

- Tuzun E, Dalmau J. Limbic encephalitis and variants: classification, diagnosis and treatment. *Neurologist*. 2007;13:261–271.

METHOTREXATE LEUKOENCEPHALOPATHY
CASE 71
- Fisher MJ, Khademian ZP, Simon EM, Zimmerman RA, Bilniuk LT. Diffusion weighted MR imaging of early methotrexate related neurotoxicity in children. *AJNR Am J Neuroradiol*. 2005;26:1686–1689.
- Inaba H, Khan RB, Laningham FH, Crew KR, Pui CH, Daw NC. Clinical and radiological characteristics of methotrexate-induced acute encephalopathy in pediatric patients with cancer. *Ann Oncol*. 2008;19:178–184.

PERIVENTRICULAR NODULAR GRAY MATTER HETEROTOPIA
CASE 72
- Barkovich AJ, Kjos BO. Gray matter heterotopias: MR characteristics and correlation with developmental and neurologic manifestations. *Radiology* 1992;182:493–499.
- Barkovich AJ, Kuzniecky RI. Gray matter heterotopia. *Neurology* 2000;55:1603–1608.

HYDRANENCEPHALY
CASE 73
- Quek YW, Su PH, Tsao TF, et al. Hydranencephaly associated with interruption of bilateral internal carotid arteries. *Pediatr Neonatol*. 2008;49:43–47.
- Sepulveda W, Cortes-Yepes H, Wong AE, Dezerega V, Corral E, Malinger G. Prenatal sonography in hydranencephaly: findings during the early stages of disease. *J Ultrasound Med*. 2012;31:799–804.

SCHIZENCEPHALY
CASE 74
- Oh KY, Kennedy AM, Frias AE Jr, Byrne JL. Fetal schizencephaly: pre- and postnatal imaging with a review of the clinical manifestations. *Radiographics* 2005;25:647–657.
- Packard AM, Miller VS, Delgado MR. Schizencephaly: correlations of clinical and radiologic features. *Neurology* 1997;48:1427–1434.

TUBEROUS SCLEROSIS COMPLEX
CASE 75
- Simao G, Raybaud C, Chuang S, Go C, Snead OC, Widjaja E. Diffusion tensor imaging of commissural and projection white matter in tuberous sclerosis complex and correlation with tuber load. *AJNR Am J Neuroradiol*. 2010;31:1273–1277.
- Umeoka S, Koyama T, Miki Y, Akai M, Tsutsui K, Togashi K. Pictorial review of tuberous sclerosis in various organs. *Radiographics* 2008;28;e32.

NEUROFIBROMATOSIS TYPE 2
CASE 76
- Dirks MS, Butman JA, Kim HJ, et al. Long term natural history of neurofibromatosis type 2-associated intracranial tumors. *J Neurosurg*. 2012;117:109–117. Epub Apr 13, 2013.
- Hoa M, Slattery WH 3rd. Neurofibromatosis 2. *Otolaryngol Clin North Am*. 2012;45:315–332.

RATHKE CLEFT CYST

CASE 77

- Byun WM, Kim OL, Kim D. MR imaging findings of Rathke's cleft cysts: significance of intracystic nodules. *AJNR Am J Neuroradiol*. 2000;21:485–488.
- Osborn AG, Preece MT. Intracranial cysts: radiologic-pathologic correlation and imaging approach. *Radiology* 2006;239:650–664.

MALIGNANT PITUITARY MACROADENOMA

CASE 78

- Gürlek A, Karavitaki N, Ansorge O, Wass JA. What are the markers of aggressiveness in prolactinomas? Changes in cell biology, extracellular matrix components, angiogenesis and genetics. *Eur J Endocrinol*. 2007;156:143–153.
- Zemmoura I, Wierinckx A, Vasiljevic A, Jan M, Trouillas J, Francois P. Aggressive and malignant prolactin pituitary tumors: pathological diagnosis and patient management. *Pituitary* 2013;16:515–522.

HAMARTOMA OF TUBER CINEREUM

CASE 79

- Amstutz DR, Coons SW, Kerrigan JF, et al. Hypothalamic hamartomas. correlation of MR imaging and spectroscopic findings with tumor glial content. *AJNR Am J Neuroradiol*. 2006;27:794–798.
- Maixner W. Hypothalamic hamartomas—clinical, neuropathological and surgical aspects. *Childs Nerv Syst*. 2006;22:867–873.

CAROTID CAVERNOUS FISTULA (II)

CASE 80

- Ellis JA, Goldstein H, Connolly ES Jr, Meyers PM. Carotid-cavernous fistulas. *Neurosurg Focus* 2012;32(5):E9.
- Gemmete JJ, Ansari SA, Gandhi D. Endovascular treatment of carotid cavernous fistulas. *Neuroimaging Clin N Am*. 2009;19:241–255.

ABERRANT NEUROHYPOPHYSIS

CASE 81

- Di Iorgi N, Allegri AE, Napoli F, et al. The use of neuroimaging for assessing disorders of pituitary development. *Clin Endocrinol (Oxf)*. 2012;76:161–176.
- Spampinato MV, Castillo M. Congenital pathology of the pituitary gland and parasellar region. *Top Magn Reson Imaging* 2005;16:269–276.

PITUITARY HEMORRHAGE

CASE 82

- Onesti ST, Wisniewski T, Post KD. Clinical versus subclinical pituitary apoplexy: presentation, surgical management, and outcomes in 21 patients. *Neurosurgery* 1990;26:980–986.
- Rogg JM, Tung GA, Anderson G, et al. Pituitary apoplexy: early detection with diffusion weighted MR imaging. *AJNR Am J Neuroradiol*. 2002;23:1240–1245.

VASCULAR SUPPLY TO THE HEAD: THE AORTIC ARCH VARIANTS

CASE 83

- Layton KF, Kallmes DF, Cloft HJ, Lindell EP, Cox VS. Bovine aortic arch variant in humans: Clarification of a common misnomer. *AJNR Am J Neuroradiol*. 2006;27:1541–1542.

- Rekha P, Senthilkumar S. A study on branching pattern of human aortic arch and its variations in south Indian population. *J Morphol Sci*. 2013;30:11–15.

AZYGOS ANTERIOR CEREBRAL ARTERY

CASE 84

- Huh JS, Park SK, Shin JJ, Kim TH. Saccular aneurysm of the azygos anterior cerebral artery: three case reports. *J Korean Neurosurg Soc*. 2007;42:342–345.
- Lemay M, Gooding CA. The clinical significance of the azygos anterior cerebral artery. *AJR Am J Roentgenol*. 1966; 98: 602–610.

CYLINDRICAL AND FUSIFORM ANEURYSMS

CASE 85

- Kamiyama H, Ueki K, Kirino T, et al. Clinicopathological study of intracranial fusiform and dolichoectatic aneurysms: insight on the mechanism of growth. *Stroke* 2000;31:896–900.
- Park SH, Yim MB, Lee CY, Kim F, Son EI. Intracranial fusiform aneurysms: it's pathogenesis, clinical characteristics and managements. *J Korean Neurosurg Soc*. 2008; 44: 116–123.

MIDDLE CEREBRAL ARTERY ANEURYSM WITH CEREBRAL VASOSPASM

CASE 86

- Kolias AG, Sen J, Belli A. Pathogenesis of cerebral vasospasm following aneurysmal subarachnoid hemorrhage: putative mechanisms and novel approaches. *J Neurosci Res*. 2009; 87:1–11.
- Nehls DG, Flom RA, Carter LP, Spetzler RF. Multiple intracranial aneurysm: determining the site of rupture. *J Neurosurg*. 1985;63:342–348.

SUPERIOR SAGITTAL SINUS THROMBOSIS

CASE 87

- Coutinho JM, Stam J. How to treat cerebral venous and sinus thrombosis. *J Thromb Haemost*. 2010;8:877–883.
- Kimber J. Cerebral venous sinus thrombosis. *QJM*. 2002;95:137–142.

VEIN OF GALEN ANEURYSMAL MALFORMATION

CASE 88

- Jones BV, Ball WS, Tomsick TA, Millard J, Crone KR. Vein of Galen malformation: diagnosis and treatment of 13 children with extended clinical follow up. *AJNR Am J Neuroradiol*. 2002;23:1717–1724.
- Lasjaunias PL, Chng SM, Sachet M, Alvarez H, Rodesch G, Garcia-Monaco R. The management of vein of Galen aneurysmal malformations. *Neurosurgery* 2006;59(Suppl 3): S184–S194.

REVERSIBLE CEREBRAL VASOCONSTRICTION SYNDROME

CASE 89

- Ducros A. Reversible cerebral vasoconstriction syndrome. *Lancet Neurol*. 2012;11:906–917. doi:10.1016/ S1474-4422(12)70135-7.
- Singhal AB. Cerebral vasoconstriction syndromes. *Top Stroke Rehabil*. 2004;1:1–6.

ARTERIOVENOUS MALFORMATION

CASE 90

• Geibprasert S, Pongpeck S, Jiarakongmun P, Shroff MM, Armstrong DC, Krings T. Radiologic assessment of brain arteriovenous malformations: what clinicians need to know. *Radiographics* 2010;30:483–501.

• Omojola MF, Fox AJ, Viñuela F, Debrun G. Stenosis of afferent vessels of intracranial arteriovenous malformations. *AJNR Am J Neuroradiol.* 1985;6:791–793.

VASOGENIC EDEMA

CASE 91

• Ho ML, Rojas R, Eisenberg RL. Cerebral edema. *AJR Am J Roentgenol.* 2012;199:W258–W273.

• Kaal EC, Vecht CJ. The management of brain edema in brain tumors. *Curr Opin Oncol.* 2004;16:593–600.

ADRENOLEUKODYSTROPHY

CASE 92

• Loes DJ, Hite S, Moser H, et al. Adrenoleukodystrophy: a scoring method for brain MR observations. *AJNR Am J Neuroradiol.* 1994;15:1761–1766.

• Melhem ER, Loes DJ, Georgiades CS, et al. X-linked adrenoleukodystrophy: the role of contrast-enhanced MR imaging in predicting disease progression. *AJNR Am J Neuroradiol.* 2000;21:839–844.

METACHROMATIC LEUKODYSTROPHY

CASE 93

• Eichler F, Grodd W, Grant E, et al. Metachromatic leukodystrophy: a scoring system for brain MR imaging observations. *AJNR Am J Neuroradiol.* 2009;30:1893–1897.

• Kim TS, Kim IO, Kim WS, et al. MR of childhood metachromatic leukodystrophy. *AJNR Am J Neuroradiol.* 1997;18:733–738.

ALEXANDER DISEASE

CASE 94

• Farina L, Pareyson D, Minati L, et al. Can MR imaging diagnose adult-onset Alexander disease? *AJNR Am J Neuroradiol.* 2008;29:1190–1196.

• van der Knaap MS, Naidu S, Breiter SN, et al. Alexander disease: diagnosis with MR imaging. *AJNR Am J Neuroradiol.* 2001;22:541–552.

TRAUMATIC INTRACEREBRAL HEMATOMA

CASE 95

• Álvarez-Sabín J, Turon A, Lozano-Sánchez M, Vázquez J, Codina A. Delayed posttraumatic hemorrhage. *Stroke* 1995;26:1531–1535.

TRAUMATIC BRAIN INJURY/DIFFUSE AXONAL INJURY

CASE 96

• Huisman TAGM, Schwamm LH, Schaefer PW, et al. Diffusion tensor imaging as potential biomarker of white matter injury in diffuse axonal injury. *AJNR Am J Neuroradiol.* 2004; 25:370–376.

• Toyama Y, Kobayashi T, Nishiyama Y, Satoh K, Ohkawa M, Seki K. CT for acute stage of closed head injury. *Radiat Med.* 2005;23:309–316.

ACUTE SUBDURAL HEMATOMA

CASE 97

• McBride W. Subdural hematoma in adults: prognosis and management. www.uptodate.com ©2013 UpToDate® sighted 8/15/2013.

• Osborne AG. *Osborn's Brain, Imaging, Pathology, and Anatomy.* 1st ed. Philadelphia, PA: Amirsys/Lippincott Williams & Wilkins; 2013.

SUBFALCINE HERNIATION

CASE 98

• Coburn MW, Rodriguez FJ. Cerebral herniations. *Appl Radiol.* 1998;27:10–16.

• Jung HJ, Kim DM, Kim SW. Paradoxical transtentorial herniation caused by lumbar puncture after decompressive craniectomy. *J Korean Neurosurg Soc.* 2012;51:102–104.

TRAUMATIC SUBDURAL HYGROMA

CASE 99

• Kumar R, Singhal N, Mahapatra AK. Traumatic subdural effusions in children following minor head injury. *Childs Nerv Syst.* 2008;24:1391–1396.

• Zanini MA, de Lima Resende LA, de Souza Faleiros AT, Gabarra RC. Traumatic subdural hygromas: proposed pathogenesis based classification. *J Trauma Inj Infect Crit Care* 2008;64:705–713.

CHRONIC CALCIFIED SUBDURAL HEMATOMA

CASE 100

• Kaplan M, Akgun B, Secer HI. Ossified chronic subdural hematoma with armored brain. *Turk Neurosurg.* 2008; 18:420–424.

• Per H, Gumus H, Tucer B, Akgun H, Kurtsoy A, Kumandas S. Calcified chronic subdural hematoma mimicking calvarial mass. *Brain Dev.* 2006;28:607–609.